T

WO
100

Clinical Surgery

THE LIBRARY

ALEXANDRA HOUSE,
CHELTENHAM GENERAL HOSPITAL
SANDFORD ROAD
CHELTENHAM
GL53 7AN

D0434691

C2083795

WO
100

Clinical Surgery:
A Practical Guide

Edited by

Qassim F Baker MRChB Diploma (Gen Surgery) FRCS
Clinical Tutor, Iraqi Board of Medical Specialisation
Assistant Professor, Baghdad College of Medicine
Formerly Consultant Surgeon, Baghdad Teaching Hospital, Baghdad, Iraq

Munther I Aldoori PhD FRCS(Glas) FRCS(Eng) FRCS(Ed) FACS
Consultant General and Vascular Surgeon, Huddersfield Royal Infirmary,
Huddersfield
Senior Clinical Lecturer, University of Leeds
Examiner for RCS Glasgow, Edinburgh and England
Member of the Intercollegiate Board in General Surgery, UK
Visiting Professor, University of Baghdad, Iraq

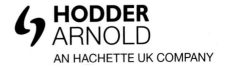

HODDER
ARNOLD
AN HACHETTE UK COMPANY

First published in Great Britain in 2009 by
Hodder Arnold, an imprint of Hodder Education,
an Hachette UK company, 338 Euston Road, London NW1 3BH

http://www.hoddereducation.com

© 2009 Edward Arnold (Publishers) Ltd

All rights reserved. Apart from any use permitted under UK copyright law, this publication may only be reproduced, stored or transmitted, in any form, or by any means with prior permission in writing of the publishers or in the case of reprographic production in accordance with the terms of licences issued by the Copyright Licensing Agency. In the United Kingdom such licences are issued by the Copyright licensing Agency: Saffron House, 6–10 Kirby Street, London EC1N 8TS.

Hachette UK's policy is to use papers that are natural, renewable and recyclable products and made from wood grown in sustainable forests. The logging and manufacturing processes are expected to conform to the environmental regulations of the country of origin.

Whilst the advice and information in this book are believed to be true and accurate at the date of going to press, neither the author[s] nor the publisher can accept any legal responsibility or liability for any errors or omissions that may be made. In particular, (but without limiting the generality of the preceding disclaimer) every effort has been made to check drug dosages; however it is still possible that errors have been missed. Furthermore, dosage schedules are constantly being revised and new side-effects recognized. For these reasons the reader is strongly urged to consult the drug companies' printed instructions before administering any of the drugs recommended in this book.

British Library Cataloguing in Publication Data
A catalogue record for this book is available from the British Library

Library of Congress Cataloging-in-Publication Data
A catalog record for this book is available from the Library of Congress

ISBN-13   978-0-340-94084-6

1 2 3 4 5 6 7 8 9 10

Commissioning Editor:	Gavin Jamieson
Project Editor:	Francesca Naish
Production Controller:	Joanna Walker
Cover Design:	Helen Townson

Typeset in 9.5 on 12pt Goudy by Phoenix Photosetting, Chatham, Kent
Printed and bound in India

What do you think about this book? Or any other Hodder Arnold title?
Please visit our website: www.hoddereducation.com

We dedicate this book to the memory of our honoured teachers and trainers, who lit the path of knowledge to so many generations of doctors.

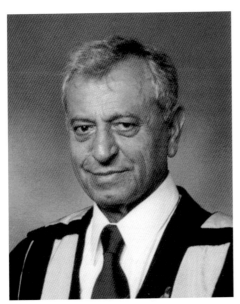

Professor Khalid Naji

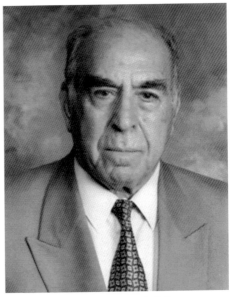

Professor Aziz Shukri

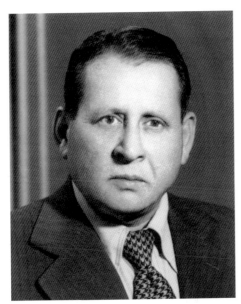

Professor Yousif Al-Numan

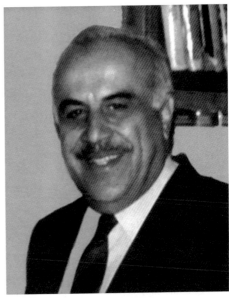

Professor Khalid Al-Qassab

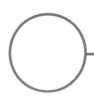

Contents

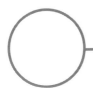

Contributors

Samir A Abdulla MBChB FRCS
Associate specialist in general surgery with
interest in upper GI and laparoscopic surgery
Queens Hospital, Burton on Trent, UK

Assad Aghahoseini FRCS
Staff grade surgeon
York Hospital NHS Trust, York, UK

William Ainslie MD FRCS(Glas) FRCS(Gen Surgery)
Consultant upper GI surgeon
Calderdale and Huddersfield NHS
Foundation Trust, Huddersfield, UK

Ahmed Al-Bahrani MBChB FRCS(Glas)
Specialist registrar
Ipswich Hospital, Ipswich, UK

Munther I Aldoori PhD FRCS(Glas) FRCS(Eng)
FRCS(Ed) FACS
Consultant general and vascular surgeon
Huddersfield Royal Infirmary, Huddersfield
Senior clinical lecturer, University of Leeds
Examiner for RCS Glasgow, Edinburgh and
England
Member of the Intercollegiate Board in
General Surgery, UK
Visiting Professor, University of Baghdad,
Baghdad, Iraq

Amer Aldouri MBChB MD MRCS FRCS
(Hepatobiliary)
Specialist registrar in surgery
St James's University Hospital, Leeds, UK

David J Alexander MBBs FRCS MS
Consultant colorectal surgeon and Clinical
director of cancer service
York Hospital NHS Trust, York, UK

Steve Allen MBBS MRCS FRCS
Consultant radiologist
Royal Marsden Hospital, London, UK

Ahmed Al-Mukhtar MBChB FRCS(Ed) FRCS
(Transplantation)
Specialist registrar in hepatobiliary and
transplant surgery
St James's University Hospital, Leeds, UK

Walid Al-Wali MBChB FRCPath
Professor of microbiology, Consultant
medical microbiologist, Lead infection
control doctor, Director for infection
prevention and control, Medical director
Department of Medical Microbiology,
Rotherham NHS Foundation Trust,
Rotherham, UK

Abdulhalim Al Zein MD FAS LAS
Consultant laparoscopic general and upper
GI surgeon
Gloucester Royal Hospital,
Great Western Road,
Gloucester, UK

Basil J Ammori MB ChB FRCS(Ed) FRCS(Eng) MD
Consultant hepatobiliary surgeon, Honorary
senior lecturer and examiner for RCS
Edinburgh
University of Manchester and Manchester
Royal Infirmary, Manchester, UK

Vikram J Anand
Consultant surgeon
Kalra Hospital and Sri Ram Cardio-Thoracic
& Neurosciences Centre,
New Delhi, India
Supervisor for postgraduate surgical studies
The National Board of Examinations,
New Delhi, India
Surgical tutor and examiner
The Royal College of Surgeons of Edinburgh,
Scotland, UK
Professor of surgery and former director,
department of surgery
Maulana Azad Medical College and
Associated Hospitals, New Delhi, India

Saleh Baghdadi MD MRCS
Registrar in cardiothoracic surgery,
Manchester Royal Infirmary, Manchester, UK

Qassim F Baker MBChB Diploma (Gen Surgery)
FRCS
Clinical tutor
Iraqi Board of Medical Specialisation
Assistant professor, Baghdad College of
Medicine, Baghdad
Formerly Consultant surgeon
Baghdad Teaching Hospital, Baghdad, Iraq

H Devalia MBBS MS(Bombay) DNB (gold medalist)
FRCS(Ed) FRCS(Gen Surg)
Specialist registrar, Breast Unit,
Royal Marsden Hospital, London, UK

Simon Dexter DM FRCS(Gen) FCSHK
Consultant upper GI surgeon
St James's University Hospital, Leeds, UK

Suhail AR Doi PhD FRCP
Consultant in endocrinology
Mubarak Al-Kabeer Teaching Hospital and
Faculty of Medicine, Kuwait University,
Kuwait

Naif El-Barghouti MBChB MSc PhD DIC FRCS(Ed)
(Gen) FRCS
Consultant general and vascular surgeon,
Scarborough General Hospital, Scarborough
Honorary Senior Clinical Lecturer, Hull York
Medical School
Examiner for RCS England and Member of
the Intercollegiate Board in General Surgery,
UK

JEF Fitzgerald BA MBChB MRCS
Research and teaching fellow
Department of Gastrointestinal Surgery,
Nottingham University Hospital, Nottingham,
UK

Sheila M Fraser MRCS
Specialist registrar in general surgery
Leeds Teaching Hospitals NHS Trust, Leeds,
UK

Laura Harvey MBChB FRCA
Specialist registrar in anaesthetics
Leeds Teaching Hospitals Trust, Leeds, UK

Refaat Kamel MBChB MCH FACS FICS(Hon)
Professor of surgery, past World President of
ICS
Faculty of Medicine, Ain Shams University,
Cairo, Egypt

Ramanathan Kandasamy DA FRCA FCARCS
Consultant in anaesthesia and ICU
Huddersfield Royal Infirmary, Huddersfield
Honorary senior lecturer
University of Leeds
Examiner for RCS Edinburgh, UK

Kevin G Kerr BSc MBChB MD FRCPath
Consultant microbiologist and Honorary
Clinical Professor (Microbiology)
Harrogate and District NHS Foundation
Trust, Harrogate, UK

CG Nanda Kumar MBBS FRCA
Consultant anaesthetist, Calderdale and
Huddersfield NHS Foundation Trust,
Huddersfield
Honorary senior lecturer, University of Leeds,
Examiner for RCS Glasgow, UK

Mark Lansdown MCh FRCS
Consultant surgeon
Leeds Teaching Hospitals NHS Trust
Honorary senior lecturer, University of Leeds,
Leeds, UK

Mike Larvin BSc MBBS FRCS MD
Professor of surgery, Consultant upper GI
and pancreatic surgeon and Head of division
Academic Division of Surgery, School of
Graduate Entry Medicine and Health, Derby
City General Hospital, Derby, UK

Andrew JP Lewington BSc MD FRCP
Consultant renal physician
St James's University Hospital
Honorary senior lecturer
University of Leeds, Leeds, UK

Andrew Lockey FRCS(Ed) FCEM
Consultant in emergency medicine
Calderdale and Huddersfield NHS
Foundation Trust, Halifax, UK

Peter Lodge MD FRCS
Professor of surgery, Consultant surgeon in
hepatobiliary and transplant surgery
St James's University Hospital, Leeds, UK

Karl S Mainprize
Consultant colorectal surgeon
Scarborough General Hospital,
Scarborough, UK

Hassan Malik MD FRCS (General surgery)
Consultant surgeon
Royal Liverpool University Hospital,
Liverpool, UK

Andrew Mavor MD FRCS(Ed)
Consultant vascular surgeon
Leeds General Infirmary, Leeds
Honorary senior lecturer, University of Leeds
Examiner for RCS Edinburgh, UK

Amjid Mohammed FRCSI FCEM
Consultant in emergency medicine
Calderdale and Huddersfield NHS
Foundation Trust, Halifax, UK

Chas G Newstead BSc FRCP
Consultant renal physician
St James's University Hospital
Honorary senior lecturer
University of Leeds, Leeds, UK

Julie O'Riordan MBChB FRCA
Consultant anaesthetist and Clinical director
for Anaesthetics and Critical Care
Huddersfield Royal Infirmary, Huddersfield,
UK

Deirdre Pallister
Associate specialist breast clinician
Jarvis Breast Screening Centre, Guildford
and Royal Marsden Hospital, London, UK

E Philip Perry MBChB FRCS
Consultant general and vascular surgeon
Scarborough District Hospital, Scarborough
Honorary senior lecturer, Hull York Medical
School
Examiner for RCS England, UK

Samie Safar DS FRCP(Ed) FRCS(Eng, Ed, Glas)
FACS
Consultant general surgeon, Newham
University Hospital, London, UK
Formerly Professor of surgery, University of
Baghdad, Baghdad, Iraq

Kishore Sasapu MBBS FRCS
Specialist registrar in surgery
Calderdale and Huddersfield NHS
Foundation Trust, Huddersfield, UK

Nigel A Scott MD FRCS
Consultant colorectal surgeon
Lancashire Teaching Hospitals Trust,
Preston, UK

Peter Sedman MBChB FRCS
Consultant surgeon
Hull and East Yorkshire NHS Trust, Hull
Honorary senior lecturer, Hull York Medical
School
Tutor in laparoscopic surgery
Royal College of Surgeons of England,
London, UK

Tharwat I Sulliaman FRCSI CABS
Professor of surgery
Baghdad College of Medicine
Consultant surgeon
Baghdad Teaching Hospital, Baghdad, Iraq

Giles Toogood MA DM FRCS
Consultant hepatobiliary and transplantation
surgeon
St James's University Hospital
Honorary senior lecturer, University of Leeds
Examiner for RCS England, Member of the
Intercollegiate Board in General Surgery, UK

Timothy R Wilson BSc MB ChB PhD MRCS
Specialist registrar in general surgery
Yorkshire Deanery, Leeds, UK

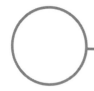

Foreword

This monograph does exactly what its title implies. Not intended by the two editors as a comprehensive surgical postgraduate textbook, it is a practical guide to the key aspects of clinical patient management in modern surgical practice; and although at first glance, some of the topics discussed appear unconnected, they add up to contribute to a holistic account addressing the various *practical* aspects of surgical management. The material is arranged in 31 chapters which address the essentials of modern general surgical practice: surgical care and monitoring, organ failure and support, acute abdominal emergencies and gastrointestinal bleeding, trauma, critical limb ischaemia, surgical treatment of the elderly, obese and patients with co-morbid disorders, surgical approaches and techniques, day case surgery, principles of oncology and common tropical disorders – of increasing relevance to surgical practice in Western countries.

The quality of the information provided is concise and up-to-date, and although the authors come from various disciplines and include non-consultant staff, the structure and layout of the various chapters of the monograph are uniform, well illustrated and to the point. The two editors, Mr Qassim F Baker and Mr Munther I Aldoori, have, with the help of their co-authors, produced a very useful monograph for postgraduate trainees sitting examinations in the generality of surgery and, for this reason, I am sure that this monograph will be well received and prove to be a useful instrument in surgical education.

Professor Sir Alfred Cuschieri MD DSc FRSE FRCS FACS F Med Sci FIBiol

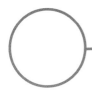

Preface

Although this is not meant to be a textbook of surgery it covers a wide range of surgical topics. It is written primarily for postgraduate trainees undertaking examinations, including IMRCS, Speciality FRCS and similar postgraduate degrees.

The majority of the senior authors are teachers, trainers and postgraduate examiners. Their endeavour has been to present complex topics in a succinct and accessible manner.

In the current global village, tropical diseases do not respect geographical boundaries; therefore we included surgery of some of the more common tropical diseases. We also included questions at the end of each chapter as we believe in their value in offering readers an opportunity for self assessment.

We are very grateful to our contributors, all of whom are very busy practicing doctors.

Our special thanks go to Professor Sir Alfred Cuschieri.

Qassim F Baker, Munther I Aldoori

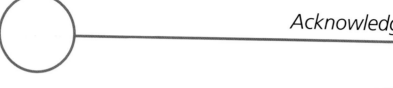

Acknowledgements

We are greatly indebted to Professor Sir Alfred Cuschieri for his kindness and generosity with his time in writing the Foreword for this book, which is greatly appreciated. We are also indebted to Rebecca Reid and Mark Lansdown for their great support and assistance in acting as English editors of this book. We acknowlege with sincere thanks the staff of the Medical Illustration department of the Huddersfield Royal Infirmary.

INTRODUCTION

Preoperative care begins as soon as a patient agrees to undergo an operation. It involves history taking, clinical examination, appropriate investigations, risk assessment and informed consent. The purpose of preoperative assessment is to improve outcomes. A simple set of measures could reduce the number of complications following surgery and reduce the average length of hospital stay (Improving Surgical Outcomes Group, 2005). Good preoperative care should reduce costs, increase efficiency of operating theatres, reduce the number of patients who do not attend for surgery or who are cancelled on the day for clinical reasons, and provide an opportunity for advising patients on their risk factors, including smoking and weight control. Good preoperative care can benefit the patient, the surgical team and the health service.

In the quest for efficient and less costly surgery, preoperative assessment has shifted increasingly from the period of time between admission and operation to the out-patient setting. Patients are often assessed by a multidisciplinary team and admitted only hours before their operation. Only for some complex major procedures, and occasionally due to individual circumstances, do patients need to be admitted a day or more before surgery in order to allow the anaesthetic and surgical team to make final preparations.

On the day of surgery, the anaesthetist and surgeon responsible for the operation must satisfy themselves from the notes and a short consultation with the patient that all appropriate steps have been taken to prepare the patient for theatre. Although much of the preoperative assessment has been delegated, the decision to proceed with the operation remains the responsibility of the surgeon and anaesthetist. The quality of preoperative assessment can directly determine the risk of morbidity or mortality and reduce the risk that a patient will have to be cancelled on the day of surgery because appropriate investigations have not been performed. To admit a patient for an operation and find that the preoperative assessment has been inadequate is an enormous waste of resources and irritating to both the surgical team and the patient.

> ◾ KEY POINT
> On the day of surgery, the anaesthetist and surgeon responsible for the operation must satisfy themselves from the notes and a short consultation with the patient that all appropriate steps have been taken to prepare the patient for theatre.

What follows in this chapter is an outline of the sometimes complex process of preoperative care. The chapter does not proscribe how this care should be organised, as this varies according to the specialty and the circumstances pertaining locally in each hospital. A useful document is *Improving Your Elective Patient's Journey* (Royal College of Surgeons of England, 2007).

● IN THE SURGICAL CLINIC

Once a patient agrees to undergo surgery, they are given a provisional date or put on a waiting list. At this point, the patient should be given some indication about how long they may need to wait and what to do if their condition changes while they are waiting. If the patient agrees to surgery and the hospital has a pre-assessment clinic, the patient is given an appointment to attend. Sometimes patients need time to discuss the advice with friends or relatives or require a second opinion. This is a good time to offer patient information leaflets.

In the surgical clinic it is best to ask a few key questions about the patient's general fitness and any conditions that might affect their suitability for an anaesthetic. There may be a pro forma to complete with details such as the underlying condition, proposed operation, laterality and expected operating time. Some consultants prefer to seek the patient's consent at this stage as well.

● IN THE PRE-ASSESSMENT CLINIC

Staffing of pre-assessment clinics varies widely between specialties and hospitals. Many have an anaesthetist and surgical and nursing staff available. Some clinics, especially in major vascular units, have a cardiologist. The National Confidential Enquiry into Patient Outcome and Death (NCEPOD, 2005, 2008) has drawn attention to the staffing of pre-assessment clinics in its reports on abdominal aortic aneurysms and coronary artery bypass grafts.

The role of the anaesthetist in pre-assessment has been outlined by the Association of Anaesthetists of Great Britain and Ireland (2001). For minor procedures, however, pre-assessment may be entirely within the remit of a trained nurse.

At first sight, the patient may appear to be fit and healthy, but a focused history should be taken to determine whether there are any factors that might impact on the patient's risk for a particular procedure. A pre-screening questionnaire completed by the patient before they see the doctor can speed up the consultation.

The history should include details of any previous surgery or procedures and their outcomes. You may need to discuss the patient's experience of previous surgery, and any concerns they still have regarding the proposed operation.

Previous surgery can influence the plan for the proposed operation and increase the risk of complications. In the abdomen, the presence of adhesions can prove troublesome, and old scars may mean that a stoma has to be sited in a different area compared with what you have read in a textbook. In the neck the increased risk of complications in reoperative thyroid surgery is well known.

It is particularly important to ask about any previous reaction to an anaesthetic, and any family history of anaesthetic problems. The anaesthetist should also enquire about this. Other relevant aspects of family history include haemoglobinopathies, such as thalassaemia and sickle cell disease. The patient should be asked specifically about latex and other allergies.

Although respiratory and cardiac health are often considered paramount, there are many other health problems that may be detected in the pre-assessment clinic. For instance, if mild symptoms of prostatic hypertrophy are detected, the patient can be warned about the small risk of urinary retention after inguinal hernia repair. Other groups of patients with particular operative risks include people who are elderly, morbidly obese or immunocompromised (e.g. as a result of human immunodeficiency virus (HIV) infection or following a transplant). Also consider the risk to the surgical team if the patient is carrying a dangerous pathogen. The country in which you are working, and your knowledge of the patient's background and travel, should alert you to diseases that are uncommon in Europe but endemic elsewhere, such as bilharzias and malaria (see also Advisory Committee on Dangerous Pathogens, 2007).

The patient's social history may raise your suspicions about the risk of potential comorbidity, and you should always ask about smoking, drinking and drug abuse.

Social circumstances are very important for patients who are to be discharged while still needing some support. For day-case surgery, it is usual to ensure that the patient will not be discharged to an empty house and that they have access to a telephone in case any complications develop.

■ KEY POINT
For day-case surgery, ensure that the patient will not be discharged to an empty house and that they will have access to a telephone in case any complications develop.

The physical examination should be appropriate to the patient and the procedure, taking into account any suspicion of health problems detected in the history. Intimate examinations should be performed only when relevant and in the presence of a chaperone and, wherever possible, should be carried out with sensitivity to the cultural expectations of the patient. If a translator is required, then a professional engaged by the hospital may be more reliable than a relative of the patient.

Investigations as appropriate are performed (see below) and the patient is asked whether they need any further information about the planned procedure before admission. If a condition is discovered that should be treated before admission (e.g. hypertension), the patient should be referred for specialist consultation or initiation of treatment by the patient's general practitioner. Similarly, preoperative treatment of anaemia based on the underlying causes can reduce the need for perioperative transfusion. In situations where a decision to delay surgery is taken, it is vital that the surgeon responsible for the patient is also informed because the risks and benefits of delaying the operation must be assessed and the operation re-scheduled appropriately. A system is also needed to inform the surgical team when the patient has been treated satisfactorily.

At the time of pre-assessment it is also appropriate to check what arrangements are required by the surgical team for the particular operation planned, such as antibacterial prophylaxis, bowel preparation or preoperative vocal cord examination. Request 'group and save' or cross-match blood according to local guidelines for the anticipated procedure. You may also need to book a high dependency or intensive care bed in advance.

Finally, patients need explicit and preferably written instructions about when they can eat and drink before the surgery, and which medications they should take on the day of surgery. If the patient is on anticoagulants, clear advice on when to stop is required.

● ROUTINE PREOPERATIVE TESTS FOR ELECTIVE SURGERY

National Clinical Guidelines for the use of preoperative tests have been developed by the National Collaborating Centre for Acute Care (2003) at the Royal College of Surgeons of England. The aim is to reduce the costs associated with unnecessary tests, which includes the investigation of false positive results.

> ■ KEY POINT
>
> The National Collaborating Centre for Acute Care at the Royal College of Surgeons of England has developed national clinical guidelines for the use of preoperative tests.

The guideline is approved by the National Institute for Health and Clinical Excellence (2003) and makes recommendations about the appropriateness of carrying out the following tests:

- Plain chest X-ray (radiograph)
- Resting electrocardiogram (ECG)
- Full blood count (e.g. to test for anaemia)
- Haemostasis (to test how well the blood clots)
- Renal function
- Random blood glucose (to test for diabetes)
- Urine analysis (e.g. to test for urinary infections or kidney problems)
- Blood gases (to test for cardiovascular or lung problems)
- Lung function tests
- Pregnancy test
- Sickle cell test.

The appropriateness of testing depends on the patient's age and other illnesses and the type of surgery that is planned. The recommendations are set out in look-up tables that are cross-referenced by the type and grade of surgery (Table 1.1), common chronic illnesses and age (Table 1.2 gives an example). The guidelines can be downloaded from the website of the Royal College of Surgeons (www.rcseng.ac.uk).

An added incentive to look at these tables is that sometimes they form the basis of questions in tests of surgical knowledge, e.g. 'Discuss what preoperative tests would be appropriate in a 65-year-old man admitted for an inguinal hernia repair.'

As well as ordering tests for the patient, it is worth checking that the results of tests already performed are available and make sense in the context of the proposed procedure. For example, if a mastectomy is proposed, is there a pathology report that unequivocally confirms the presence of cancer in a breast biopsy or fine-needle aspiration?

● OPTIMISING THE PATIENT'S PREOPERATIVE CONDITION

Pulmonary dysfunction

Patients with an American Association of Anesthesiologists (ASA) grade greater than 2 (see Table 1.3) have double the risk of pulmonary complications compared with patients with ASA

Table 1.1 Surgery grades*

Grade	Examples
1 (minor)	Excision of lesion of skin, drainage of breast abscess
2 (intermediate)	Primary repair of inguinal hernia, tonsillectomy, knee arthroplasty
3 (major)	Total abdominal hysterectomy, lumbar discectomy, thyroidectomy
4 (major+)	Total joint replacement, lung operations, colonic resection, radical neck dissection

*Neurosurgery and cardiovascular surgery are considered separately.

Table 1.2 Example of a look-up table: American Association of Anesthesiologists (ASA) grade 1 – adults ≥ 16 years

Test	Age (years)			
	16 to < 40	40 to < 60	60 to < 80	≥ 80
Chest X-ray	No	No	No	No
ECG	No		Yes	
FBC	No	Yes	Yes	
Haemostasis	No	No	No	No
Renal function	No	No		
Random glucose	No			
Urine analysis*				

*Dipstick urine testing in asymptomatic individuals not recommended (UK National Screening Committee).
ECG, electrocardiogram; FBC, full blood count.
Taken from National Collaborating Centre for Acute Care (2003). *Preoperative Tests: The Use of Routine Preoperative Tests for Elective Surgery.* London: National Collaborating Centre for Acute Care and the Royal College of Surgeons of England.

grade 1. Chronic obstructive pulmonary disease is a particular risk factor. Ask the patient about their smoking habits and any known pulmonary disease such as asthma or bronchitis. Upper abdominal operations carry a greater risk of pulmonary complications than do lower abdominal or laparoscopic operations. Ask about cough, excessive sputum production, wheezing and exercise tolerance. Ask about any medication that is being used, or has been used, for respiratory disorders. If the patient has asthma, enquire particularly about their previous use of oral corticosteroids (which can lead to adrenal suppression) and inhalers. You should also explore symptoms that might suggest sleep apnoea, which is sometimes predictive of difficult intubation and unplanned or prolonged ventilation postoperatively.

Table 1.3 American Association of Anesthesiologists (ASA) grading system

ASA1	Normal healthy patient without clinically important comorbidity and without clinically significant past/present medical history
ASA2	Patient with mild systemic disease
ASA3	Patient with severe systemic disease
ASA4	Patient with severe systemic disease that is a constant threat to life

■ KEY POINT
Upper abdominal operations carry a greater risk of pulmonary complications than do lower abdominal or laparoscopic operations.

Observe the patient's breathing pattern: is it faster than normal or laboured? Is the patient breathless at rest? Is the chest examination normal?

Patients with suspected pulmonary dysfunction may require further investigation, depending on the nature of the proposed surgery. This may include a chest X-ray, full pulmonary function tests and sometimes blood gases to determine whether carbon dioxide (CO_2) retention is present. If surgery is necessary in the presence of severe pulmonary dysfunction, every effort should be made to optimise pulmonary function before surgery. Smokers should be encouraged to stop: more than a few weeks of abstinence will reduce their risks. Bronchodilators, physiotherapy and postural drainage may help clear inspissated secretions from the airway; steroids are sometimes indicated. A physiotherapist should teach the patient techniques of deep breathing and coughing before surgery so that the patient does not have to learn the techniques after their operation. Postoperative physiotherapy can be booked in advance.

Postoperative pain control is very important, balancing the benefits of allowing the patient to breath deeply with the risk of respiratory suppression if opiates are necessary. Consider with the anaesthetist whether an epidural will be of benefit during the postoperative period. Remember also that, in patients with severe pulmonary dysfunction, overuse of oxygen in the postoperative period can aggravate respiratory acidosis and lead to CO_2 retention.

Cardiac function

Question the patient for evidence of angina or limited exercise tolerance due to chest pain or breathlessness. Ask about previous heart disease and any treatment received. Non-urgent elective surgery is usually deferred for at least 6 months after myocardial infarction. Age over 60 years, evidence of peripheral vascular disease and major surgery (e.g. aortic aneurysm repair) are among the major risk factors for cardiac complications.

■ KEY POINT

Age over 60 years, evidence of peripheral vascular disease and major surgery (e.g. aortic aneurysm repair) are among the major risk factors for cardiac complications.

Is the patient still on medication, and will this affect the surgery? If the patient is on warfarin, consider whether warfarin should be replaced with a heparin infusion before and after surgery until warfarin is restarted. Most surgeons stop clopidrogel a week before elective surgery. The risk of increased bleeding with low-dose aspirin is less than that associated with clopidrogel, but the surgeon should at least be aware that the patient is taking aspirin. Check the patient's blood pressure and check the pulse for abnormal rhythm and rate. Is there evidence of peripheral vascular disease or diabetes? Examine the patient for evidence of congestive cardiac failure (including jugular venous pressure (JVP) and adventitial heart sounds), and consider whether formal cardiac assessment is required. An ECG and echocardiogram are relatively easy to organise, but more invasive investigations such as cardiopulmonary exercise testing (CPX), isotope scanning or cardiac angiography may be required. A useful method of risk stratification is based on functional class (Table 1.4) as defined by the New York Heart Association (Reginelli and Mills, 2001).

Table 1.4 New York Heart Association functional classes

Class 1	No limitation of regular physical activities
Class 2	Mild limitation of physical activities, comfortable at rest Normal physical activity results in dyspnoea, fatigue or angina
Class 3	Major limitation of physical activity, comfortable at rest Minimal physical activity results in dyspnoea, fatigue or angina
Class 4	Inability to perform any physical activity without symptoms Symptoms present at rest and worsened by any activity

Surgical risk in patients with heart failure can be minimised by delaying elective surgery until performance has been optimised using appropriate medication, but remember the impact of the delay on the patient's psychological and physical wellbeing.

Renal disease

Renal dysfunction is often asymptomatic, but chronic renal failure has widespread effects on the patient, which may impact on the postoperative course, particularly cardiac morbidity. As well as its association with hypertension and attendant complications, uraemia can lead to anaemia and impaired platelet function. This can increase the risk of perioperative haemorrhage. If the patient has recently been anticoagulated during haemodialysis, remember to check their clotting preoperatively. Patients may have hypocalcaemia or hypercalcaemia, which can be exacerbated by dehydration in the perioperative period.

> ■ KEY POINT
> Chronic renal failure has widespread effects on the patient, which may impact on their postoperative course.

Special consideration should be given to patients on dialysis. You may need to liaise with the renal team in order to schedule dialysis the day before surgery. Extra care is required with fluid replacement during and after surgery. Does the patient have a functional shunt? If so, remember not to put a blood pressure cuff on that arm.

Renal metabolism of drugs such as muscle relaxants is important. Patients who have had a kidney transplant may be on immunosuppressants.

Liver failure

If the patient has had hepatitis or has a history of excessive alcohol consumption, consider the possibility that they may have cirrhosis and portal hypertension. This may not have been diagnosed previously but could have significant implications for their procedure. Examine the patient for signs of liver disease, including spider naevi, palmer erythema and Dupuytren's contractures. A history or signs of liver disease are indications for checking liver function tests and blood clotting and, in some patients, hepatitis status. There are increasing numbers of patients with successful liver transplants, and they will be on immunosuppressants.

Check clotting in jaundiced patients and correct if necessary. Take care to avoid dehydration in the perioperative period, which can lead to renal impairment (hepato-renal syndrome). Malnutrition as assessed by hypoalbuminaemia is also an independent predictor for poor outcome: is a period of enteral supplementation indicated?

> ■ KEY POINT
> Check clotting in jaundiced patients and correct if necessary.

> ■ KEY POINT
> Hypoalbuminaemia is an independent predictor for poor outcome.

Endocrine system

Diabetes mellitus, especially type II, is common and sometimes discovered only when patients are assessed for surgery. In patients with established diabetes, consider the impact this may have had on their cardiovascular system and renal function. Autonomic neuropathy can impair the patient's response to cardiovascular stress.

Most patients with type II diabetes can be managed by omitting their oral medication on the day of surgery. Patients with type I diabetes require a sliding-scale insulin infusion. Ideally diabetic patients should be scheduled early on the operating list. Wound healing in uncontrolled diabetes can be impaired by volume depletion and hyperosmolar states, and there is an increased risk of wound infection.

Always look out for previously undiagnosed hypothyroidism and hyperthyroidism. Most patients who have been euthyroid for some time on medication should not pose any particular problem. However, patients who are hypothyroid may be more sensitive to some anaesthetic agents, while those who are hyperthyroid may be at risk of a thyroid storm or milder complications such as increased risk of cardiac arrhythmias and myocardial infarction.

Patients who have been taking corticosteroids may have adrenal suppression. Additional steroids, usually as hydrocortisone, in the perioperative period may be required.

> ■ KEY POINT
> Patients who have been taking corticosteroids may have adrenal suppression and may require additional steroids, usually as hydrocortisone, in the perioperative period.

If there is a family history of any endocrine disorder, or if the patient is known to have multiple endocrine neoplasia, reflect on whether a phaeochromocytoma has been adequately excluded. In some centres it is now usual to request plasma metanephrines and 24-h catecholamines.

Medication

Adverse drug interactions in the perioperative period should be foreseen and, if at all possible, prevented. Consider whether any of the patient's medications may have a pharmacodynamic or pharmacokinetic effect on the drugs used for their anaesthetic. A pharmacodynamic interaction is where a drug potentiates or antagonises another drug, usually by acting at receptors. A pharmacokinetic interaction is due to altered absorption, distribution, metabolism or excretion of a drug, and this can potentiate or antagonise the effects of another drug. A patient should be asked about any hypersensitivity or reaction to previous medications, especially antibiotics. Ask the patient what medication they are currently taking and what they have taken previously. If in doubt about which drugs should be continued and which should be stopped before anaesthetic, consult with the anaesthetist.

> ■ KEY POINT
> Interactions between a patient's medications and the drugs used in anaesthesia may be pharmacodynamic (where one potentiates or antagonises the other) or pharmacokinetic (due to altered absorption, distribution, metabolism or excretion).

The risk of losing disease control after stopping long-term medication before surgery is often greater than the risk posed by continuing medication during surgery. However, monoamine oxidase inhibitors should be stopped 2 weeks before surgery. Lithium can usually be stopped 24 hours before major surgery, but it may be continued if surgery is anticipated to be minor – that is, unlikely to lead to disturbance of fluid balance or electrolytes. Potassium-sparing diuretics should be omitted on the morning of surgery because a rise in serum potassium may be precipitated if there is impaired renal perfusion or tissue damage. Warfarin may be stopped temporarily if it was prescribed for a previous deep vein thrombosis or arrhythmias, but if the patient has a mechanical heart valve it may be necessary to convert the patient to heparin, stopping this a few hours before surgery and restarting it a few hours after surgery, before the patient is subsequently re-warfarinised.

The oral contraceptive pill should, ideally, be stopped 4 weeks before major elective surgery, any surgery to the legs and surgery involving prolonged immobility of a lower limb. The benefit of stopping the pill must be balanced against the risk of unwanted pregnancy. The pill should be recommenced at the first menses occurring at least 2 weeks after surgery. If this is impractical – for instance, because the patient is admitted as an emergency – then other steps should be taken to reduce the risk of deep vein thrombosis. This advice also applies to hormone replacement therapy and tamoxifen.

> ■ KEY POINT
> The oral contraceptive pill should be stopped 4 weeks before major elective surgery, any surgery to the legs and surgery involving prolonged immobility of a lower limb.

Pregnancy

It is usual to ask whether the patient is pregnant, but sometimes it is appropriate to request a pregnancy test as well. For the obviously pregnant patient, remember the potential impact on the patient's anatomy and physiology. The middle trimester is considered to be the safest time to operate. If surgery must be performed during pregnancy, then you should discuss the possible complications with the patient, in terms of both her own health and that of her unborn child. In the later stages of pregnancy there will be some circumstances when induction will be appropriate. You should not hesitate to ask an obstetrician for advice.

● ON THE DAY OF SURGERY

The surgeon and anaesthetist may or may not have met the patient before in the surgical or pre-assessment clinic. The full case notes and the results of any tests requested should be available. The surgeon needs all relevant X-rays in theatre.

It is important to check that no further health problems have arisen since the pre-assessment clinic and that the patient has been taking medication as advised before admission. If the patient has developed a cold it may be best to put off an elective operation, but if the decision is to proceed this must be made in conjunction with the anaesthetist.

> ■ KEY POINT
> On admission, check that no further health problems have arisen since the pre-assessment clinic and that the patient has been taking medication as advised before admission.

The operative site may need to be marked with an indelible marker. In many hospitals, correct site surgery documentation is also required. The Royal College of Surgeons of England and National Patient Safety Agency (2005) jointly launched guidance, and most hospitals have now introduced checklists that have to be filled in on the ward and in theatre, generally by nominated members of the team.

Advice on prevention of deep vein thrombosis and pulmonary embolus has been published by the National Institute for Health and Clinical Excellence (2007). The patient must be assessed to identify their risk factors and must be given information about their risks and effectiveness of prophylaxis. Consider for each patient which combination of preventive measures is appropriate, for example calf compression stockings, intermittent calf compression or subcutaneous low-molecular-weight heparin.

Shaving the operative site before theatre may increase the risk of surgical site infection: again, check local policy.

● CONSENT

If it was not done in clinic, the patient's consent must be recorded on admission by a surgeon capable of performing the procedure or trained to take consent for that procedure. Ultimately, the surgeon carrying out the operation is responsible for ensuring that the patient is genuinely consenting to what is being done, and this surgeon will be held responsible in law if this is later challenged (Department of Health, 2001).

The General Medical Council website (www.gmc-uk.org) is a rich resource of information on the process of taking informed consent (e.g. General Medical Council, 2008). You should be aware of these guidelines and how to proceed in cases where the patient cannot give consent legally or because their illness has rendered them incapable. The legal requirements vary between countries but, whatever the circumstances, you should act in a way that you can justify fully if your decision is questioned in the future.

You should explain potential complications in terms that the patient can understand. Some complications are very uncommon but, because of the morbidity that they incur, they must be discussed; examples include nerve injury during surgery on the thyroid and parotid glands, and erectile dysfunction after male pelvic surgery.

■ KEY POINT

You should explain potential complications in terms that the patient can understand. Some complications are very uncommon but, because of the morbidity that they incur, they must be discussed.

Remember to warn patients undergoing laparoscopic surgery that the procedure may be converted to an open one.

The list of potential complications is vast: if you can imagine something going wrong, then at some time it probably has. If you are not sure what to discuss with the patient, then you should not be taking the consent – liaise with a more senior doctor.

● SUMMARY

Preoperative care involves history-taking, clinical examination, appropriate investigations, risk assessment and informed consent. The process of preoperative care begins in the surgical clinic when the patient agrees to undergo surgery and continues in the pre-assessment clinic and when the patient is admitted. In order to minimise the risk of adverse outcomes, any concurrent conditions must be considered and treated appropriately, and surgery delayed if appropriate. Guidelines should be followed in order to choose the preoperative tests that are required and to gain the patient's consent. Prescribing antibiotic prophylaxis and prophylaxis against thromboembolic complications is also part of the process. Final checks, e.g. completing a correct site surgery document, occur in the anaesthetic room and theatre.

● QUESTIONS

1   What preoperative tests would be appropriate in a 65-year-old man admitted for an inguinal hernia repair?
2   Define the ASA grades.
3   What are the major risk factors for cardiac complications?
4   Which patients need supplements of corticosteroids after major surgery? What would you use and in what dose?
5   What methods do you know of for reducing the risk of thromboembolic complications? What are the advantages and disadvantages of each?
6   If a complication is rare, do you need to discuss it when asking for the patient's consent?

● REFERENCES

Advisory Committee on Dangerous Pathogens (2007). Infection control of CJD and related disorders in the healthcare setting (revised TSE guidance, part 4). In: *Transmissible Spongiform Encephalopathy Agents: Safe Working and the Prevention of Infection*. London: ACDP/Department of Health. www.advisory-bodies.doh.gov.uk/acdp/tseguidance/tseguidancepart4-30mar07.pdf (accessed 20 July 2007).

Association of Anaesthetists of Great Britain and Ireland (2001). *Pre-operative Assessment: The Role of the Anaesthetist*. London: Association of Anaesthetists of Great Britain and Ireland. www.aagbi.org/publications/guidelines/docs/preoperativeass01.pdf (accessed 20 July 2007).

Department of Health (2001). *Good Practice in Consent Implementation Guide: Consent to Examination or Treatment*. London: Department of Health. www.dh.gov.uk/en/Publicationsandstatistics/Publications/PublicationsPolicyAndGuidance/DH_4005762 (accessed 20 July 2007).

General Medical Council (2008). *Consent: Patients and Doctors Making Decisions Together*. www.gmc-uk.org/guidance/ethical_guidance/consent_guidance/index.asp (accessed 11 June 2008).

Improving Surgical Outcomes Group (2005). *Modernising Care for Patients Undergoing Major Surgery: Improving Patient Outcomes and Increasing Clinical Efficiency*. London: Improving Surgical Outcomes Group. www.reducinglengthofstay.org.uk/doc/isog_report.pdf (accessed 20 July 2007).

National Collaborating Centre for Acute Care (2003). *Preoperative Tests: The Use of Routine Preoperative Tests for Elective Surgery*. London: National Collaborating Centre for Acute Care/ Royal College of Surgeons of England. www.rcseng.ac.uk/publications/docs/preop_test.html (accessed 20 July 2007).

National Confidential Enquiry into Patient Outcome and Death (NCEPOD) (2005). *Abdominal Aortic Aneurysm: A Service in Need of Surgery? Summary Report*. London: National Confidential Enquiry into Patient Outcome and Death. www.ncepod.org.uk/2005report2/Downloads/summary.pdf (accessed 20 July 2007).

National Confidential Enquiry into Patient Outcome and Death (NCEPOD) (2008). *Death Following a First Time Coronary Artery Bypass Graft*. London: National Confidential Enquiry into Patient Outcome and Death. www.ncepod.org.uk/2008report2/Downloads/CABG_report.pdf (accessed 8 June 2008).

National Institute for Health and Clinical Excellence (2003). *Preoperative Tests: The Use of Routine Preoperative Tests for Elective Surgery*. Clinical guideline 3. London: National Institute for Health and Clinical Excellence. www.nice.org.uk/page.aspx?o=CG003 (accessed 20 July 2007).

National Institute for Health and Clinical Excellence (2007). *Venous Thromboembolism: Reducing the Risk of Venous Thromboembolism (Deep Vein Thrombosis and Pulmonary Embolism) in Inpatients Undergoing Surgery*. Clinical guideline 46. London: National Institute for Health and Clinical Excellence. www.nice.org.uk/guidance/CG46 (accessed 20 July 2007).

Reginelli JP, Mills RM (2001). Non-cardiac surgery in the heart failure patient. *Heart* **85**: 505–7.

Royal College of Surgeons of England (2007). *Improving Your Elective Patient's Journey*. London: Royal College of Surgeons of England. www.rcseng.ac.uk/publications/docs/patient_journey.html (accessed 20 July 2007).

Royal College of Surgeons of England, National Patient Safety Agency (2005). *Correct Site Surgery*. Patient safety alert 06. London: Royal College of Surgeons of England and the National Patient Safety Agency. http://www.npsa.nhs.uk/patientsafety/alerts-and-directives/alerts/correct-site-surgery (accessed 20 July 2007).

Perioperative care

Andrew Mavor and Qassim F Baker

INTRODUCTION

This chapter considers the safe transfer of the patient from the ward to the operating theatre, and some of the safety measures designed to limit the risks to the anaesthetised patient.

PATIENT IDENTIFICATION AND SAFETY MEASURES

It is unfortunate that the process of bringing the correct patient to theatre, and performing the planned operation on the correct side, should fail so often. Data from the National Patient Safety Agency (NPSA; www.npsa.nhs.uk) in the UK suggest that almost 25 000 cases of incorrect patient identification occurred in a single year of reporting. This figure is probably a low estimate. The hazards of patient misidentification do not need listing, but mismatched transfusions and surgery on the wrong limb are two of the higher-profile consequences of this fundamental error. Analysis of near-misses in commercial aviation suggest that the actual disaster – whether an air crash or an incorrect operation – is the end result of a series of errors, none of which may seem particularly dangerous in isolation but which in combination lead to a life- or limb-threatening situation.

Patient identification is one of several areas where mistakes may be made. Problems may arise when two patients on the ward have the same or similar names. The wrong case notes may accompany a patient and, unless the patient is specifically asked to confirm his or her name and details, information from the wrong notes may be used to plan surgery and decide on the site and side. Do not assume that patients will point out mistakes: hearing impairment, apprehension and pain may all prevent patients picking up on the fact that they are being addressed incorrectly. It is the responsibility of the operating surgeon to confirm before surgery that the patient in the anaesthetic room is the one expected and is having the operation indicated on the consent form.

Most of the steps to confirm a patient's identity involve manual checking of labels, consent forms, clinic letters, etc., combined with verbal confirmation by the patient. Manual checking is subject to human error, and mistakes such as misreading names and incorrectly stating hospital numbers are relatively common. In an attempt to reduce this sort of error, a number of newer techniques have emerged. These include the use of barcodes, which can be read by a machine and are in regular use by the blood transfusion service; radio-tagging, which allows data to be read electronically; magnetic strip 'credit-card' technology, which allows a recording of when and where the identification was made; and biometric methods such as fingerprint recognition, already widely used in personal digital assistants (PDAs). There are numerous barriers to the introduction of these new technologies – cultural, behavioural, economic and others. Nevertheless, the persistently and unacceptably high rate of incorrect procedures means that, in future, it will be quite normal to back up the routine verbal and manual checking of identity with electronic information. As mentioned above, problems arise when a series of errors occur, and adding in more checks means that the chance of everything going wrong at the same time is reduced.

● PREOPERATIVE WARD CHECKLIST

This is a standard list that would be checked by the ward nurse with the patient before leaving the ward for theatre:

- Name, date of birth, hospital number
- Allergy status (red wrist bands)
- Consent – planned operation with side, signed and dated
- Site of operation marked with indelible pen and as per the NPSA guidelines (see Further reading)
- Time of last meal and drink
- Clothing, jewellery, makeup, nail varnish and body piercings removed
- Dentures removed, and capped or crowned teeth noted
- Pregnancy
- Presence of any prostheses, e.g. joint replacement, implants, pacemaker
- Bladder emptied
- Bowel preparation if appropriate
- Blood and X-ray results
- Observations – blood pressure, pulse, oxygen saturation.

Once the patient is in the anaesthetic room, these checks are repeated partially or completely. In addition, in the UK, the NPSA has recommended a preoperative verification checklist, which includes details of the patient, the proposed operation, and the site and side of surgery. There are four checks; and these are completed by the operating surgeon and the ward staff and also involve the anaesthetist and theatre team. The final check is performed when the patient is in theatre, and the surgeon asks the anaesthetist and theatre team to confirm verbally that the correct patient is having the planned procedure on the intended site or side.

● INTRAOPERATIVE RISKS AND HAZARDS

The anaesthetised patient is especially vulnerable. Protective reflexes are lost, meaning that noxious stimuli (e.g. diathermy burns) do not induce the normal withdrawal reaction. Active movement is abolished, so that pressure (e.g. on a peripheral nerve) is not relieved. The normal indications that things are going wrong (e.g. the physiological changes seen early in hypoglycaemia) are absent. As well as hazards to patients, there are of course hazards to theatre staff during surgery, such as needlestick or sharps injury, infection (especially viral), diathermy burns and exposure to ionising radiation.

Common examples of hazards to patients include the following:

Injuries during movement of the patient

The anaesthetised patient must be supported carefully during the move from the anaesthetic trolley to the operating table, and abnormal extension of, for example, the limbs should be avoided. It is particularly important that the patient's head is supported well during such moves, in order to avoid injury to the cervical spine. The relevant padding, supports (e.g. neck rings) and table attachments should be available before the patient is moved so that there is no delay in supporting the patient once on the operating table.

Nerve injuries (neurapraxia)

Intraoperative nerve injuries result from failure to support the limbs properly and to prevent abnormal movements while the patient is paralysed, or from failure to protect vulnerable nerves from pressure from the operating table or its attachments. The following scenarios illustrate some of the hazards:

- Lithotomy (e.g. for procedures on the perineum) or reverse Trendelenburg position (e.g. for anterior resection of the rectum) may lead to pressure on the common peroneal nerve as it winds around the neck of the fibula if this area is protected inadequately.
- In lateral positions (e.g. for thoracotomy), if the arm is not supported properly, the radial nerve may be compressed against the humerus, leading to a wrist-drop, or the ulnar nerve may be compressed against the medial epicondyle.
- Hyperabduction of the arm during axillary surgery may lead to traction injury of the brachial plexus.

Retained swabs, instruments and needles

This is particularly likely during a long, complicated operation, which may involve a change of nursing staff, many atraumatic needles, and multiple packs or swabs placed within the abdomen during the procedure. It is standard practice to carry out a double-check of swabs, needles and instruments at the end of the procedure, but it is the surgeon's responsibility to ensure that all foreign objects have been removed before closing the wound. It may seem like a chore at the end of a major procedure, but this is exactly when the risk is highest.

● DIATHERMY

Diathermy involves the passage of a high-frequency alternating current (AC) through body tissues, where the current is locally concentrated, resulting in heating of the tissues. This is also known as electrosurgery.

Types of diathermy

Monopolar diathermy

The current is delivered from the generator to the diathermy knife or probe (active electrode) held by the surgeon (Figure 2.1). The current passes through the tissues to the return electrode (an adhesive metallic pad usually placed on the trunk or proximal part of a limb) and back to the generator. The current density is highest near the probe, and so this is where the greatest heating of the tissues occurs. Monopolar diathermy is used for cutting and coagulation of tissues.

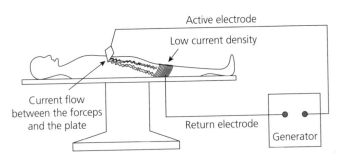

Active electrode

Low current density

Current flow between the forceps and the plate

Return electrode

Generator

Figure 2.1 ● Monopolar diathermy.

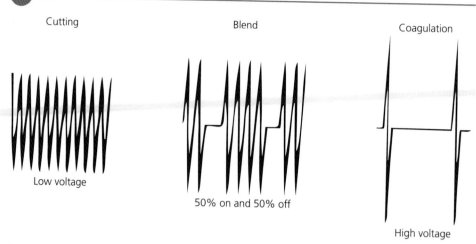

Cutting

Blend

Coagulation

Low voltage

50% on and 50% off

High voltage

Figure 2.2 ● Diathermy waveforms.

The effect depends on the waveform generated. Cutting is produced by generating a continuous wave. If the wave is discontinuous, then energy transfer to the tissues is reduced. The effect is a less rapid rise in temperature, and coagulation (rather than the vaporisation seen in cutting mode) occurs (Figure 2.2).

■ KEY POINT

The surgeon should avoid excessive use of diathermy on tissues, especially skin flaps, where local necrosis can easily occur. Monopolar diathermy should be avoided on the penis and digits: these have a relatively narrow attachment to the body where current density may be concentrated, resulting in heating of the tissues and coagulation of vessels.

Bipolar diathermy

This method involves passing a current between the tips of a pair of forceps or the blades of a pair of scissors (Figure 2.3). It avoids the need for a return electrode and uses less power, so causing less local thermal damage.

Figure 2.3 ● Bipolar diathermy.

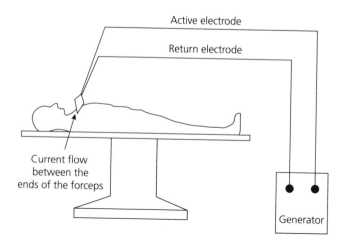

Active electrode

Return electrode

Current flow between the ends of the forceps

Generator

> ■ KEY POINT
> Bipolar diathermy cannot be used to cut tissues, and the bleeding point has to be held between the tips of the forceps. If the tips of the forceps are closed together on the tissue, the current will flow directly between the tips and not through the tissue.

Hazards of diathermy

Monopolar diathermy may produce a burn at the site of the return electrode if this is not applied correctly to the patient. Burns may also occur if there is contact between the patient and earthed metal objects such as drip stands and exposed metal parts of the operating table.

Beware of using diathermy on or inside the gut: intestinal gas contains hydrogen and methane, and the result is often inflammable and explosive.

Beware of using monopolar diathermy on appendages (salpinx, penis) and isolated tissue such as the testis (during herniotomy or orchidopexy leading to atrophy of the testis later on). The use of diathermy during circumcision in children can result in penile gangrene.

Patients with pacemakers or implantable cardioverter defibrillators (ICD) may be affected adversely by diathermy because of the electrical interference generated. Bipolar diathermy should be used wherever possible, although even this mode can generate sufficient interference to affect the implants. A patient with a pacemaker or ICD should be managed in conjunction with the cardiology department, which will advise on the most appropriate action – for example, deactivating the ICD so that it does not attempt to defibrillate the heart as a result of interference from diathermy. Guidance is available from the Medicines and Healthcare Products Regulatory Agency (MHRA) in the UK.

● TOURNIQUETS

Historically tourniquets were used on the battlefield to control bleeding before amputations. The modern use of tourniquets in surgical practice is primarily to produce a bloodless field. This allows accurate identification of structures and facilitates safe and accurate surgery. The tourniquet has an intrinsic and unavoidable drawback – bleeding on release of the tourniquet, which may be more difficult to control than if it were managed as the operation progressed. This is compounded by the hyperaemia that occurs on reperfusion of the ischaemic tissues. Tourniquets are most often used in orthopaedic surgery, but they may have a role in any surgery involving the extremities.

Types of tourniquet

Simple (non-inflatable) tourniquets

These include tourniquets used for phlebotomy and insertion of intravenous cannulae and, rarely, tourniquets used in traditional fashion for the emergency control of bleeding from a limb. This latter use is largely responsible for the tourniquet falling into disfavour in emergency medicine, as limbs have been lost because tourniquets were inadvertently left applied.

Pneumatic tourniquets

These are used to produce a bloodless field for surgery, usually in conjunction with an exsanguinating device, which displaces blood from the limb by compression. For surgery on the arm and lower leg, the recommended maximum inflation pressure is 250–300 mmHg applied for not more than 1 h. For the thigh, the recommended maximum inflation pressure is 300–350 mmHg applied for not more than 90 min. It is vital to record the inflation pressure and the time that the tourniquet was inflated and deflated.

Uses of the pneumatic tourniquet

- Surgery on the knee or elbow, including knee arthroscopy
- Surgery on the foot (e.g. removal of a ganglion) and hand (e.g. carpal tunnel decompression)
- Less commonly, intravenous regional anaesthesia, in which a special tourniquet with a double cuff is used in order to minimise the risk of accidental deflation.

Contraindications

The tourniquet is relatively or absolutely contraindicated under the following conditions:

- Sickle cell disease (risk of thrombosis)
- Presence of infection or cellulitis
- Presence of significant peripheral vascular disease (ankle brachial pressure index (ABPI) ≥ 0.7)
- Vascular graft, such as a femoropopliteal bypass (very high risk of graft thrombosis).

Complications

- *Tourniquet palsy:* spectrum of severity from neuropraxia to permanent irreversible damage; the radial nerve in the upper arm is the most commonly affected.
- *Local tissue necrosis and compartment syndrome:* especially likely following prolonged use. In severe cases, may result in crush syndrome (rhabdomyolysis) and acute renal failure.
- *Ischaemic damage due to arterial thrombosis:* most likely in patients with pre-existing arterial insufficiency. A typical example is an elderly patient with peripheral vascular disease who undergoes a knee replacement. It is vital to note and record the vascular status in all at-risk (e.g. elderly, diabetic) patients and, if necessary, to seek a vascular opinion before any orthopaedic surgery is carried out.
- *Failure to release the tourniquet:* particularly likely when a tourniquet such as a rubber or silastic catheter is applied to a digit, usually a toe. Part or all of the tourniquet may accidentally be left in place under a dressing.
- *Unplanned deflation of the tourniquet:* this can lead to troublesome intraoperative bleeding or (in the case of intravenous regional anaesthesia) potentially toxic systemic levels of local anaesthetic agent.

● INADVERTENT PERIOPERATIVE HYPOTHERMIA

Hypothermia is a common consequence of general anaesthesia unless certain precautions are taken. Reduction in body temperature should be avoided unless it is desired specifically to lower metabolic requirements, such as during some cardiac and neurosurgical procedures. The inadvertent cooling of a patient produces a number of physiological abnormalities; the most obvious to the operating surgeon will be the development of a coagulopathy. There are other, more subtle effects, including longer recovery from anaesthesia, alteration in the metabolism of drugs and anaesthetic agents, and increased incidence of wound infections.

Hypothermia is defined as a core temperature of less than 36 °C. The prevention of inadvertent hypothermia should begin on the ward before surgery. Patients are at particular risk of developing hypothermia if they are high-risk surgical candidates (American Surgical Association (ASA) grade II+), are undergoing major surgery, or have a risk of developing cardiovascular complications. Such patients should be kept warm before theatre; this may involve simple measures such as wrapping up well, but it could also include active heating, for example with forced air warming.

It is important to record the patient's temperature throughout the operation and to take action if hypothermia is developing. Basic precautions such as keeping the theatre warm and not leaving the patient exposed while waiting for surgery to begin will reduce heat loss. There are a number of intraoperative strategies that prevent or reduce hypothermia. These include intraoperative warming devices such as the Bair Hugger®, which circulates warm air over the patient; warming intravenous fluids; and minimising heat loss by ensuring that the patient, including the head if appropriate, is covered. The precautions should extend into the postoperative phase and the patient should not be returned to the ward unless the core temperature is at least 36 °C.

● SUMMARY

Safe and effective perioperative management will reduce the incidence of complications. Systems are in place to make surgery safer and every member of the theatre team should be familiar with the procedures. It is the surgeon's responsibility to ensure that the patient is correctly positioned for surgery and that the risks of injuries during surgery are minimised. It is important to have a working knowledge of technical aids, such as diathermy and tourniquets, so that they can be used effectively and with minimal risk. Finally, if any member of the team spots a potential risk in theatre, it is his or her duty to take appropriate action a soon as possible – even if this means stopping the proceedings. It is too late once the complication has occurred.

● QUESTIONS

1 What types of check are used to confirm that the correct patient is being sent to theatre on the ward? What are the potential hazards of this approach?
2 What precautions would you take in order to avoid incompatible blood transfusion in the anaesthetised patient?
3 Which nerves are particularly vulnerable to intraoperative injuries as a result of bad positioning or pressure?
4 What are the main indications for tourniquets in surgical practice?
5 What complications may occur as a result of applying a tourniquet?
6 What complications may occur from the use of diathermy?
7 What measures may be taken in order to prevent perioperative hypothermia?

● FURTHER READING

McEwen JA (2007). www.tourniquets.org. A very comprehensive website about surgical tourniquets.

Medical and Healthcare Products Regulatory Agency. www.mhra.gov.uk. Safety information about pacemakers and defibrillators during surgery.

National Institute for Health and Clinical Excellence (NICE). www.nice.org.uk/guidance/CG65. NICE guidelines on inadvertent peroperative hypothermia.

National Patient Safety Agency (2005). Correct site surgery. www.npsa.nhs.uk/patientsafety/alerts-and-directives/alerts/correct-site-surgery. Gives information about correct site surgery and the preoperative verification checklist.

03 Postoperative care

CG Nanda Kumar, Ahmed Al-Mukhtar and Munther I Aldoori

● THE POSTOPERATIVE CARE UNIT

For the patient to reap the full benefits of a surgical procedure, good postoperative care is of the utmost importance. Postoperative care is a continuum that begins at the end of surgery, with immediate care in the recovery or post-anaesthesia care unit (PACU). In this unit, the patient's level of consciousness, airway, breathing and circulation are observed carefully. Temperature is also measured, since hypothermia and pyrexia have their own problems and need to be corrected. Hypothermia can lead to shivering, which increases oxygen consumption and can lead to hypoxaemia.

The need for postoperative care is influenced by the severity of underlying illness, the duration and complexity of the anaesthetic and surgical procedures, and the potential for postoperative complications (Barash *et al.*, 1992). This needs specific care from the surgical point of view (e.g. for wound care, antibiotics, change of dressing) and also more general care (e.g. for pain relief, fluid and electrolyte balance, nutrition, oxygenation).

The postoperative period is a vulnerable time when things can go wrong very quickly. It is imperative that the PACU is close to the operating theatres in order to ensure a speedy return to theatre and rapid intervention if required.

The patient is handed over to the recovery unit staff by providing a concise summary of the patient's pre-existing medical condition, surgical procedure performed (including drains, bladder catheters, etc.) and intraoperative problems (including blood loss and urine output). Details of anaesthetic, fluids administered (including blood and blood products), analgesics, other drugs given (e.g. steroids, antibiotics) and estimated blood loss are given on handing over care. Clear instructions are given regarding any investigations that need to be undertaken, such as blood glucose and haemoglobin.

Appropriate prescription charts, e.g. for oxygen, fluids, blood and antibiotics, are completed and checked, and postoperative instructions, both surgical and regarding acceptable parameters, should be issued.

Potential problems and interventions must be laid out clearly. Trained personnel should monitor the patient for all the parameters mentioned above and ensure haemodynamic stability, adequate oxygenation and normothermia. Any major problems should be rectified before discharging the patient to the ward by handing over to the ward nurse.

Essential equipment

Certain essential equipment should be readily available in the recovery area:

- The trolley on which the patient is transported to the recovery area should have a mechanism for a rapid, easy head-down tilt.
- An oxygen supply and appropriate means of administering the gas (e.g. masks, nasal cannulae) must be available.
- Suction for maintaining a patent airway must be available.

Monitoring

All patients should be monitored for pulse oximetry and blood pressure. In addition, the following monitoring should be available:

- *Electrocardiogram (ECG)*: particularly in patients with cardiac abnormalities and arrhythmias, either pre-existing or perioperative
- *Airway equipment*: e.g. for endotracheal tubes, oro/nasopharyngeal airways, laryngoscopes, emergency cricothyrotomy kits
- *Invasive monitoring equipment*: for direct arterial pressure and central venous pressure (CVP) monitoring.

PROBLEMS IN THE POSTOPERATIVE CARE UNIT AND INTERVENTION

- *Hypoventilation*: this is one of the main problems in the immediate postoperative period (Box 3.1). Hypoventilation is an important cause of hypoxaemia and postoperative respiratory problems.
- *Drowsiness*: a decrease in the level of consciousness postoperatively is usually due to residual effects of anaesthetic agents and opiates, leading to depression of the central nervous system (CNS).
- *Nausea and vomiting*: this may be a distressing side effect of anxiety, pain, anaesthesia or the various adjuncts used, e.g. opiates, inhalational agents, antibiotics. Hypoxia and hypotension can also cause nausea.
- *Hypotension*: this is usually due to inadequate fluid replacement or increased fluid or blood loss, or it may be secondary to the effects of anaesthetic agents, particularly with regional techniques; occasionally it is secondary to arrhythmias.
- *Hypertension*: occasionally patients are hypertensive due to release of catecholamines, usually secondary to pain.
- *Pain*: see below.
- *Urinary retention*: this is secondary to pre-existing problems (prostatic hypertrophy), pain, opiates or regional techniques (e.g. spinal, epidural). If a bladder catheter is already in situ, blockage of the catheter must be ruled out; this is a common, but often overlooked, cause of postoperative restlessness.

PAIN

Pain is an unpleasant sensation perceived by the patient in response to nociceptive stimuli. Untreated pain can lead to several problems that can be detrimental to the patient (Table 3.1). Pain can cause sympathetic stimulation, which in turn may result in tachycardia, hypertension, sweating, anxiety, poor compliance with treatment and hypoventilation.

Pain after abdominal surgery can lead to splinting of the diaphragm, resulting in hypoventilation, hypoxaemia and atelectasis of the lungs, and predispose to postoperative retention of pulmonary secretions and pneumonia (reduced ability to cough).

Pain also causes the release of endogenous catecholamines, with cardiovascular sequelae.

Box 3.1 Causes of hypoventilation

Airway obstruction
- Tongue (falling back) or laryngeal spasm
- Foreign bodies (e.g. tooth, gauze), secretions, blood (due to trauma), vomit (including particulate matter), tumours
- Oedema or haematoma following surgery (particularly surgery involving the airway, e.g. ear, nose and throat (ENT), thyroid surgery).

Central respiratory depression
- Residual inhalational or intravenous anaesthetic agents
- Strong analgesics, particularly opioids (e.g. morphine)
- Hypocapnia
- Hypothermia
- Intracranial event (e.g. stroke).

Impaired mechanics of breathing
- Pain (particularly after abdominal surgery), leading to splinting of the diaphragm
- Residual effects of muscle relaxants
- Pneumothorax, haemothorax
- Obesity, leading to splinting of the diaphragm.

Table 3.1 Effects of postoperative pain

System	Effect
Central nervous	Anxiety, restlessness, lack of cooperation, stress response, hyperglycaemia
Cardiovascular	Tachycardia, hypertension, hypotension, (less commonly) due to vasovagal episodes
Respiratory	Hyperventilation, hypoventilation (particularly after abdominal surgery), hypoxaemia
Renal	Urinary retention (due to pain and certain regional analgesic techniques)
Gastrointestinal	Delayed gastric emptying, nausea and vomiting, constipation (following anal surgery)

Pain pathways

The following ascending pathways carry nociceptive impulses from the receptors to the sensory cortex:

- *First-order neurons:* free nerve endings carry sharp pain (fast pain) through myelinated Aδ fibres and slow pain (dull, aching) through unmyelinated C fibres to the dorsal horn, where the first-order neurons end and the second-order neurons begin (Figure 3.1).
- *Second-order neurons:* these cross over (over one to two segments) and ascend in the anterior (touch) and lateral (temperature and pain) spinothalamic tracts (Figure 3.2).
- *Third-order neurons:* these are differentiated in the thalamus (posteroventrolateral nuclei) and ascend to the sensory cortex (post-central gyrus).

This elicits the appropriate response, e.g. for withdrawal from a painful stimulus.

In our recovery unit, pain is commonly scored on a visual analogue scale of 0 to 10, with 0 being no pain and 10 being the worst possible pain. This is a crude guide to the patient's

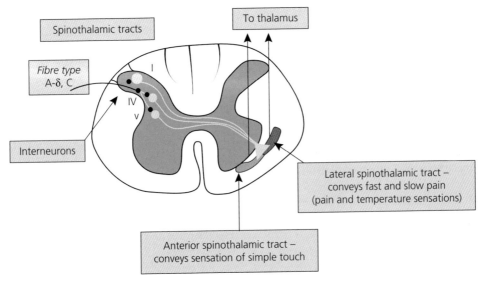

Figure 3.1 ● Pain pathway.

Reproduced with permission from AnaesthesiaUK (www.anaesthesiauk.net).

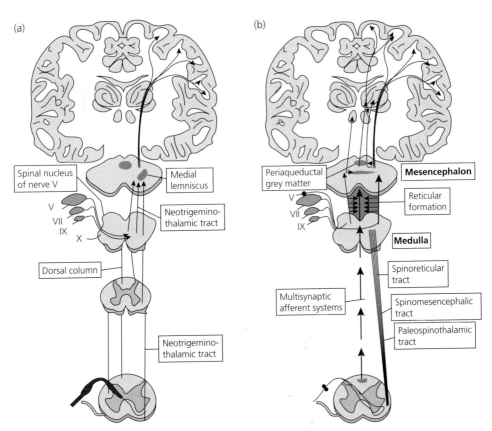

Figure 3.2 ● Temperature (a) and pain (b) pathways.

Reproduced with permission from AnaesthesiaUK (www.anaesthesiauk.net).

individual perception, since there is a great deal of individual variation in pain perception. The aim is to have a pain score of less than 4 before discharging the patient to the ward.

Objective assessment includes observing the patient's expression (grimacing, wincing), purposeful movements towards the surgical site, and parameters such as heart rate (usually increases but occasionally decreases), blood pressure (increases) and respiratory rate (increases except when depressed due to opiates).

Urinary retention and a full bladder are common causes of postoperative restlessness but are often overlooked. Beware the blocked urinary catheter!

Gate theory of pain

According to the gate control theory of Melzack and Wall (1965), the transmission of impulses conducting pain is regulated by a 'gate' and mediated through large afferent Aα fibres that inhibit transmission of pain from other afferents.

The 'gate' is believed to be located in the inhibitory neurons of lamina II in the dorsal horn of the spinal cord. This is the basis of transcutaneous electrical nerve stimulation (TENS) and probably acupuncture. A continuous stream of afferent impulses closes the 'gate' and prevents more painful impulses from being transmitted. Since the pain is not transmitted, it is not felt.

Pain is mediated by stimulation of the free or naked nerve endings and is accompanied by release of one of several mediators of inflammation, including prostaglandins, histamine, bradykinin, substance P and 5-hydroxytryptamine (5-HT, serotonin).

Mesencephalic pain inhibitory system

This is a descending inhibitory pathway that arises from the mesencephalic grey matter (periaqueductal grey matter, substantia nigra, dorsal raphe nucleus in the medulla) and descends to the dorsal horn cells (rexed laminae IV and V) in the spinal cord in the dorsolateral funiculus. Opiate receptors are found in the brain and spinal cord (dorsal horn neurons and on the terminals of the nociceptors within the dorsal horn).

Stimulation of the mesencephalic pain inhibitory system (e.g. by electrical stimulation or stress) produces intense analgesia.

Endogenous peptides such as substance P can be nociceptive or can produce analgesics such as endorphins and encephalins (see below).

Postoperative pain relief

Pain cascade/pain ladder

Figure 3.3 shows the three-step pain ladder of the World Health Organization (WHO):

Step 1: simple oral analgesics (non-opioid)
Step 2: stronger oral analgesics (opioid)
Step 3: strong oral or parenteral opioids.

Pain relief is assessed and administered appropriately (usually based on local protocols), postoperative nausea and vomiting are treated, the surgical wound (including drains, dressings, underwater seals, etc.) is inspected, and the appropriate specialists are alerted immediately if there are any concerns.

There are several methods of providing analgesia in the postoperative period. It must be borne in mind that postoperative analgesia can start in the preoperative period.

Preoperative administration

For short procedures where postoperative pain is anticipated, particularly in the day surgery unit, analgesics such as paracetamol and diclofenac can be included as part of the premedication. They

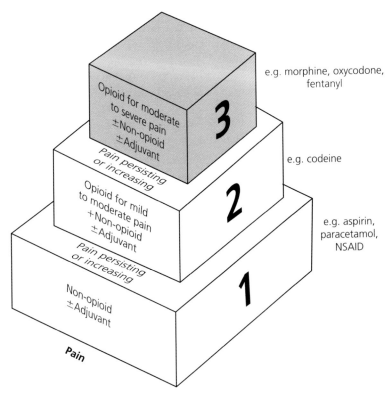

e.g. morphine, oxycodone, fentanyl

e.g. codeine

e.g. aspirin, paracetamol, NSAID

3 Opioid for moderate to severe pain ±Non-opioid ±Adjuvant

Pain persisting or increasing

2 Opioid for mild to moderate pain +Non-opioid ±Adjuvant

Pain persisting or increasing

1 Non-opioid ±Adjuvant

Pain

Figure 3.3 ● World Health Organization three-step pain ladder.

NSAID, non-steroidal anti-inflammatory drug.

can be administered orally or rectally (after informed consent). This proves useful in the post-operative period by reducing the requirements for postoperative analgesia.

Local anaesthetics

Local anaesthetics are generally administered intraoperatively or occasionally preoperatively, particularly for surgery undertaken under local anaesthesia.

Simple local anaesthetic techniques include wound infiltration, instillation at the operative site, field blocks (for inguinal hernia), nerve blocks (e.g. penile block for circumcision), plexus block (brachial plexus at different sites, e.g. for shoulder surgery), and central neuraxial block-ade (spinal/epidural) for intra- and postoperative analgesia.

Commonly used local anaesthetics are lidocaine (lignocaine) and bupivacaine.

Lidocaine is short-acting and in repeated doses is known to lead to tachyphylaxis (particu-larly when used for epidural blocks). The safe dose of lidocaine is 3–4 mg/kg when used plain and up to 6 mg/kg when used with adrenaline (epinephrine). Lidocaine is commonly available as 1% and 2% solutions, and for spinal use as 5% (heavy) solution; this is now not used fre-quently due to concerns regarding transient neurological syndrome (TNS).

The safe dose of *bupivacaine* is 2 mg/kg. Bupivacaine is commonly available as 0.25% and 0.5% solutions. For spinal (subarachnoid) injection, 0.5% solution rendered hyperbaric (heavy) by addition of dextrose is commonly used. Plain 0.5% bupivacaine (normally preser-vative-free) can also be used and is known to be slightly hypobaric (specific gravity less than that of cerebrospinal fluid, CSF). The baricity (specific gravity in relation to CSF) determines the preferential spread of local anaesthetics injected into the subarachnoid space. Hyperbaric solutions settle down into the most dependent part (since they are 'heavy'), while hypobaric solutions tend to rise up to the non-dependent area.

A 1% solution refers to a concentration of 10 mg/mL. Therefore, a 0.5% solution has a concentration of 5 mg/mL and a 0.25% solution has a concentration of 2.5 mg/mL. This is very important when calculating the amount of local anaesthetic that can be used safely for infiltration.

Care must be taken when injecting into areas with good blood flow, since more rapid absorption results in higher serum levels being attained more rapidly, increasing the likelihood of developing toxicity (see Chapter 17) – hence the mandatory precaution of aspirating the syringe before injecting local anaesthetics.

Bupivacaine has systemic toxicity refractory to treatment when serum levels exceed therapeutic limits, particularly related to the heart. Bupivacaine is thus contraindicated for intravenous (IV) regional analgesia, e.g. Bier's block.

Prilocaine (an ester local anaesthetic) is preferred for Bier's block. In doses larger than 600 mg, prilocaine can cause methaemoglobinaemia. The quest for safer isomers of its racemic mixture has led to the advent of two preparations that are believed to be safer, especially in relation to cardiac toxicity: ropivacaine and levobupivacaine use the safer, pharmaceutically isolated isomers of bupivacaine, greatly reducing the risk of cardiac toxicity and rendering them amenable to treatment if toxicity does occur.

Epidural and spinal anaesthesia can be used as the sole technique for the operation, e.g. for peripheral limb surgery, hernia repairs, and orthopaedic procedures on the hip and knee joints (Barash et al., 1992).

Epidural and spinal anaesthesia can also be used as an adjunct to general anaesthesia, particularly epidural analgesia coupled with general anaesthesia for major abdominal surgery. This helps to minimise the use of parenteral opiates, allows the patient an earlier return to consciousness at the end of surgery, and provides better quality of analgesia with minimal depression of consciousness, better ventilatory mechanics, minimal or no respiratory depression and the ability to cough and breathe without pain.

Potential side effects of epidural and spinal anaesthesia are hypotension, hindered ventilation (particularly with respect to the contribution of abdominal and intercostal muscles) with higher levels of blockade, and occasionally decreased sensation, which can interfere with ambulation (seen only with higher concentrations of epidural local anaesthetics). It is more common to find that the good pain relief actually aids and encourages ambulation.

Patients on anticoagulants need to be treated with extreme caution. Generally patients on low-molecular-weight heparin (LMWH) or fractionated heparin should not receive an epidural within 12 h of heparin administration. This is due to the definite risk of an epidural haematoma, which, although uncommon, is potentially dangerous and can lead to paraplegia if not treated urgently (usually surgically). Another risk is the formation of an epidural abscess.

Epidural analgesia is usually given by a continuous technique, using a clearly labelled custom-built infusion pump (Figure 3.4) and dedicated infusion lines that cannot be confused with IV infusion tubing. The epidural catheter is inserted into the epidural space. The epidural infusion consists of either local anaesthetic alone, or a combination of local anaesthetic and opiate.

Opiates

Endorphins (e.g. β-endorphin) and encephalins (enkephalins) are endogenous ligands for the opiate receptors. The precursor of adrenocorticotrophic hormone (ACTH) gives rise to β-endorphin and melanocyte-stimulating hormone (MSH). β-Endorphin is also released from the hypothalamus.

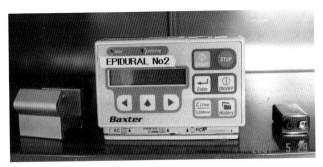

Figure 3.4 • Epidural infusion pump.

Encephalins are pentapeptides. They are distributed widely in the neurons of the CNS and in the intrinsic neurons of the gastrointestinal tract.

Opiates commonly used for spinal and epidural analgesia are *fentanyl* (2–4 µg/mL for epidural), *alfentanil* (20–40 µg/mL for epidural) and *diamorphine* (300–400 µg for spinal). All are highly lipid-soluble, bind to the opiate receptors in the spinal cord and reduce the requirement of local anaesthetics. These opiates help not only by enhancing the analgesia provided and the duration of blockade but also by reducing the dose requirements and side effects.

Morphine is poorly lipophilic. The usual dose is 0.1–0.2 mg. Morphine stays free in the CSF and can ascend up the spinal cord and produce delayed respiratory depression as much as 12 h later by depressing the respiratory centre. Since by this time the patient is usually on the ward, it could lead to potential problems. Therefore, morphine should be used with caution; alternatively, diamorphine should be used instead.

Local anaesthetic/opiate mixtures reduce the degree of hypotension. Since lower concentrations of local anaesthetic can be used, these mixtures also reduce the degree of motor blockade, permitting early ambulation and reducing the risk of deep vein thrombosis (DVT).

A potential problem of adding opiates to epidural infusions, particularly in abdominal surgery, is the possibility of reduced gut motility.

Parenteral analgesics range from subcutaneous and intramuscular to IV opiates. They are used both intraoperatively and postoperatively. The preferred route is intravenous.

Patient-controlled analgesia (PCA) is used increasingly in appropriate people. A device delivers a small dose of IV opiate (commonly morphine) on activation of a push-button that has to be pressed deliberately by the patient. The device is connected through custom-made IV tubing to a (preferably dedicated) IV cannula (Figure 3.5).

The bolus dose delivered is commonly 1 mg morphine. The device self-locks for a programmed period (usually 5 min) in order to prevent the patient from overdosing. Commonly, 100 mg of morphine sulphate is diluted in 50 mL of 0.9% sodium chloride.

The programming is checked by two staff members in order to avoid errors. The device is locked and is therefore tamper-proof. Reprogramming requires the device to be unlocked with a special key.

Problems of PCA include the following:

- The pump can fail and deliver a wrong dose.
- Occasionally the delivery tubing is disconnected and the patient does not receive the analgesic.
- Intravenous access may be occluded or extravasate into the subcutaneous tissue.
- The patient may be unduly sensitive to the doses administered or may not get any relief – the programming may then need to be altered.

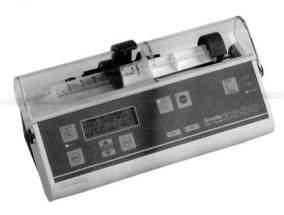

Figure 3.5 ● Graseby 3300 pump.

Reproduced with permission from AnaesthesiaUK (www.anaesthesiauk.net).

- If the key is misplaced, the programming cannot be altered.
- Errors in programming are possible – two nurses usually work together in order to avoid such errors.

Opiates and opioids have side effects. Naloxone is a specific antagonist, but it must be remembered that administration of naloxone not only reverses the side effects such as respiratory depression but also reverses the analgesia, leading to pain.

● FLUID BALANCE

Postoperative fluid balance is important in order to maintain circulating intravascular volume, isotonicity and adequate oxygen-carrying capacity. Fluid balance involves giving enough fluids and giving fluids appropriately based on the individual patient's needs.

Total fluid loss in the average adult is about 2500 mL/day. This includes 100–200 mL/day through the gastrointestinal tract, insensible fluid losses (through the lungs and skin) of about 500–1000 mL/day, and urine output of about 1000 mL/day.

The fluid volume required, therefore, is generally about 2500 mL/day for a 70-kg adult, with Na^+ of 30 mEq/L and K^+ of 15–20 mEq/L.

The fluids available are crystalloids, colloids, blood and blood products. Generally crystalloids containing electrolytes normally found in plasma are administered. Depending on the degree of blood loss (estimated and measured), blood and/or blood products might be required. Table 3.2 lists the types of fluids commonly used, and Figure 3.6 shows the volumes of distribution of isotonic colloid, saline and glucose solutions.

As a general rule, maintenance requirements to compensate for preoperative starvation and insensible loss amount to about 2 mL/kg/h (Barash *et al.*, 1992). In addition to maintenance requirements and measured loss, note the following:

- For most *major surgical procedures*, an additional 4 mL/kg/h should be added, giving a total of 6 mL/kg/h.
- For *major abdominal procedures and trauma*, an additional 6 mL/kg/h should be added, giving a total of 8 mL/kg/h.

- For *major thoracic and complex procedures*, 8 mL/kg/h is added to the maintenance regime, giving a total of 10 mL/kg/h.

In addition to maintaining general hydration and circulating volume, electrolytes, particularly potassium, have to be replaced and maintained. Lactated Ringer's solution contains potassium and is generally the preferred solution. The lactate is converted by a functioning liver into bicarbonate.

Table 3.2 Types of fluids commonly used

Fluid	pH	Osmolarity/osmolality (mosmol/L)	Electrolytes (mmol/L)	Duration in circulation (h)
Compound sodium lactate	Approx. 6	278	Na⁺ 131, K⁺ 5, Ca²⁺ 2, Cl⁻ 111, lactate 29	1–2
0.9% sodium chloride	6.5	300	Na⁺ 154, Cl⁻ 154	1–2
5% dextrose	4.1	278 (glucose is metabolised to leave water – hypotonic)	0	1–2
Haemaccel® (degraded gelatin)	7.3	350	Na⁺ 145, K⁺ 5, Ca²⁺ 6.2, Cl⁻ 145	2–4
Gelatins, e.g. Volplex®	7.4	284 (mean molecular weight 30 000)	Na⁺ 154, Cl⁻ 125	> 6
Dextran (40 or 70)	6–7	300–303 (mean molecular weight 70 000)	Na⁺ 154, Cl⁻ 154	4–6
Starches (penta- or hexa-), e.g. Voluven®	4.0–5.5	308 (mean molecular weight 130 000)	Na⁺ 154, Cl⁻ 154	> 6

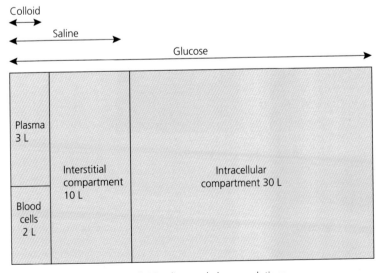

Figure 3.6 ● Distribution of isotonic colloid, saline, and glucose solutions.

Colloids stay in circulation for much longer and are broadly divided into gelatins (e.g. Haemaccel®, Gelofusine®) and starches (penta- or hexa-starches). Starches have varying molecular weights; larger-molecular-weight starches are broken down into smaller particles and hence last longer than small-molecular-weight starches in the intravascular compartment.

Dextrans are available in various molecular weights. Dextran 40 predisposes to interference with coagulation and dextran 110 can lead to renal problems. Dextran 70 seems to have fewer side effects.

Blood loss is estimated and if possible measured (gravimetric and colorimetric methods). Blood in suction bottles, drapes and other areas (e.g. on the floor) should be taken into account. Simple bedside tests, e.g. using the Hemocue® photometer, can give a quick and fairly accurate measure of the haemoglobin concentration (Figure 3.7).

Gravimetric methods involve weighing the blood-soaked gauze used during surgery and estimating the difference in weight between dry and soaked gauzes. This gives an approximate idea of blood loss. Older methods involved weighing the patient before and during or after surgery in order to estimate blood loss.

Colorimetric methods involve estimating the haemoglobin concentration of blood-soaked fluid and washing the blood-soaked gauzes in a known volume of isotonic fluid. This gives the approximate blood loss. Photometric methods, e.g. using the Hemocue discussed above, measure the haemoglobin from a tiny blood sample from the patient and are very accurate.

Indications for blood transfusion

The type of blood transfusion required depends on the severity and rapidity of blood loss:

- *Packed cells:* acute loss (e.g. surgical) where the haemoglobin concentration drops below 7–8 g/dL.
- *Fresh frozen plasma (FFP), clotting factor concentrates, cryoprecipitate (high concentration of factor VIII, fibrinogen and von Willebrand factor):* massive blood loss and haemodilution, where clotting factors are depleted.
- *Platelets:* generally if platelet count drops below $50 \times 10^9/L$ or below and/or if there is active bleeding despite surgical haemostasis with a platelet count below $100 \times 10^9/L$.

For further details, see Table 3.3 and Chapter 6.

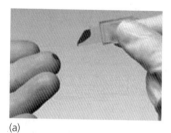
(a)

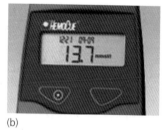
(b)

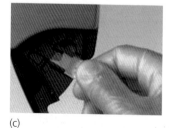
(c)

Figure 3.7 ● Using the Hemocue® haemoglobinometer.
(a) Apply the micro-cuvette to the specimen. Draw the correct volume into the cuvette by capillary action. (b) After wiping off any excess of the specimen from the sides of the cuvette, place it in the cuvette holder and insert it into the instrument.
(c) The laboratory-quality result is displayed automatically.

Table 3.3 Blood loss and blood transfusion

Class	I	II	III	IV
Blood loss				
%	< 15	15–30	30–40	> 40
Volume (mL)	< 750	750–1500	1500–2000	> 2000
Blood pressure				
Systolic	Unchanged	Normal	↓	↓↓↓
Diastolic	Unchanged	≠ (narrow pulse pressure)	↓	↓↓↓
Heart rate (beats/min)	< 100	↑	↑↑	↑↑↑
Capillary refill	Normal (< 2 s)	Delayed	Very slow	Undetectable
Respiratory rate (breaths/min)	Normal (< 20)	↑	↑↑	↑↑↑
Urine output (mL/h)	Normal (> 30)	20–30	10–20	< 10
CNS	Normal or slightly anxious	More anxious	Restless, agitated, confused	Drowsy, lethargic, unconscious
Management	Crystalloids	Crystalloids/colloids	Blood transfusion in addition to class II	Blood and blood products (clotting factors, platelets, etc.)

● POSTOPERATIVE PYREXIA

Pathophysiology

Fever is a regulated increase in body temperature. It is one part of a complex host defence response to infection and non-infectious disease (Negishi and Lenhardt, 2003). Fever develops when cytokines – such as interleukins 1, 2 and 6 (IL-1, IL-2, IL-6), interferons (IFN) and tumour necrosis factor alpha (TNF-α) – are released as a response of the body to inflammation and tissue damage. These endogenous cytokines, including macrophages and inflammatory proteins, increase the thermostatic set point in the hypothalamus by inducing prostaglandin (PGE2) in the cells lining the brain ventricles, which in turn results in increased heat production and decreased heat dissipation.

These cytokines do not pass the blood–brain barrier, and the molecular aspects of how these cytokines send signals to the brain to induce prostaglandins are not fully understood.

Fever, like other parts of the acute response to inflammation, is mediated by the immune, endocrine and neuronal systems.

During the course of fever, various mediators are released to decrease the set point and prevent the body temperature from rising to dangerous levels. These endogenous antipyretics include interleukin 10 (IL-10), glucocorticoids, vasopressin, MSH, nitric oxide (NO) and TNF-α.

The role of tumour TNF-α in fever is controversial. Some studies indicate that it acts as a cryogen to inhibit fever, while others suggest that it is an endogenous pyrogen that mediates fever.

Fever may up-regulate some host defence mechanisms and inhibits the growth of bacteria under specific conditions. It has been shown that there is positive correlation between survival and maximum temperature in Gram-negative sepsis.

Harmful effects of pyrexia

Fever can have harmful effects, especially for elderly people and patients with poor cardiac or pulmonary function. In fever, the heart rate is increased by about 9 beats/min and oxygen consumption is increased by about 7 per cent per 1 °C rise in temperature.

The increases in heart rate and oxygen consumption reflect a higher metabolism, which in the short term is probably relatively harmless; if prolonged, however, this can lead to breakdown of skeletal muscles for energy, with concomitant increased water loss (300–500 mL/m^2/day per 1 °C) and alveolar hyperventilation, which leads to alkalosis.

Fever in the postoperative period greatly aids the detection of complications.

Common causes of postoperative pyrexia

There are four causes of postoperative fever that should always be considered first (Leaper, 2000):

- Deep and superficial wound infection
- Pulmonary infection
- Deep and superficial venous thrombosis
- Urinary tract infection.

The sooner the fever appears after an operation, the more serious is the complication.

Relationship between the cause and the timing of postoperative pyrexia

The time when pyrexia is observed postoperatively may give a clue to the cause:

- At *24–48 h* postoperatively, one should consider pulmonary atelectasis, the non-specific metabolic response to trauma, a transfusion reaction, and pyrogen-containing IV fluids.
- At *2–7 days* postoperatively, consider chest infection, urinary infection (particularly if there is an urinary catheter), IV or central line infection, and wound infection.
- At *5–10 days* postoperatively, consider anastomotic leak, wound abscess and DVT.

Relationship between the cause and the degree and type of postoperative pyrexia

The level of postoperative fever is variable:

- *Postoperative pneumonia* can occur during any stage of the postoperative period. Atelectasis and decreased cough efforts increase the risk considerably.
- The fever may reach different levels on different days. The fever accompanying *postoperative thrombosis* is commonly of low grade but increasing slowly and steadily.
- In the *postoperative urinary tract infection*, the higher the temperature, the more dangerous the infection.
- A sudden increase in fever to 40 °C combined with localised symptoms indicates *urinary tract sepsis*, which may be fatal in elderly or debilitated patients if not treated promptly with IV fluids, antibiotics and relief of urinary outflow obstruction.
- Patients who present with high fever on the first or second day after abdominal or thoracic anastomosis should be considered to have *anastomotic leak* until proven otherwise.
- *Necrotising fasciitis* can occur earlier than other wound infection and is associated with high fever.

The pattern of fever may indicate the cause of pyrexia. Spiking, 'church-spire' fever up to 39–40 °C may indicate the presence of intra-abdominal abscess following an anastomotic leak, whereas a 'grumbling' pyrexia of about 37.5–38 °C indicates an early atelectasis or perhaps a later wound infection.

Postoperative fever may also be due to an unrelated common infection such as tonsillitis or to drug reactions.

● VENOUS THROMBOEMBOLISM

The term 'venous thromboembolism' (VTE) encompasses DVT and pulmonary embolism (PE). Venous thromboembolism has a high prevalence among surgical patients. During the perioperative period DVTs in both proximal and distal deep veins are often clinically silent. By the time a proximal DVT has been diagnosed, PE has occurred in around 50 per cent of patients, although only 30–40 per cent are symptomatic. Without treatment PE has a mortality rate of approximately 30 per cent. Different types of surgery are associated with varying risks of VTE. Up to 60 per cent of patients undergoing major orthopaedic surgery and 25 per cent undergoing general surgery will develop DVTs without prophylaxis (Rogers *et al.*, 2007).

Pathophysiology

The pathophysiology of VTE formation is multifactorial. Virchow proposed his celebrated triad of thrombosis – blood stasis, endothelial wall damage, and a local or systemic state of hypercoagulability – over a century ago.

Venous thrombosis commonly originates in veins with slow blood flow. These are typically the calf and thigh veins, accompanying valve pockets and at the bifurcation of veins. Slow blood flow is aggravated by postoperative immobilisation. Poor blood flow alone is not sufficient to cause thrombosis because of the presence of natural anticoagulants.

Vessel wall damage is essential to thrombus formation. Vascular endothelial damage activating the clotting system and contributing to the hypercoagulable state is a reason for the high DVT rate in major hip and knee orthopaedic surgery.

There is a recognised link between VTE and hypercoagulable state. There is usually a balance between procoagulant factors and opposing anticoagulant factors, together with the fibrinolytic system, to prevent abnormal thrombosis formation. Any variation in this intricate coordination can result in a procoagulant state. If this imbalance is secondary to an inherited defect, then the patient has a lifelong risk for thrombosis. However, if the hypercoagulable state is a temporary state, then the risk will decrease after cessation of the situation (Solymoss, 2000).

Risk factors

All patients admitted to hospital should be assessed for their individual risk of a thromboembolic event (Rogers *et al.*, 2007; Solymoss, 2000). This should take into account:

- personal risk factors for VTE;
- previous history of VTE;
- the type of surgery or trauma.

> ■ KEY POINT
> All patients admitted to hospital should be assessed for their individual risk of a thromboembolic event.

Acquired risk factors

- Age

- Obesity (BMI > 30) – thought to cause decreased fibrinolytic activity and anti-thrombin III levels
- Surgery or trauma
- Pregnancy and the postpartum period
- Cancer and chemotherapy:
  - patients with cancer have a four to eight times increased chance of an acute thromboembolic event compared with the general population;
  - patients with cancer are often in a procoagulant state, due to increased production of tissue factor
- Oral contraceptive pill (OCP) and hormone replacement therapy (HRT):
  - spontaneous risk in young females of a thromboembolic event is less than 1 in 10 000 per year; it is three times higher in women taking a low-dose modern OCP
  - OCP has only a small impact in surgery, increasing the VTE risk from 0.5 per cent to 0.9 per cent
  - stopping the OCP 4–6 weeks before surgery may reduce this risk, but there is currently no consensus on this policy
- Prolonged immobilisation
- Significant comorbidity, including recent myocardial infarction (MI), cerebrovascular accident (CVA) or congestive cardiac failure (CCF)
- Antiphospholipid syndrome:
  - autoimmune condition of unknown cause
  - diagnostic autoantibodies are lupus anticoagulant, anticardiolipin or anti-$\beta 2$-glycoprotein I
  - causes inhibition of natural anticoagulants and the fibrinolytic system and activation of endothelial cells, monocytes, platelets and complement
  - characterised by venous and arterial thrombosis and fetal loss
  - affects up to 40 per cent patients with systemic lupus erythematosus (SLE), but can also present in isolation
  - not all patients with antiphospholipid antibodies develop antiphospholipid syndrome, and therefore diagnosis is also based on clinical findings
  - risk of recurrent thrombosis if antibody levels remain high, necessitating warfarin to maintain an international normalised ratio (INR) of 3–4.

Genetic risk factors

Inherited thrombophilias are a group of conditions that predispose patients to thromboembolic events.

Common genetic factors include the following:

- Activated protein C resistance
- Factor V Leiden – due to a single point mutation in the factor V gene; prevalence is about 5 per cent, although varies with race
- Elevated factor VIII levels
- Mutation of prothrombin gene – present in 2 per cent of healthy individuals and 8 per cent of patients with VTE.

Uncommon genetic factors include the following:

- Hyperhomocysteinaemia – autosomal recessive disorder of homocysteine metabolism that promotes thrombosis through damage to endothelium, and indirectly inhibits protein C activation
- Anti-thrombin III deficiency – rare autosomal dominant condition that is not a direct cause but provides an environment that allows development of thrombosis when other risk factors are present

- Protein C and S deficiencies – vitamin-K-dependent proteins that inactivate procoagulant cofactors; prevalence of protein C deficiency is 0.4 per cent; protein S prevalence is unknown
- Elevated factor IX, X and XI levels.

Diagnosis

In many patients DVTs are asymptomatic or present with non-specific symptoms. The remainder present with pain, erythema and tenderness. The most significant sign is pitting oedema, which correlates with a diagnosis of DVT in 70 per cent of cases.

Substantial thrombosis of the femoral vein can result in a white, painful swollen leg, phlegmasia alba dolens, as a consequence of capillary compression by gross tissue oedema. A blue painful leg as a consequence of thrombosis of the iliac veins is called phlegmasia caerulea dolens, venous gangrene (Figure 3.8).

Well's prediction rule for deep vein thrombosis

Patients are classified as low, moderate or high risk for DVT after a clinical assessment of risk factors and clinical findings (Scarvelis and Wells, 2006). Each of the following clinical characteristics is assigned one point:

- Active cancer (or treatment within the past 6 months)
- Paralysis, paresis or recent plaster immobilisation of the lower extremities
- Recently confined to bed for more than 3 days or major surgery within the past 12 weeks requiring general or local anaesthetic
- Localised tenderness along the distribution of the deep venous system

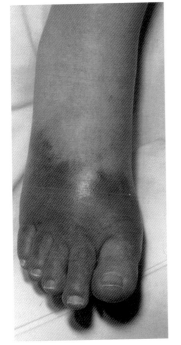

Figure 3.8 ● Phegamasia caerulea dolens.

- Swelling of entire leg
- Calf swelling more than 3 cm larger than asymptomatic side (measured 10 cm below tibial tuberosity)
- Pitting oedema confined to the symptomatic leg
- Collateral superficial veins (non-varicose).

Two points are subtracted for any alternative diagnosis at least as likely as DVT.
The probability of DVT is as follows:

High: ≥ 3 points
Moderate: 1–2 points
Low: < 1 point.

In addition, patients with a suspicion of DVT should undergo D-dimer testing. D-Dimer is released as the breakdown product from a fibrin blood clot. Although high readings are seen with acute thrombosis, D-dimer levels are also raised in a variety of conditions, such as trauma, surgery, haemorrhage, cancer and pregnancy. D-Dimer elevation is a sensitive but non-specific test (Scarvelis and Wells, 2006).

> ■ KEY POINT
> All patients with a suspicion of DVT should undergo D-dimer testing.

In patients with a low risk of DVT on clinical assessment and a negative D-dimer, the diagnosis of DVT can be excluded without further tests. D-Dimer assay results should not be used to rule out a DVT in patients with a high clinical probability.

In patients with a moderate to high clinical risk, both D-dimer testing and Doppler ultrasound examination should be performed. Acute DVT is recognised on ultrasound as occlusive, non-echogenic, continuous thrombosis. If there are doubts over the ultrasound examination, serial testing should be performed and the patient treated with low-molecular-heparin doses in the interim period. The sensitivity of ultrasound is high (over 95%) for the detection of proximal vein DVTs but much lower (73%) in detecting DVTs in the distal calf, upper limb veins and asymptomatic patients.

Computed tomography pulmonary angiography (CTA) is now usually the first imaging test on a clinical suspicion of a PE and has a reported sensitivity of 83–100 per cent. If the possibility of a DVT has not been investigated previously by ultrasound, then computed tomography (CT) venography can be combined with CTA. This increases the detection rate of thromboembolic disease compared with CTA alone but has no major advantage if Doppler ultrasound has been performed previously.

Treatment

The aim of treatment for a lower-limb DVT is to stop the propagation of thrombus, prevent PE, optimise fibrinolysis and prevent recurrence.

Initial treatment

Either unfractionated heparin (UFH) or LMWH is recommended as first-line treatment. A fixed LMWH daily dose does not require laboratory monitoring and has fewer complications compared with an adjusted dose of UFH. Current practice is to administer heparin for 5–7 days while implementing oral anticoagulant therapy.

Long-term treatment

Warfarin, a vitamin K antagonist, is the standard and effective treatment for the prevention of a recurrent thrombotic event. Therapy is usually continued for 3–6 months, when the risk of a thrombotic recurrence reduces. In patients with a combined genetic defect, long-term warfarin treatment should be considered beyond 6 months. Warfarin is recommended as prophylaxis for patients with multiple genetic defects and a high risk of thromboembolic complications.

Other interventions

Thrombolysis has been trialled in addition to standard anticoagulation therapy. Unfortunately thrombolysis has not been shown to affect the rate of PEs and also confers a major risk of haemorrhage, including intracranial haemorrhage. Therefore, the routine use of thrombolytic therapy is not recommended, except in cases of a massive DVT resulting in phlegmasia caerulea dolens, which can threaten the survival of the affected limb.

Another treatment used in conjunction with anticoagulant therapy is an inferior vena cava filter. This has been demonstrated to reduce the risk of PE; conversely, however, the filter increases the risk of recurrent DVT formation. Retrievable filters are possibly indicated in patients with a newly diagnosed DVT and a contraindication to anticoagulation therapy.

Prevention of venous thromboembolism

The National Institute for Health and Clinical Excellence (NICE) guidelines suggest that every patient admitted for surgery should be assessed for their risk factors for a thromboembolic event.

General advice

- All patients undergoing surgery should be offered thigh-length graduated compression stockings (unless contraindicated).
- Regional anaesthesia reduces the risk of a thrombotic event compared with general anaesthesia and should be offered if it is an appropriate alternative.
- Young females are advised to stop the OCP 4 weeks before surgery.
- All patients should be encouraged to mobilise as soon as possible after surgery.
- Care should be taken to prevent patients becoming dehydrated.

Orthopaedic surgery

- Patients should be offered mechanical prophylaxis and either LMWH or fondaparinux.
- Patients undergoing hip surgery (both elective replacement surgery and acute surgery) are advised to continue their LMWH or fondaparinux for 4 weeks after surgery.

General, cardiac, gynaecological, vascular and neurological surgery

- All patients should be offered mechanical prophylaxis.
- If one or more risk factors (apart from surgery) for a thrombotic event is present, the patient must be offered LMWH or fondaparinux in addition.
- The exception is that neurosurgical patients with ruptured cranial or spinal vascular malformations should not be offered pharmacological prophylaxis until the lesion has been secured.

Fondaparinux is a synthetic compound and a newer anticoagulant that catalyses antithrombin mediated inhibition of factor Xa. Fondaparinux has so far demonstrated equal results when compared with LMWH.

● SUMMARY

- Venous thromboembolic disease is common in surgical patients.
- All patients should be assessed for underlying risk factors and given appropriate prophylaxis.
- Clinical symptoms vary. Any patient with a suspicion of thrombosis should be clinically evaluated, D-dimers performed and ultrasound performed if warranted.
- Treatment is usually initially with heparin before longer-term warfarin.

● QUESTIONS

1. Define hypothermia, and list its causes and problems.
2. What is stridor? What are the causes and management of upper airway obstruction?
3. Discuss postoperative fluid and electrolyte replacement.
4. What are the indications for postoperative ventilatory support (elective/emergency)?
5. Discuss intra-abdominal sepsis and postoperative pyrexia.
6. Discuss atelectasis.
7. Discuss the methods of postoperative pain relief available.
8. What is D-dimer and what is fondaparinux?

● REFERENCES

Barash P, Cullen B, Stoelting R (1992). *Clinical Anesthesia*, 2nd edn. Philadelphia, PA: Lippincott.

Leaper DJ (2000). Postoperative care. In: Toouli J, Russell C, Devitt P, Ingham Clark C. *Integrated Basic Sciences*. London: Arnold, pp. 679–84.

Melzack R, Wall PD (1965). Pain mechanisms: a new theory. *Science* **150**: 971–9.

Negishi C, Lenhardt R (2003). Fever during anaesthesia. *Best Pract Res Clin Anaesthesiol* **17**: 499–517.

Rogers SO Jr, Kilaru RK, Hosokawa P, *et al.* (2007). Multivariable predictors of postoperative venous thromboembolic events after general and vascular surgery: results from the patient safety in surgery study. *J Am Coll Surg* **204**: 1211–21.

Scarvelis D, Wells PS (2006). Diagnosis and treatment of deep-vein thrombosis. *Can Med Assoc J* **175**: 1087–92.

Solymoss S (2000). Risk factors for thromboembolism: pathophysiology and detection. *Can Med Assoc J* **163**: 991–4.

04 | Cardiovascular monitoring

CG Nanda Kumar

● INTRODUCTION

Cardiovascular monitoring is a mandatory component of patient monitoring and starts before induction of anaesthesia. The onset of anaesthetic care of the patient starts from the time the anaesthetist institutes patient monitoring.

> ■ KEY POINT
> Cardiovascular monitoring is a mandatory component of patient monitoring.

● THE IMPORTANCE OF CARDIOVASCULAR MONITORING

Why monitor the cardiovascular system?

- To assess the function of the heart and the circulation of blood, which carries oxygen (O_2) to the tissues and eliminates carbon dioxide (CO_2) from the tissues.
- Surgery can produce fluid shifts, blood loss and alterations to tissue perfusion.
- Anaesthesia can produce haemodynamic changes and alterations to tissue perfusion.
- With advances in technology and in anaesthetic techniques, we are undertaking more complex surgical procedures in older and sicker patients. These patients are likely to have greater comorbidity, particularly related to the cardiovascular system.
- Inadequate tissue perfusion results in decreased oxygen delivery to the tissues. (Oxygen delivery to tissues depends on oxygen content of arterial blood and tissue blood flow.) This leads to anaerobic metabolism, lactic acidosis and shock.

What do we monitor?

- Electrocardiogram (ECG)
- Arterial blood pressure (non-invasive and invasive)
- Central venous pressure (CVP)
- Oxygen saturation of arterial blood (SpO_2)
- Capnograph (measurement of CO_2 breathed out by the patient)
- Cardiac output (non-invasive and invasive)
- Tissue perfusion (indirectly), e.g. urine output, gastric pH
- Acid–base balance (lactic acidosis is an indicator of anaerobic metabolism).

What are the benefits of monitoring?

- Optimum tissue perfusion and oxygenation
- Better haemodynamic stability
- Better wound-healing
- Better outcome.

How do we monitor?

- Equipment
- Techniques
- Complications
- Recent trends.

The Association of Anaesthetists of Great Britain and Ireland (AAGBI, 2000) has set minimum monitoring standards:

The presence of an appropriately trained and experienced anaesthetist is the main determinant of patient safety during anaesthesia. However, human error is inevitable, and many studies of critical incidents and mortality associated with anaesthesia have shown that adverse incidents and accidents are frequently attributable, at least in part, to error by anaesthetists.

The following minimum monitors need to be present and used before induction of anaesthesia:

- *Pulse oximeter:* measures the percentage oxygen saturation of the arterial blood using a finger probe and light-emitting diodes using the absorption of red and infrared radiation by haemoglobin (Hb).
- *Non-invasive blood pressure monitor:* blood pressure can be monitored using a Riva–Rocci sphygmomanometer and the use of Korotkoff sounds (if recording manually) or measured automatically.
- *Direct arterial blood pressure monitor:* a cannula is inserted into a peripheral artery, usually the radial artery, to measure continuous arterial blood pressure (Figures 4.1 and 4.2). This is also useful for taking repeated samples for arterial blood gas analysis.

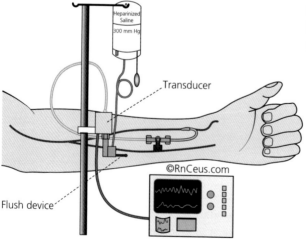

Figure 4.1 • Direct arterial blood pressure monitor.

From http://rnceus.com/hemo/artline.htm

Figure 4.2 ● Normal arterial wave form.

From http://rnceus.com/hemo/artline.htm

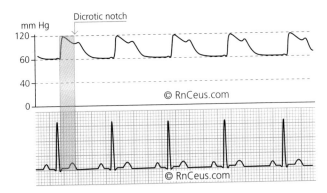

● *Capnograph:* measures the CO_2 breathed out by the patient (end tidal CO_2). This is the only medicolegally acceptable evidence of correct placement of an endotracheal tube within the trachea. This also indicates indirectly the arterial carbon dioxide tension ($PaCO_2$) and therefore the adequacy of ventilation (Figures 4.3 and 4.4).

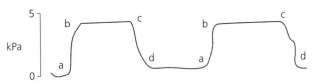

Figure 4.3 ● Normal capnogram. (a) Near-zero baseline – exhalation of CO_2-free gas contained in dead space. (a–b) Rapid, sharp rise – exhalation of mixed dead space and alveolar gas. (b–c) Alveolar plateau – exhalation of mostly alveolar gas. (c) End tidal value – peak CO_2 concentration – normally at the end of exhalation. (c–d) Rapid, sharp down stroke – inhalation.

Figure 4.4 ● Capnogram in a patient with delayed expiration, e.g. in chronic obstructive pulmonary disease (COPD).

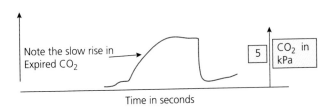

● ECG: monitors the electrical activity of the heart. Gives an idea about the heart's rhythm and rate and can give information about myocardial ischaemia.
● *Cardiac output monitor:* determines tissue perfusion and oxygenation (see later). Tissue perfusion is also assessed indirectly by measurement of urine output, and occasionally splanchnic perfusion is assessed by gastric tonometry (estimation of pH of gastric acid).
● *Acid–base balance:* generally determined by arterial blood gas analysis, which gives useful parameters such as the arterial oxygen and carbon dioxide tensions, pH, base excess and bicarbonate.
● *Additional monitoring:* determined by the patient's comorbidity.

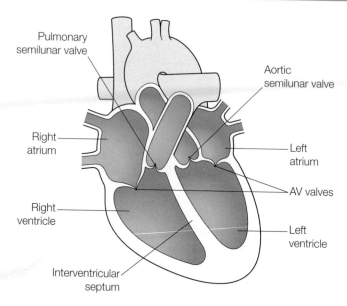

Figure 4.5 • Diagram of the heart chambers.

● CARDIAC PHYSIOLOGY

The heart and the blood vessels comprise the cardiovascular system. The heart acts to ensure that blood is delivered to the organs and tissues of the body. The heart can be considered as two parallel pumps, each with an atrium and ventricle, acting in synchrony to pump blood into the pulmonary (from the right side) and systemic (from the left side) circulations (Figure 4.5).

Blood contains Hb, which carries oxygen to the tissues, and also contains plasma, which contains dissolved oxygen. The Hb carries 97 per cent of the oxygen (1.34 mL of oxygen per 1 g of Hb), while the plasma carries 0.003 mL/mmHg of oxygen/100 mL of blood. The arterial oxygen content is measured as volume per cent and is about 20 mL/100 mL of blood.

Carbon dioxide is transported in the plasma mainly as bicarbonate (HCO^{3-}). This accounts for 80 per cent of the CO_2: most of the rest is carried by the Hb as carbamino compound, while a small quantity (about 3 mL/100 mL) is dissolved in the plasma.

Gas exchange occurs at the level of the lungs and the tissues. In the lungs, oxygen from the atmosphere is taken up by the blood in the alveolar capillaries, which also gives up the CO_2 carried from the tissues. In the tissues, the oxygen carried by the plasma and Hb are delivered, and the CO_2 produced is taken up.

Oxygen delivery from the atmosphere to the tissues follows the oxygen cascade (Figure 4.6).

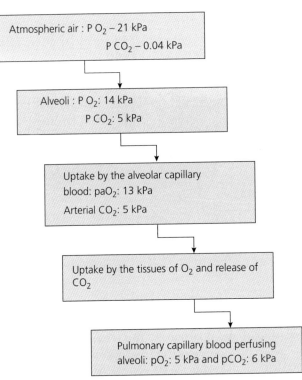

Figure 4.6 ● Partial pressures in gas exchange.

Atmospheric air : $P O_2 - 21$ kPa
$P CO_2 - 0.04$ kPa

Alveoli : $P O_2$: 14 kPa
$P CO_2$: 5 kPa

Uptake by the alveolar capillary blood: paO_2: 13 kPa
Arterial CO_2: 5 kPa

Uptake by the tissues of O_2 and release of CO_2

Pulmonary capillary blood perfusing alveoli: pO_2: 5 kPa and pCO_2: 6 kPa

● ELECTROCARDIOGRAPHY

Continuous ECG monitoring (Figure 4.7) is a non-invasive way of observing immediate evidence of changes in the heart rate and detecting and diagnosing arrhythmias. Changes in the ECG morphology may indicate the presence of myocardial ischaemia or electrolyte disturbances such as hypo- or hyperkalaemia.

> ■ KEY POINT
> Changes in the ECG morphology may indicate the presence of myocardial ischaemia or electrolyte disturbances.

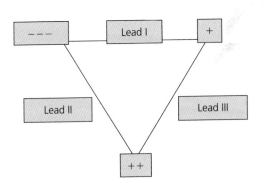

Figure 4.7 ● Einthoven's triangle, showing standard limb leads.

Lead I

Lead II   Lead III

Figure 4.8 ● Components of a normal electrocardiogram (ECG).

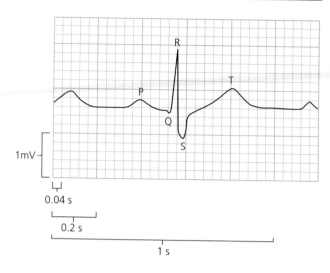

Basic electrocardiography

The components of a normal ECG are shown in Figure 4.8.

In the normal heart, the sequence of depolarisation is initiated in the sinoatrial (SA) node in the right atrium and then spreads through the atrial muscle. This is seen as the *P wave*. The depolarisation wave is channelled through the atrioventricular (AV) node and the His–Purkinje system and passes into the right and left ventricles through the corresponding bundle branches (specialised conducting tissue). This is seen as the *P–R interval* on the ECG.

Ventricular depolarisation corresponds to the *QRS complex* and triggers ventricular contraction. Provided depolarisation originates above the ventricles and passage through the conducting system is normal, the QRS complex will be narrow (< 100 ms). If conduction is aberrant or delayed, or if the focus originates below the AV node, then the QRS complex will be broad (> 100 ms).

The *T wave* on the ECG represents ventricular repolarisation. The normal cardiac rate is 60–100 beats/min (bpm). A rate of < 60 bpm is defined as bradycardia and > 100 bpm as tachycardia. The intrinsic rate of the SA node is around 120 bpm, but this is toned down by the parasympathetic activity of the vagus.

Standard lead II is best for monitoring rhythm disturbances, as P waves are seen most clearly in this position. Placement of leads in the so-called CM5 position, however, gives the most reliable evidence of myocardial ischaemia (alterations to the ST segment) and demonstrates most dysrhythmias. The right arm electrode of lead I is placed over the centre of the manubrium sterni (CM) and the left arm electrode over the left fifth intercostal space in the anterior axillary line (5). The indifferent electrode is placed on the left shoulder.

The display on a cardiac monitor is suitable only for rhythm recognition, and not for analysis of ST segment abnormalities or more detailed interpretation. A printout of the rhythm allows better interpretation of the rhythm.

How to read a rhythm strip

Figure 4.9 indicates the PR and QRS intervals of an ECG. Application of the following basic principles will help interpret most rhythms:

● Ventricular (QRS) rate can be calculated by counting the number of large squares between complexes.

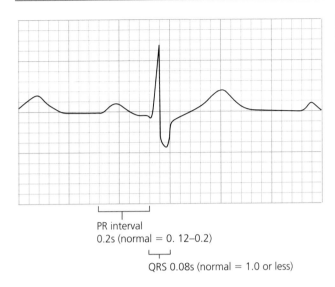

Figure 4.9 ● PR and QRS intervals of an electrocardiogram (ECG).

PR interval
0.2s (normal = 0. 12–0.2)

QRS 0.08s (normal = 1.0 or less)

- Heart rate is 300/number of large squares.
- Is the QRS rhythm regular or irregular?
- Is atrial activity present, i.e. are P waves visible?
- How is atrial activity related to ventricular activity? Is there a constant relationship between P waves and the ensuing QRS complex? A normal P–R interval should be < 0.2 s (one large square).
- Is the QRS complex normal or prolonged?

The rhythm strips also form a useful record of the event. In the case of a difficult arrhythmia or evidence of ischaemia, a 12-lead ECG may contain additional diagnostic information.

Figure 4.10 shows the haemodynamics of the cardiac cycle as seen on an ECG.

Points to remember

- ECG monitoring provides no indication of the adequacy of the circulation and can lead to a false sense of security.
- ECG should be used in conjunction with other forms of monitoring that indicate the presence and adequacy of the circulation.
- A normal-looking ECG is no guarantee that the patient is not profoundly hypoxic or hypovolaemic or that the patient even has a pulse. It is quite possible to have normal electrical activity without adequate contractility (e.g. in pulseless electrical activity, PEA).

> ■ KEY POINT
> ECG should be used in conjunction with other forms of monitoring that indicate the presence and adequacy of the circulation.

● CENTRAL VENOUS PRESSURE

The measurement of CVP involves inserting a catheter into a central vein, connecting the catheter to a transducer (a device that converts one form of energy to another) via a fluid-filled (heparinised saline) column, and zeroing the transducer so that it is at the level of the right atrium

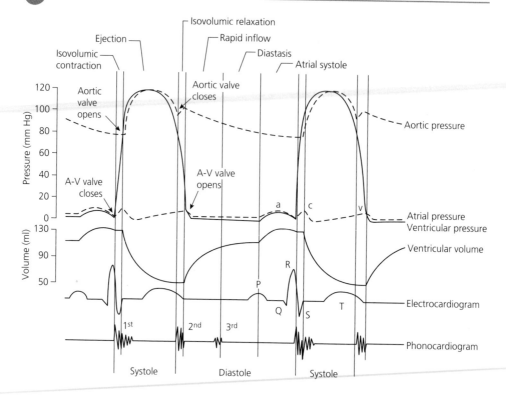

Events of the cardiac cycle for left ventricular function, showing changes in left atrial pressure, left ventricular pressure, aortic pressure, ventricular volume, the electrocardiogram, and the phonocardiogram.

Figure 4.10 ● Electrocardiogram (ECG) and associated haemodynamics in the cardiac cycle.

(mid-axillary line at the level of sternal angle). The transducer is connected to a monitor, which displays the waveform and the numerical values in terms of millimetres of mercury (mmHg).

Normal CVP values are 5–10 cmH_2O (or a very similar value in mmHg, since specific gravity of mercury is 13.6, and 10 mm = 1 cm).

Methods of insertion of a CVP catheter are shown in Figure 4.11.

The CVP trace has three positive and two negative waveforms (Figure 4.12):

- The a wave corresponds to atrial systole (and the P wave on ECG).
- The c wave corresponds to isovolumetric contraction of the right ventricle, causing a bulge of the tricuspid valve into the right atrium (correlates with the end of QRS on ECG).
- The v waves are due to filling of the right ventricle leading to a lifting of the tricuspid valve (correlates with the end of the T wave on ECG).
- The x descent is due to ventricular contraction pulling down the tricuspid valve.
- The y descent is due to ventricular diastole (opening of the tricuspid valve).

The relationship between ECG and CVP is shown in Figure 4.13.

Left atrial pressure is measured indirectly by using a pulmonary artery catheter (Swan–Ganz). This is a multi-lumen balloon floatation catheter introduced through a central vein and advanced until the tip of the catheter is in the pulmonary artery. The inflated balloon wedges

A. Catheter over needle

(a) insert into vein

(b) remove needle

Figure 4.11 ● Insertion of a central venous pressure catheter.

B. Catheter over guidewire (Seldinger technique)

(a) insert wire through needle in vein

(b) remove needle

(c) pass catheter over wire

(d) remove wire

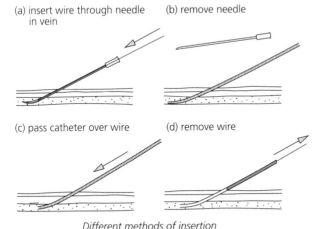

Different methods of insertion

Figure 4.12 ● Waves associated with central venous pressure trace.

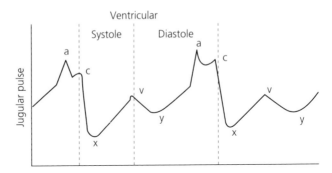

against the pulmonary artery and gives a wedge pressure, which indicates the left atrial pressure. This technique has been largely replaced by less invasive methods.

The saline used to fill the pressure tubing and transducer assembly is anticoagulated (heparin 1–2 units/mL) to prevent thrombus formation. The measurement is both analogue (in the form of a pressure wave) and digital (numbers indicating systolic, diastolic and mean arterial pressures).

● CARDIAC OUTPUT

Cardiac output is the volume of blood pumped by the heart per minute. For an average adult (70 kg) at rest, cardiac output is about 5 L/min. During severe exercise, cardiac output can increase to over 30 L/min (although not unfit people).

The three main determinants of cardiac output are preload, cardiac contractility and afterload.

Figure 4.13 •
Relationship between
electrocardiogram and
central venous pressure
waveform.

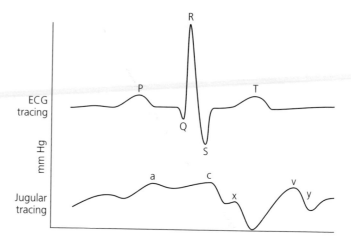

Preload reflects ventricular filling and is determined chiefly by venous return.

Contractility is determined by the force of ventricular contraction and in the normal heart is determined largely by the initial fibre length, which is determined by the ventricular filling (preload). Within physiological limits, greater initial ventricular filling (preload) results in greater contractility and hence increased cardiac output.

When the ventricular filling exceeds the ability of the heart to increase its contractility, decreased cardiac output results. This is believed to be due to stretching of the sarcomeres beyond their optimal length, such that actin and myosin do not overlap enough in order to produce an effective contraction.

Afterload is the resistance that comes into play after the onset of cardiac contraction and is determined largely by the systemic vascular resistance (SVR) and the pulmonary vascular resistance (PVR) for the left and right sides of the heart, respectively.

The *stroke volume* is the volume of blood pumped out of each ventricle during each contraction. It increases as the initial fibre length increases, within physiological limits. This initial fibre length of the heart muscle is represented as 'filling pressure' on the x-axis of the graph in Figure 4.14 and corresponds to the filling of the heart or 'preload'.

Cardiac output is often divided by body surface area to take into account the size of the subject. Cardiac output is then expressed as $L/min/m^2$ and is known as the 'cardiac index'. This is much more accurate, since there is a large variation in individual values of cardiac output, which can create a wrong impression of its true significance.

Oxygen delivery is the product of the cardiac output and the arterial oxygen content and represents the amount of oxygen delivered to the tissues in the arterial supply.

Oxygen flux is the volume of oxygen delivered by the left ventricle per minute and is usually about 1000 mL/min. This includes the volume of oxygen carried by the Hb and plasma and is influenced by the amount of Hb present, the per cent saturation of Hb and the cardiac output.

Why measure cardiac output?

- It is frequently necessary to assess the state of a patient's circulation.
- The simplest measurements, such as heart rate and blood pressure, may be adequate for many patients, but more detailed measurements are needed if there is a cardiovascular abnormality.
- Cardiac output and, more reliably, cardiac index provide a better indication of tissue perfusion and oxygen delivery than blood pressure or central venous pressure.

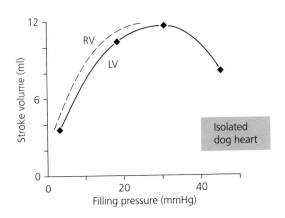

Figure 4.14 ● Starling's curve for the heart.

■ KEY POINT

Cardiac index provides a better indication of tissue perfusion and oxygen delivery than blood pressure or central venous pressure.

Methods of measuring cardiac output

The Fick principle

According to the Fick principle:

Cardiac output = oxygen consumption/arteriovenous oxygen content difference

The original method described by Fick in 1870 is difficult to carry out. Several variants of the basic method have been devised, but usually they are less accurate. There are many other methods of measuring cardiac output nowadays, but the most accurate are those that use some form of indicator dilution.

Bio-impedance

This method was described by Kubicek and colleagues in 1966 and has been reviewed by Critchley and Critchley (1999).

A small, high-frequency current is passed through the thorax from a pair of spot electrodes stuck to the skin. Sensing electrodes are used to measure the changes in impedance within the thorax; the normal value for an adult is 20–48 Ω at a frequency of 50–100 Hz. Contraction of the heart produces a cyclical change in transthoracic impedance. Although the method has been reported to give accurate results in normal subjects, several studies show some inaccuracy in critically ill patients.

Echocardiography

Transoesophageal echocardiography (TOE) provides diagnosis and monitoring of a variety of structural and functional abnormalities of the heart. It can be used to derive cardiac output from measurement of blood flow velocity by recording the Doppler shift of ultrasound reflected from the red blood cells.

The instantaneous blood flow velocity during one cardiac cycle is obtained for the blood flow in the left ventricular outflow tract (other sites can also be used). This is multiplied by the cross-sectional area and the heart rate to give cardiac output.

LiDCO

The LiDCO™ system is a bolus indicator dilution method of measuring cardiac output. A small dose of lithium chloride is injected via a central or peripheral venous line; the resulting arterial lithium concentration–time curve is recorded by withdrawing blood past a lithium sensor attached to the patient's existing arterial line.

The LiDCO™*plus* haemodynamic monitor is intended for monitoring continuous blood pressure and cardiac output in patients with pre-existing peripheral arterial line access.

The PulseCO™ algorithm computes the heart beat period and stroke volume from the entire blood pressure waveform.

● ORGAN AND TISSUE PERFUSION

Organ and tissue perfusion is the ultimate goal of the cardiovascular system and blood circulation. Vital organs have autoregulatory mechanisms to regulate their blood flow, e.g. the renin–angiotensin–aldosterone mechanism in the kidneys. Autoregulation occurs within a range of mean arterial pressures (MAP) and maintains organ perfusion. Myogenic and metabolite theories are the most commonly postulated mechanisms for autoregulation.

Direct and indirect assessment of organ perfusion can be achieved by assessment of blood flow to the organs and by assessment of organ function. Simple measurements such as urine output give an idea of adequate hydration, MAP and adequate perfusion to the kidneys.

Adequate oxygen should be carried by blood to the tissues. This depends on the amount of Hb (g/100 mL of blood) available, the percentage of Hb fully saturated with oxygen, the inspired concentration of oxygen and an adequate circulation of the blood for it to reach the tissues.

Control of the blood pressure is central, via the vasomotor centre, and peripheral, via the feedback mechanism from the baroreceptors in the carotid sinus and aortic arch (Figure 4.15).

Figure 4.15 ● Baroreceptors.

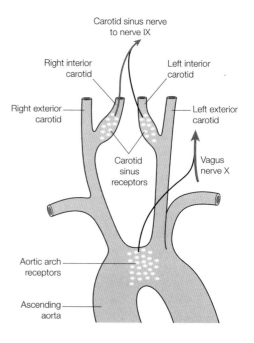

Carotid sinus nerve to nerve IX

Right interior carotid

Left interior carotid

Right exterior carotid

Left exterior carotid

Carotid sinus receptors

Vagus nerve X

Aortic arch receptors

Ascending aorta

● SUMMARY

- Based on the baseline parameters of the individual patient, the urgency and the complexity of the planned surgical procedure, monitoring, particularly for the cardiovascular system, needs to be established sufficiently early.
- The goal is to optimise the patient's preoperative status to the best extent possible in the time available for surgery, without causing further deterioration to the patient's pathophysiology. This may involve wide-bore peripheral intravenous access, monitoring of fluid intake and output, CVP monitoring if required, and occasionally direct arterial pressure monitoring.
- In more complex cases, cardiac output monitoring is also established before surgery.
- The main determinants of cardiac output are preload, contractility and afterload. These are optimised by adequate volume replacement and, if required, pharmacological agents. This optimisation is continued throughout and after the surgical procedure so that the patient has the best chance of coming through the surgery and anaesthesia successfully.
- Induction of general anaesthesia and regional blocks, e.g. for epidural (sympathetic blockade), can affect the venous return (preload), contractility (some anaesthetic agents are myocardial depressants) and afterload (sympathetic blockade, vasodilation).
- General anaesthesia can result in arrhythmias, which, if severe, can affect cardiac function.
- Splanchnic circulation may be decreased during general anaesthesia.
- Prolonged hypotension can lead to vital organ dysfunction, particularly of the kidneys.
- Blood loss is a common cause of hypovolaemia. Blood loss should be assessed carefully and replaced with fluids and, if severe, blood and blood products.
- The patient's regular medications, e.g. angiotensin-converting enzyme (ACE) inhibitors, beta-blockers and calcium channel blockers, can not only aggravate the hypotension produced by anaesthetic agents but also make the hypotension more difficult to correct.
- The chief goal of patient management is to maintain the cardiovascular parameters around 15–20 per cent of their baseline values (Tables 4.1. and 4.2).

● QUESTIONS

1 How is cardiac output controlled?
2 How is central venous pressure measured?
3 How is arterial blood pressure regulated?
4 How is left atrial pressure measured?
5 What is shock?

● REFERENCES

Association of Anaesthetists of Great Britain and Ireland (2000). Recommendations for Standards of Monitoring During Anaesthesia and Recovery. London: Association of Anaesthetists of Great Britain and Ireland.

Critchley LAH, Critchley JAJH (1999). A meta-analysis of studies using bias and precision statistics to compare cardiac output measurement techniques. *J Clin Monit* **15**: 85–91.

Kubicek WG, Karnegis JN, Patterson RP (1966). Development and evaluation of an impedance cardiac output system. *Aerosp Med* **37**: 1208–12.

Table 4.1 Normal haemodynamic parameters (adult)

Parameter	Equation	Normal range
Arterial blood pressure (BP)	Systolic (SBP) Diastolic (DBP)	90–140 mmHg 60–90 mmHg
Mean arterial pressure (MAP)	$SBP + [(2 \times DBP)/3]$	70–105 mmHg
Right atrial pressure (RAP) (corresponds to CVP)		2–6 mmHg
Right ventricular pressure (RVP)	Systolic (RVSP) Diastolic (RVDP)	15–25 mmHg 0–8 mmHg
Pulmonary artery pressure (PAP)	Systolic (PASP) Diastolic (PADP)	15–25 mmHg 8–15 mmHg
Mean pulmonary artery pressure (MPAP)	$[PASP + (2 \times PADP)]/3$	10–20 mmHg
Pulmonary artery wedge pressure (PAWP)		6–12 mmHg
Left atrial pressure (LAP)		6–12 mmHg
Cardiac output (CO)	$HR \times SV/1000$	4.0–8.0 L/min
Cardiac index (CI)	CO/BSA	2.5–4.0 L/min/m^2
Stroke volume (SV)	End diastolic volume (EDV) – end systolic volume (ESV)	60–100 mL/beat
Systemic vascular resistance (SVR)	$80 \times [(MAP - RAP)/CO]$	800–1200 dynes s/cm^5
Pulmonary vascular resistance (PVR)	$80 \times [(MPAP - PAWP)/CO]$	< 250 dynes s/cm^5
Ventricular ejection fraction (VEF)	SV/EDV	40–60%

Table 4.2 Oxygenation parameters (adult)

Parameter	Equation	Normal range
Partial pressure of arterial oxygen (Pa_{O_2})		80–100 mmHg
Partial pressure of arterial CO$_2$ (Pa_{CO_2})		35–45 mmHg
Bicarbonate (HCO_3)		22–28 mEq/L
pH		7.38–7.42
Arterial oxygen saturation (Sa_{O_2})		95–100%
Mixed venous saturation (Sv_{O_2})		60–80%
Arterial oxygen content (Ca_{O_2})	$(0.0138 \times Hgb \times Sa_{O_2}) + (0.0031 \times Pa_{O_2})$	17–20 mL/dL
Venous oxygen content (Cv_{O_2})	$(0.0138 \times Hgb \times Sv_{O_2}) + (0.0031 \times Pv_{O_2})$	12–15 mL/dL
AV oxygen content difference ($C(av)_{O_2}$)	$Ca_{O_2} - Cv_{O_2}$	4–6 mL/dL
Oxygen delivery (D_{O_2})	$Ca_{O_2} \times CO \times 10$	950–1150 mL/min
Oxygen consumption (V_{O_2})	$(C(av)_{O_2}) \times CO \times 10$	200–250 mL/min

05 | *Shock, blood transfusion and coagulation*

Sheila M Fraser, Amer Aldouri and Giles Toogood

- Introduction
- Shock
- Blood transfusion in the surgical patient
- Coagulation
- Bleeding disorders
- Thrombophilia
- Summary
- Questions
- References

● INTRODUCTION

This chapter reviews the pathophysiology, clinical signs and treatment of shock, concentrating on hypovolaemic or haemorrhagic shock and considers issues connected with blood transfusion and bleeding in the surgical patient, including the processes of coagulation and haemostasis and the situations in which these processes are disrupted – bleeding disorders and thrombophilia.

● SHOCK

Shock is defined as impaired tissue oxygenation. In most classes of shock, this is due to the inadequate perfusion of tissues. In septic shock, cells are unable to utilise the oxygen supply. There are five categories of shock (Table 5.1).

> ■ KEY POINT
> Shock is defined as inadequate tissue perfusion and oxygenation.

Hypovolaemic shock (haemorrhagic shock) is usually secondary to rapid blood loss. It remains a leading cause of death in trauma patients and is important in surgical practice. It is the main cause of shock considered in this chapter.

> ■ KEY POINT
> Hypovolaemic shock is usually most significant in surgical practice.

Pathophysiology of hypovolaemic shock

Severe haemorrhage produces a pathological state resulting in an inadequate supply of oxygen to the cells. The reduction in tissue perfusion and oxygen availability leads to a predominantly anaerobic metabolism. Compared with aerobic metabolism, this is extremely energy-inefficient, requiring high amounts of glucose to produce a small quantity of adenosine triphosphate (ATP), a nucleotide that functions as the intracellular energy store. Instead of carbon dioxide being produced as a by-product of the reaction, lactate and hydrogen ions are released. These rapidly cause a metabolic acidosis with associated cellular swelling and further loss of extracellular fluid into the cells. Lactate is metabolised in the liver, which does not function efficiently to clear the acidosis due to decreased perfusion and generalised hypoxia.

Table 5.1 Categories of shock

Category	Notes
Hypovolaemic	Usually secondary to rapid blood loss
Cardiogenic	Usually due to acute myocardial infarction (MI) with at least 40% damage or death of left ventricle
	Majority of patients have had previous MI with associated stenosis of all main coronary vessels
Septic	Divided into hyperdynamic (warm) and hypodynamic (cold) septic shock
	Hyperdynamic shock is early; main physiological problem is impaired cell metabolism, preventing efficient oxygen utilisation to form adenosine triphosphate (ATP)
	Hypodynamic shock occurs when sepsis persists without adequate fluid resuscitation
	Increased capillary permeability occurs very early in septic shock
	Fluid moves from intravascular to interstitial space, causing profound hypotension requiring aggressive fluid resuscitation
Anaphylactic	Usually history of initiating event
	Penicillin is most common iatrogenic cause; bee and wasp stings and shellfish are other frequent causes
	Stridor, wheeze and swelling of mouth, tongue or around bite sites may be evident
	Due to immunoglobulin E (IgE) production, with subsequent release of histamine and slow-reacting substances of anaphylaxis
Neurogenic	Typically caused by blockade of sympathetic nervous system by trauma or pharmacological agents
	Produces vasodilation of arterioles in affected area and increased vascular capacity, with subsequent relative hypovolaemia and hypotension

ATP is vital for cells to maintain the plasma membrane sodium–potassium pump. The intracellular concentration of sodium is normally low (10–12 mmol/L) compared with the extracellular fluid concentration (135–145 mmol/L). Ischaemia or cell damage stops the pump functioning, allowing sodium to diffuse into the cell, while potassium is lost into the interstitial fluid. More fluid is then drawn into the cells from the extracellular space by the high sodium concentration.

Severe hypovolaemic shock leads to the rapid depletion of intracellular ATP, with subsequent anaerobic metabolism and acidosis, plus a dysfunctional inflammatory response. This can progress to the activation of the systemic inflammatory response syndrome (SIRS) and acute respiratory distress syndrome (ARDS), eventually resulting in multiple organ dysfunction syndrome (MODS), sepsis and death.

The physiological response to hypovolaemia is to preserve blood flow to vital organs, including the brain, heart, kidneys and liver, with compensatory vasoconstriction of cutaneous and other peripheral blood vessels. Activation of the coagulation system occurs promptly in response to an acute haemorrhage.

There are three stages of the physiological response to a reduction in the circulating blood volume (Worthley, 2000):

1 *Immediate response:*
- Fall in blood pressure decreases the rate of discharge of arterial baroreceptors, composed of the carotid sinuses and the aortic arch baroreceptor.

- Fewer signals are transmitted to the vasomotor centre in the medulla and pons, activating the sympathetic nervous system and vagus nerves.
- The effect of the baroreceptors is to restore stroke volume, cardiac output and mean arterial pressure towards normal values.
- Further baroreceptors found in the walls of the atria and ventricles and pulmonary veins provide extra sensitivity.
- Additional stimuli triggering an increase in blood pressure include reduced arterial oxygen concentration, increased CO_2 concentration, diminished blood flow to the brain, and pain originating in the skin.
- The baroreceptor response is short-term: baroreceptors adapt to continued stimulation and reset at a new pressure.

2 *Intermediate response:*
- Occurs 12–24 hours after haemorrhage; can restore blood volume to virtual normal levels after a moderate bleed.
- Reduced blood pressure and increased arteriolar constriction cause a reduction in capillary hydrostatic pressure.
- Fluid is therefore absorbed from the interstitial to the intravascular space (transcapillary refill).
- Protein follows this trend later.
- Hyperglycaemia occurs, causing a further osmotic fluid shift, secondary to (i) initial catecholamine release instigating hepatic glycogenolysis and sympathetic stimulation initiating glycogen breakdown; and (ii) insulin resistance in peripheral tissues.

3 *Long-term response:*
- Humoral response occurs within days to weeks.
- Increased circulating levels of antidiuretic hormone (ADH), renin and aldosterone raise the intravascular volume and renal retention of fluid.

Clinical signs of hypovolaemic shock

Hypovolaemic shock is divided into four classes of severity, depending on blood loss and clinical signs. Classes 3 and 4 are associated with a mortality of approximately 30 per cent.

Shock is a clinical diagnosis. Clinical signs are often non-specific, varying according to the amount of blood lost, the age of the patient and any concurrent medical conditions. Classic clinical signs include the following:

- Hypotension
- Oliguria
- Poor peripheral perfusion
- Pallor
- Tachycardia
- Dyspnoea
- Change in mental state.

> ■ KEY POINT
> The most important clinical signs are hypotension, oliguria and poor peripheral perfusion.

Systolic blood pressure is not a reliable indicator of shock. Blood loss in healthy adults is often underestimated as rapid vasoconstriction occurs, maintaining a relatively normal blood pressure until 30 per cent of the blood volume is lost. Diastolic pressure is a more sensitive indicator of hypovolaemia. Conversely, in patients with ischaemic heart disease, a relatively small loss of blood can cause a significant drop in blood pressure. Care should be taken when interpreting signs in patients taking beta-blockers, who will not develop tachycardia. It is important to realise that patients who are drowsy or unconscious secondary to hypovolaemic shock have lost at least 40 per cent of their blood volume.

Clinically, haemorrhage occurs at a variable rather than a fixed rate, which usually slows as the blood pressure drops. In a surgical or trauma situation, the source of bleeding should be established promptly. Patients who need emergency surgery have a better outcome if the time between assessment and diagnosis and theatre is minimised.

Treatment of haemorrhagic shock

The key aims are:

- to restore the circulating blood volume and haemoglobin levels;
- to arrest bleeding;
- to correct coagulopathy.

The primary objective is to expand the circulating blood volume and restore tissue perfusion. Fluid resuscitation is carried out in order to return the pulse rate and blood pressure to normal limits, to establish adequate urine output and to sustain a moderate central venous pressure (CVP).

> ■ KEY POINT
> The key aims of treatment in shock are to restore the circulating volume and to stop the cause of bleeding.

There is ongoing controversy regarding the optimal fluid treatment in hypovolaemic shock. Crystalloid fluid is usually given as an initial bolus. Isotonic crystalloids are cheap, have few side effects and replace the extracellular fluid lost into the intravascular and intracellular spaces; however, they can cause haemodilution, hypothermia, acidosis, coagulopathy and tissue oedema. Colloid solutions have a higher molecular weight and are more efficiently contained intravascularly; despite this, increased membrane permeability in haemorrhagic shock will cause extravasation of fluid. Hypertonic saline dextran has been shown to be an advantage only in patients with hypovolaemic shock and concurrent closed head injuries (Alpar and Killampalli, 2004; Moore et al., 2004).

Meta-analyses have shown no significant difference in long-term outcomes between crystalloid and colloids and have concluded that they are clinically equivalent (Moore et al., 2004; Stainsby et al., 2006).

The role of permissive hypotension is disputed in the treatment of haemorrhagic shock. It is mainly advocated in pre-hospital trauma situations with uncontrolled haemorrhage when there is a delay before surgical control of bleeding. Relatively hypovolaemic resuscitation stops or slows bleeding temporarily due to the combination of hypotension, vasoconstriction and thrombus formation. The aim is to attain the minimum perfusion pressure that will perfuse vital organs sufficiently, while resuscitating the patient to a below-normotensive blood pressure. This method may be followed in patients with penetrating torso trauma; caution should be taken with blunt injuries, due to the risk of concurrent brain injury, which is exacerbated by hypotension (Krausz, 2006; Spahn et al., 2007).

Resuscitation of patients with a ruptured aortic abdominal aneurysm (AAA) is another situation of uncontrolled haemorrhagic shock before intervention. Although vigorous fluid resuscitation can worsen bleeding, and cause clot disruption and coagulopathy, there have been no prospective trials to fully evaluate the role of permissive hypotension. In contrast to most trauma patients, patients with AAA are usually elderly with atherosclerotic disease and require higher perfusion pressures to prevent end-organ ischaemia, especially to coronary and renal vessels. A balance must be achieved during fluid resuscitation between organ ischaemia and rebleeding (Roberts *et al.*, 2006).

The transfusion trigger in haemorrhagic shock is unclear. Haemoglobin levels are a poor indicator during acute bleeding, although serial readings are helpful. Blood transfusions should be directed by a clinical evaluation of blood loss and the response to fluid resuscitation. Blood is almost always signified if the haemoglobin concentration drops below 6 g/dL and is seldom required above haemoglobin concentrations of 10 g/dL (Moore *et al.*, 2004). Blood should be used to increase oxygen delivery and tissue perfusion, but not as a volume expander.

Resuscitation of the patient with haemorrhagic shock involves prompt identification of the bleeding source. Early intervention to stop bleeding is paramount to the treatment and prevention of further complications.

● BLOOD TRANSFUSION IN THE SURGICAL PATIENT

Transfusions may be used as a source of cells (red blood cells (RBCs), platelets, granulocytes) or plasma-derived products (Table 5.2). In this section we review issues associated with the transfusion of RBC, platelets, granulocytes and fresh frozen plasma and cryoprecipitates. We consider the problems associated with blood transfusion, both in general and when massive transfusions are required, and review the alternatives.

Table 5.2 Blood products

Cellular products	Fresh frozen plasma
Red blood cells	Cryoprecipitate
Platelets	Coagulation factors
Granulocytes	Albumin
	Immunoglobulins

All blood components in the UK undergo mandatory testing for:

- human immunodeficiency virus (HIV) (antibody);
- hepatitis B (surface antigen);
- hepatitis C (antibody and RNA);
- human T lymphotropic virus type 1 (antibody);
- syphilis (antibody).

Red blood cells

ABO and rhesus (Rh D) antigen compatibility

Transfusing a compatible blood group is essential in order to avoid a haemolytic transfusion reaction. There are four major blood groups; their distributions in the UK are as follows:

O: 47 per cent
A: 41 per cent
B: 8 per cent
AB: 3 per cent.

Blood group O individuals have no antigens on the red cells but have anti-A and anti-B antibodies in the plasma. Blood group A individuals have A antigens on the red cells and anti-B antibodies in the plasma. Blood group B individuals have B antigens on the red cells and anti-A antibodies in the plasma. AB individuals have A and B antigens on the red cells but carry neither antibody. O individuals are 'universal donors': they can donate blood to all groups but receive blood only from O donors. AB individuals are 'universal recipients': they can receive blood from all blood groups but donate only to AB patients.

In the UK 85 per cent people carry the Rh D antigen and are labelled 'rhesus-positive'. Antibodies to the rhesus antigen occur only in rhesus-negative individuals exposed to rhesus-positive blood, usually secondary to transfusion or pregnancy. If a rhesus-negative woman develops antibodies and has a rhesus-positive fetus, antibodies can cross the placenta and destroy the fetal RBCs, resulting in death of the fetus or severe neurological abnormalities.

In an emergency situation, if blood is required before there is time to cross-match, it is recommended that O Rh D-negative blood is given to females of reproductive age. O Rh D-positive blood can be given to males and older females of an unidentified blood group (Stainsby *et al.*, 2006).

■ KEY POINT

Blood transfusions should always be ABO-compatible, and should be rhesus-compatible in young women.

Transfusion of red blood cells

The purpose of an RBC transfusion is to treat or prevent tissue hypoxia. Patients should be transfused on a clinical basis and not based only on the haemoglobin count. In general, patients without shock or significant cardiac disease require a transfusion at levels of 7 g/dL. Even in critically ill patients, haemoglobin levels of 7–9 g/dL are adequate to maintain oxygen-carrying capacity (Hebert *et al.*, 1999). Traditionally, patients with coronary artery disease have been transfused to keep haemoglobin levels over 10 g/dL in order to prevent myocardial ischaemia. It is now recommended that transfusions are commenced when signs of insufficient oxygenation develop, and most patients tolerate normovolaemic haemodilution well. An exception is patients with aortic or pulmonary stenosis who are unable to increase their cardiac output (Madjdpour *et al.*, 2006). In patients with ongoing blood loss, high risk of a rebleed, head injury or stroke, and in critically ill septic patients, a higher haemoglobin concentration is advocated.

■ KEY POINT

Blood transfusion is usually required with a haemoglobin ≤ 7 g/dL in order to maintain adequate tissue perfusion and oxygenation.

One RBC unit represents the red cells prepared from one standard blood donation after filtering out the white blood cells, platelets and majority of plasma. Plasma is replaced by additive fluid – saline with adenine, glucose and mannitol. Red blood cells are kept at 4 °C and can be stored for 5 weeks. Typically, transfusing a unit of blood will increase the haemoglobin concentration by 1 g/dL, the haematocrit by 3 per cent and the blood volume by 500 mL.

Red blood cells are leucodepleted as a preventive measure against transmission of variant Creutzfeldt–Jakob disease (vCJD). Benefits of leucodepletion include:

- decreased non-haemolytic transfusion reactions;
- reduced transmission of leucocyte-associated viruses, e.g. cytomegalovirus (CMV);

- lessened immunosuppressive effects;
- decreased cytokine-mediated organ damage.

Platelets

Platelets are used for the control of bleeding in patients with thrombocytopenia or platelet dysfunction. In patients actively bleeding, the aim is to keep the platelet count above $50 \times 10^9/L$. Platelet counts are commonly kept over $100 \times 10^9/L$ after high-velocity trauma or central nervous system injuries due to the high prevalence of coagulopathy and disseminated intravascular coagulation (DIC) (Stainsby *et al.*, 2006). Disorders of platelet dysfunction that may require transfusion include during surgical bypass, renal failure and following antiplatelet treatment.

Platelets are provided either from whole blood or via aphaeresis. The usual dose is an adult dose unit, which should contain $2.5–3 \times 10^{11}$ platelets. Approximately 40 per cent of transfused platelets are sequestered in the spleen in patients with normal splenic size and function; this amount increases in splenomegaly. Platelets are stored at 22 °C with constant agitation; the higher temperature means they are more susceptible to bacterial contamination compared with RBCs. Platelets can be stored for only 5 days. ABO-compatible platelet transfusions are mandatory.

Granulocytes

The recent availability of granulocyte colony-stimulating factor (G-CSF) has rekindled interest in granulocyte transfusions. Donors receiving G-CSF, usually in combination with steroids, produce approximately $50–70 \times 10^9$ neutrophils, compared with pre-G-CSF optimal collections of $20–30 \times 10^9$ neutrophils. Transfusing G-CSF-stimulated neutrophils can restore the neutrophil count to near-normal levels.

The routine use of granulocyte infusions is not yet recommended. Preliminary trial data suggest that G-CSF-stimulated granulocyte transfusions are advantageous in severely septic neutropenic patients. However, there have been no large, well-designed prospective trials to definitively establish the clinical benefit.

Clinical scenarios where G-CSF-stimulated granulocyte transfusions may be justified include severe resistant infection in neutropenic patients (neutrophil count $< 0.2–0.5 \times 10^9$) who are not responding or progressing on appropriate antifungals or broad-spectrum antibiotics, with no recovery in neutrophil count expected for over 7 days. This is particularly relevant for patients undergoing intensive chemotherapy, stem cell transplantation, induction for acute leukaemia, and neonatal sepsis with invasive fungal infections. Patients should receive granulocytes daily for at least 4 days (Bishton and Chopra, 2004).

Granulocytes are suspended in plasma and can be stored for up to 24 h, although function and survival decrease with increased storage time. Consequently granulocytes are usually administered immediately after donation. Transfusions must be ABO-compatible. The high lymphocyte content means that severely immunosuppressed patients are at risk of graft-versus-host disease. CMV-seronegative patients should receive donation only from CMV-negative patients.

Fresh frozen plasma

Despite the wide use of fresh frozen plasma (FFP), there are few absolute indications for its utilisation. Transfusion of FFP is recommended when the prothrombin time (PT) is 1.5 times greater than normal, together with the presence of bleeding or predicted bleeding. Transfusion of FFP is indicated in patients with multiple coagulation factor deficiencies associated with severe bleeding or DIC (although not without bleeding), for plasma exchange in thrombotic thrombocytopenic purpura (TTP), and in patients with liver failure and a prolonged PT before invasive procedures (O'Shaughnessy et al., 2004). Transfusion of FFP should not be used for volume expansion, or be used to reverse a prolonged international normalised ratio (INR) in the absence of bleeding, or be transfused prophylactically in massive RBC transfusions. Where possible, patients should receive recombinant or virally inactivated coagulation factors (e.g. factors VII, VIII, IX, anti-thrombin III), and FFP should be reserved for emergency situations when concentrates are unavailable.

Pathogen-reduced plasma (PRP) is available for patients who are likely to receive large or repeated doses of FFP, and for all patients aged 16 years or younger. PRP is achieved by methylene blue and light treatment (MBFFP) or solvent detergent treatment (SDFFP). Both methods of pathogen reduction cause some reduced activity of clotting factors, mainly related to factor VIII.

Fresh frozen plasma is prepared either from whole blood or from aphaeresis and is frozen to −30 °C to maintain the haemostatic ability of coagulation factors, especially factors V and VIII. After thawing at 37 °C, FFP can be stored as thawed plasma at 4 °C for up to 24 h if there is any delay before administration. If possible, ABO-compatible FFP should be used, as plasma will still contain some ABO antibodies. Incompatible FFP should be used only if it contains no high-titre anti-A or anti-B antibodies (Stainsby et al., 2006). Adults normally require 4–7 units of FFP to correct a substantial coagulopathy.

Cryoprecipitate

This is defined as the cryoglobulin fraction of plasma and is rich in factor VIII, von Willebrand's factor, factor XIII, fibronectin and fibrinogen. Cryoprecipitate is generally used to increase fibrinogen levels in dysfibrinogenaemia, after a massive transfusion or during DIC. Cryoprecipitate may be used for factor VIII deficiency and von Willebrand's disease when factor VIII concentrate is not available. It is normally indicated when plasma fibrinogen levels are below 1 g/L. Cryoprecipitate is stored frozen and must be transfused within 6 h of thawing. Pathogen-reduced cryoprecipitate is not available in the UK.

Problems of blood transfusions

General problems of all blood transfusions include the following:

- Acute haemolytic reaction
- Delayed haemolytic transfusion reaction
- Febrile non-haemolytic transfusion reaction
- Transfusion-associated infections
- Increasing costs
- Anaphylaxis
- Immunomodulatory effects
- Iron overload
- Fluid overload.

Acute haemolytic reaction

When incompatible RBCs are transfused, they can react with anti-A or anti-B antibodies present in the plasma. If a patient receives the incorrect blood, there is roughly a one in three chance of ABO incompatibility. Typically the most serious reaction is when a patient with blood group O receives group A red cells. The most common reason for transfusing incompatible RBCs is human error, which is more frequent in emergency situations. Errors in blood transfusion usually involve faults in requesting blood or sampling patients, laboratory errors, or mistakes in collecting or administering blood. It is vital to adhere to hospital protocols for transfusion products in order to minimise risk.

Clinical signs of acute haemolytic reaction include the following:

- Hypotension
- Tachycardia
- Tachypnoea
- Chest, flank or abdominal pain
- Discomfort at the site of transfusion
- Urticaria.

If there is any suspicion of acute haemolysis, the transfusion must be stopped immediately and the reaction reported to the blood bank. A post-transfusion sample and any unused blood should be sent to the blood bank for analysis. The patient should be vigorously resuscitated with crystalloid fluids to maintain an adequate urine output and blood pressure. Inotropic support is required in prolonged hypotension. The majority of patients need intensive care support. Serious complications include renal failure and DIC; these are secondary to the production of immune complexes that lyse RBCs and subsequently release tissue factor. There is a high chance of fatality in a major ABO-incompatible reaction.

Delayed haemolytic transfusion reaction

This is more common (approximately one in 1000) than an acute haemolytic reaction and occurs more than 24 h post-transfusion. It is seen in patients in whom previous transfusions or pregnancy have primed the immune system against an antigen on transfused RBCs. This may not be detectable on routine blood bank screening. Many delayed haemolytic reactions are not recognised, but they should be suspected in patients with fever, jaundice and low haemoglobin despite transfusion. Treatment is not usually necessitated.

Anaphylaxis

A rare but potentially life-threatening complication of transfusion is anaphylaxis. Patients with a severe immunoglobulin A (IgA) deficiency and IgA antibodies have a critical allergic response if exposed to IgA in donor blood. Anaphylaxis can also occur when individuals with prior sensitisation to an antigen producing immunoglobulin E (IgE) antibodies are subsequently re-exposed in donor blood to the same antigen.

Clinical features of anaphylaxis include the following:

- Hypotension
- Tachycardia
- Bronchospasm and stridor
- Periorbital and laryngeal oedema
- Urticaria
- Cardiac arrhythmia
- Shock and cardiac arrest.

Management includes the immediate cessation of the transfusion, reporting the reaction to the blood bank, and returning any unused units. Supportive care includes intravenous chlorphenamine (chlorpheniramine), oxygen and salbutamol nebulisers. Adrenaline (epinephrine) is indicated in life-threatening hypotension. If further blood transfusions are required in patients with anti-IgA antibodies, saline-washed RBCs should be used from IgA-deficient donors and advice taken from the blood bank.

Massive blood transfusion

A massive blood transfusion due to uncontrolled bleeding is a known complication of trauma and surgery. It is defined as the replacement of the total blood volume of the patient within 24 h. An alternative definition is the replacement of 50 per cent of the total blood volume within 3 h (Hardy *et al.*, 2005). Before blood is given, initial resuscitation of the patient with crystalloid or colloid fluids and full blood sampling should be undertaken.

Although a massive blood transfusion is vital for the treatment of hypovolaemic shock and subsequent multiorgan failure, there are recognised complications, including the following:

- Acute haemolytic reaction
- Coagulopathy
- Transfusion-related acute lung injury (TRALI)
- Hyperkalaemia (storage at 4 °C significantly increases extracellular potassium)
- Ionised hypocalcaemia (due to citrate toxicity; causes reduced myocardial contractility, vasodilation and exacerbation of bleeding; corrected with intravenous calcium chloride)
- Hypothermia
- DIC.

> ■ KEY POINT
> A massive blood transfusion has multiple complications, the most significant being coagulopathy, TRALI and DIC.

Coagulopathy

During a massive blood transfusion, coagulopathy is a multifactorial event involving interactions between RBCs, fibrinogen and platelets plus fluid replacement, hypothermia and diminished coagulation factors. Hypothermia is generally seen in trauma scenarios and significantly contributes to coagulopathy. It should be treated aggressively and prevented (Spahn *et al.*, 2007).

In surgery coagulopathy is often related to decreased coagulation factors due to dilution, compared with DIC in a trauma situation. Red blood cells have an important role in coagulation as they affect platelet margination and function. To prevent coagulopathy, evidence suggests that the optimal haematocrit needs to be about 35 per cent (Hardy *et al.*, 2005). Fresh frozen plasma and cryoprecipitate are both recommended in massive transfusions to keep PT and activated partial thromboplastin time (APTT) ratios within 1.5 of normal and a fibrinogen concentration of least 1.0 g/L in plasma. Four units of FFP will usually raise the clotting factors to 30 per cent of normal. Platelets are important to control microvascular bleeding.

> ■ KEY POINT
> Fresh frozen plasma, platelets and coagulation factors are needed in massive transfusions and for the treatment of particular bleeding disorders.

Transfusion-related acute lung injury

Transfusion-related acute lung injury is defined as acute respiratory distress with hypoxia and non-cardiogenic pulmonary oedema related to plasma-containing blood products. This is the foremost cause of transfusion-related morbidity and mortality in the UK. The risk of TRALI is five times higher following the administration of FFP or platelets than after administration of RBCs (Stainsby *et al.*, 2006).

The pathogenesis of TRALI is still under debate. The activation and sequestration of neutrophils within the lungs is the primary pathological event in TRALI. Recipient factors such as recent surgery or infection cause the release of cytokines and encourage neutrophils to attach to the pulmonary vascular endothelium. Antibodies from transfusion products; the majority anti-leucocyte antibodies (anti-HLA) plus anti-granulocyte antibodies (anti-HNA) then prime neutrophils. Biologically active mediators within blood products such as soluble CD40L and bioactive lipids can also activate neutrophils (Bux and Sachs, 2007).

Donor antibodies are most commonly from multiparous women due to increased contact with paternal antigens during pregnancy. If feasible, samples from donors implicated in a case of TRALI should be tested for autoantibodies. Male donors are now used to produce FFP in the UK when possible.

Transfusion-related acute lung injury remains a clinical diagnosis supported by radiological and laboratory tests. Respiratory distress must have occurred within 6 h of a transfusion to confirm the diagnosis. Treatment is mainly supportive, aiming to maintain good oxygenation. Ventilatory support should be considered early. The majority of patients improve within 48–96 h, although mortality is still 5–10 per cent.

Transfusion alternatives

Allogeneic blood transfusions often provide life-saving treatment. There are disadvantages, however: allogeneic blood still carries a risk of disease transmission, can cause fatal haemolytic reactions, requires typing and cross-matching before use, has a limited storage time and remains in chronically short supply worldwide. Other situations when an alternative may be considered include an objection to blood transfusions for religious reasons, the use of blood that has not undergone all rigorous safety checks, and in patients with multiple antibodies or autoimmune haemolytic anaemia (Goodnough *et al.*, 2003).

■ KEY POINT

In elective situations, alternatives to allogeneic blood transfusions may be considered.

Although preoperative planning is the key way to avoid or reduce the need for allogeneic blood transfusion, alternative methods are being examined in the acute setting. Current strategies include the following:

- *Preoperative autologous blood donation:*
  - Blood is pre-donated 3–5 weeks before surgery.
  - Blood can be stored for up to 35 days.
  - A starting haemoglobin over 11.0 g/dL is necessary.
  - Additional iron supplementation should be taken preoperatively due to collecting several units of blood within a few weeks.
  - The main benefit is avoidance of viral and immunological risks.
- *Optimisation of preoperative low haemoglobin:*
  - Both erythropoietin and iron can be used.
  - Initial haemoglobin should be less than 13.0 g/dL.
  - Optimal dose and dosing schedule of erythropoietin has not been determined.
  - If there are concerns about the cause of preoperative anaemia, these should be investigated before surgery.
- *Acute normovolaemic haemodilution (ANH):*
  - Whole blood is removed and restored with crystalloid or colloid.
  - Blood is removed either before surgery or during the early stage of the operation.
  - Limited to patients with a high starting haemoglobin and who can tolerate a relatively low final haemoglobin level.

- Blood can be kept for up to 6 h at room temperature and is generally used in theatre.
- Current evidence for this technique is equivocal.
- *Autologous blood cell salvage:*
  - Blood lost during surgery is collected, filtered and returned to the patient.
  - Beneficial in operations typified by substantial blood loss.
  - Should not be used if there is bacterial contamination of the operating field.
  - Caution advised in patients undergoing oncological operations, although the risk of dissemination of malignancy is now considered minimal.
- *Pharmacological haemostatic agents:*
  - Drugs include aprotinin, tranexamic acid, desmopressin and recombinant activated factor VII (rFVIIa).
  - rFVIIa can be considered during massive transfusions when surgical control of the bleeding is not possible and coagulation factors have been replaced (Moore *et al.*, 2004).
  - Shown to reduce blood loss in elective cardiac and liver surgery.
  - Concerns remain regarding the thrombotic potential of these drugs and the risk of anaphylactic reactions.
- *Artificial oxygen-carrying solutions (RBC substitutes):*
  - Divided into two main groups – haemoglobin-based oxygen carriers (HBOCs) and perfluorocarbon-based oxygen carriers (PFBOCs) (Kim and Greenburg, 2004).
  - HBOCs utilise purified human, animal or recombinant haemoglobin.
  - PFBOCs use perfluorinated carbons, chemically and biologically inert liquids with high gas solubility.
  - Adverse events in clinical trials have generally been mild, but several severe adverse events have occurred, necessitating early termination of trials.
  - Research and clinical trials continue; currently there are no products available for clinical use in the UK.

COAGULATION

Haemostasis is a complex and dynamic physiological process that aims to stop bleeding within the body. The discontinuation of bleeding depends on the interaction of endothelial cells, platelets and coagulation factors (Dahlback, 2005). Anticoagulation factors and the fibrinolytic system oppose coagulation and remove clots.

> ■ KEY POINT
> Coagulation is instigated by disruption to endothelial cells in a vessel wall.

Platelet plug formation

The initial response of a vessel to injury is vasoconstriction, followed by the rapid formation of a platelet plug:

1. Injury to a blood vessel causes disruption of the endothelium and exposure of subendothelial collagen.
2. Von Willebrand factor (vWF) is released from endothelial cells and platelets and forms a bridge between platelets and the exposed collagen.
3. Platelet binding initiates the discharge of intracellular dense and α-granules.
4. Adenosine diphosphate (ADP) and serotonin secretion causes platelet activation and membrane modification to allow fibrinogen binding, resulting in platelet aggregation.
5. Adhesion of platelets sets converts arachidonic acid to thromboxane A_2, causing further platelet aggregation and potent vasoconstriction.

6   Platelets contain actin and myosin, which contract in aggregated platelets, compressing and strengthening the platelet plug.

7   Undamaged adjacent endothelial cells convert arachidonic acid to prostaglandin I_2 and release nitric oxide, preventing the spread of a platelet plug from the site of injury.

> ■ KEY POINT
> The initial response to vascular injury is platelet plug formation.

The coagulation cascade

Blood clotting occurs more slowly and reinforces the platelet plug. It is also initiated by disruption to vessel wall endothelium. There are two coagulation cascades in the body that lead to the creation of a fibrin clot, termed the intrinsic and extrinsic pathways (Figure 5.1).

> ■ KEY POINT
> The coagulation cascade, via the intrinsic and extrinsic pathways, forms a fibrin clot.

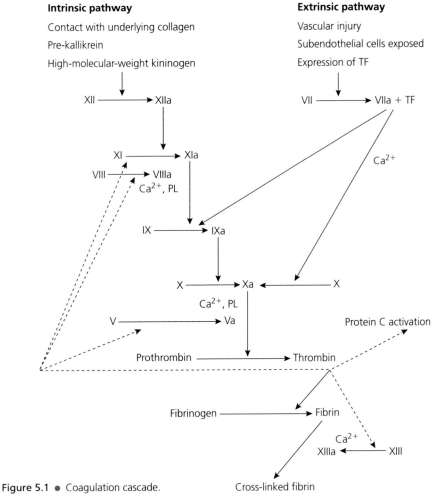

Figure 5.1 ● Coagulation cascade.

PL, phospholipids; TF, tissue factor.

The *extrinsic pathway* is activated when vessel wall damage occurs, exposing subendothelial cells. Tissue factor on these cells forms a complex with factor VII, activating it to VIIa and starting the coagulation cascade.

The *intrinsic pathway* is triggered by an abnormal vessel wall and is secondary to contact activation with the underlying collagen fibres. It begins with the activation of factor XII to XIIa, in association with pre-kallikrein and high-molecular-weight kininogen.

Both pathways converge to a common pathway with the activation of factor X to Xa, which catalyses the conversion of prothrombin to thrombin. Clotting is usually initiated via tissue factor and the extrinsic pathway, with minimal input from factor XII at the start of the intrinsic pathway. Although the extrinsic pathway produces only a small amount of thrombin, it does elicit a positive-feedback loop by thrombin production to activate factors XI and VIII and platelets in the intrinsic pathway. This then produces the large amount of thrombin that is required for adequate clotting. Thrombin activates platelets, leading to the presentation of plasma-membrane receptors, allowing coagulation reactions to occur on the surface of platelets.

Calcium ions are essential for the activation of factors II, VII, IX and X. Calcium binding alters the conformational shape of coagulation factors. This is necessary for the interaction of prothrombin (factor II) and factor X with the surface of aggregated platelets for thrombin production. Phospholipids allow binding to occur on platelet surface and are cofactors in the activation of factor X and the conversion of prothrombin to thrombin.

Prostaglandins are unsaturated carboxylic acids with a diverse range of functions, including a role in coagulation. Platelets release thromboxane A_2, which is produced from arachidonic acid in conjunction with cyclo-oxygenase 1 (COX-1) and enhances platelet adhesion and aggregation. In healthy vasculature, this is balanced by prostaglandin I_2, derived from endothelial cells in the presence of cyclo-oxygenase 2 (COX-2), which demonstrates vasodilatory and anti-thrombotic properties.

Thrombin converts fibrinogen to fibrin in the presence of factor XIII, forming a fibrin mesh or blood clot.

The anti-clotting system

Endothelial cells produce tissue factor pathway inhibitor (TFPI), a plasma protein that acts in the initial stages of clot formation. TFPI binds to the tissue factor–factor VIIa complex, preventing factor X activation and limiting thrombin production via the extrinsic pathway.

> ■ KEY POINT
> Opposing the coagulation cascade are anticoagulation factors and the fibrinolytic system.

Thrombin has a role in regulating the coagulation system by binding to thrombomodulin, an endothelial cell receptor. This complex prevents the conversion of fibrinogen to fibrin and activates protein C, a plasma protein. Together with protein S, protein C inactivates factors Va and VIIIa, controlling the extent of the coagulation cascade.

Certain plasma proteins act as natural anticoagulants and regulate the activation of thrombin from prothrombin. The most important is anti-thrombin III, which also limits the activity of factors IXa, Xa, XIa and XIIa. Anti-thrombin III is activated by heparin or heparin-like molecules on the surface of endothelial cells to prevent clots spreading.

The fibrinolytic system

A fibrin clot is a temporary solution until permanent repair of the blood vessel occurs. Fibrin clots are dissolved by plasmin, the active form of the plasma pro-enzyme plasminogen.

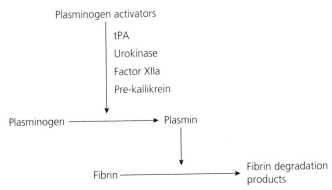

Figure 5.2 ● Fibrinolytic system.

tPA, tissue plasminogen factor.

There are multiple plasminogen activators; the most important is tissue plasminogen factor (tPA). As a clot forms, plasminogen and tPA adhere to fibrinogen and fibrin and are incorporated into the clot. The presence of fibrin increases the enzymatic ability of tPA, triggering the conversion of plasminogen to plasmin (Figure 5.2).

● BLEEDING DISORDERS

The most common cause of bleeding in a surgical patient is intraoperative technical error. This should always be excluded before investigating for coagulopathy. Common laboratory tests for bleeding disorders are summarised in Table 5.3.

> ■ KEY POINT
> A coagulation dysfunction is usually an acquired disorder.

Disseminated intravascular coagulation

A wide range of pathological conditions can result in the development of DIC. Development of DIC significantly increases patient mortality over that of the underlying disease. The clinical manifestations of DIC are haemorrhage and thrombosis. Although thrombosis is predominantly of the microvascular system and less clinically evident, it causes widespread ischaemia, multi-organ failure and disease-associated mortality. Box 5.1 describes the pathophysiology of DIC.

Disseminated intravascular coagulation is not a primary diagnosis. It is always secondary to an underlying disorder, commonly:

● sepsis;
● trauma, particularly associated with massive head injury or extensive muscle damage;
● intravascular haemolysis (e.g. haemolytic transfusion reaction, massive transfusion);
● malignancy;
● obstetric complications (e.g. amniotic fluid embolism, placental abruption, eclampsia);
● viraemia;
● vascular disorders;
● organ destruction;
● toxic/immunological reactions.

Table 5.3 Laboratory tests for coagulation disorders

Laboratory test	Purpose of test	Affected by
Prothrombin time (PT)[a,b,c]	Assesses extrinsic and common pathways	Vitamin K deficiency Liver disease Warfarin treatment DIC Factors VII, X, V, prothrombin, fibrinogen
Activated partial thromboplastin time (APTT)[b,c,d]	Assesses intrinsic and common pathways	Pre-kallikrein, HMWK Factors XII, XI, IX, VIII, X, V Prothrombin, fibrinogen Heparin DIC
Thrombin time (TT)	Tests final stage of pathway; conversion of fibrinogen to fibrin by thrombin	Heparin DIC Hypofibrinogenaemia
Platelet count[b]	Platelet number	Liver disease DIC Iatrogenic drug treatment ITP

[a]Also expressed as international normalised ratio (INR), which removes laboratory variation. [b]The most frequent laboratory tests carried out to assess bleeding are PT, APTT and platelet count. [c]Neither PT nor APTT is delayed until there is a 70% deficiency of one or more coagulation factors. [d]Von Willebrand disease can cause an extended APTT as it is a carrier for factor VIII; if suspected, specific tests should be requested for von Willebrand factor (vWF) deficiency. DIC, disseminated intravascular coagulation; HMWK, high-molecular-weight kininogen; ITP, immune thrombocytopenic purpura.

Box 5.1 Pathophysiology of disseminated intravascular coagulation

- Activation or injury of monocytes or endothelial cells exposes tissue factor, activating the extrinsic pathway of the coagulation cascade.
- Systemic intravascular thrombin formation occurs, resulting in systemic fibrin deposition, trapping platelets and contributing to thrombocytopenia.
- Systemic plasmin generation occurs in response to fibrin production and subsequent tissue plasminogen factor (tPA) release, producing fibrin degradation products (FDPs).
- FDPs degrade coagulation factors, induce platelet defects causing bleeding, and stimulate the release of pro-inflammatory cytokines from monocytes.
- Thrombin has a pro- and anticoagulant role, binding to thrombomodulin and causing protein C activation; this balance is lost in disseminated intravascular coagulation (DIC), with persistent thrombin generation.
- Depletion of anticoagulant proteins – anti-thrombin, protein C, protein S, tissue factor pathway inhibitor (TFPI) – occurs due to decreased thrombomodulin availability, anti-thrombin inactivation and FDP degradation.
- Thrombin interacts with cell-surface receptors, activating the inflammatory system and producing pro-inflammatory cytokines – interleukin 1 (IL-1), interleukin 6 (IL-6), tumour necrosis factor alpha (TNF-α) – which induce further coagulation.
- The intrinsic pathway and increased availability of negatively charged phospholipid surfaces for coagulant reactions (due to cell damage and apoptosis) cause continued thrombin generation.

Although all coagulation factors are reduced in acute DIC, levels of factors V, VIII and XIII and fibrinogen are usually exceptionally low. Laboratory tests often do not give a definitive diagnosis of DIC; diagnosis is partly clinical, although serial coagulation tests may be useful.

Classic laboratory findings include the following:

- Prolonged PT, APTT and thrombin time (TT)
- Increased fibrin degradation products and D-dimers
- Low platelet counts and fibrinogen levels
- Low plasma levels of coagulation factors and inhibitors.

The management of DIC is based on the diagnosis and treatment of the underlying disorder. The replacement of platelets, coagulation factors and inhibitors is important to stop severe haemorrhagic events. Heparin treatment remains controversial; however, it is advised in patients in whom thrombosis is the dominant feature. Treatment with exogenous antithrombin III and activated protein C (APC) remain contentious and are undergoing clinical trials (Franchini *et al.*, 2006).

Common acquired bleeding disorders

The most common acquired bleeding disorders are:

- *Anticoagulant therapy:* very common in clinical practice – usually secondary to warfarin or aspirin
- *Hypothermia:*
  - Core temperature below 35 °C impairs coagulation
  - Causes platelet dysfunction and impaired reactions of coagulation factors and the fibrinolytic system
  - Patients should be actively rewarmed; this will control bleeding in the absence of any other coagulopathy
- *Hepatic failure:*
  - The liver has an important indirect role in coagulation; reduced synthesis of coagulation factors occurs as a result of hepatocellular damage
  - Bile is needed to absorb vitamin K in the intestine, which is required to produce coagulation factors in the liver
  - Portal hypertension is associated with hypersplenism and secondary thrombocytopenia
  - Serious bleeding in cirrhotic patients is typically due to thrombocytopenia, coagulopathy and vascular abnormalities
- *Renal failure:* uraemia results in impaired platelet interaction with the vessel wall, due to increased levels of nitric oxide
- *Vitamin K deficiency:*
  - Vitamin K is necessary for the production and function of clotting factors II, VII, IX and X
  - Lack of vitamin K can result from inadequate dietary intake, malabsorption and warfarin treatment, and in critically ill patients
  - Minor bleeding is treated with parenteral vitamin K; ongoing bleeding may require FFP
- *Thrombocytopenia:*
  - Acquired platelet dysfunction is more common than inherited disorders
  - Drugs that cause platelet dysfunction include aspirin, non-steroidal anti-inflammatory drugs (NSAIDs), clopidogrel, integrin αIIbβ3 and large doses of beta-lactam antibiotics (penicillin above cephalosporins)
  - Renal and hepatic failure, myeloproliferative disorders, myeloma and surgical bypass procedures affect platelet number or function
  - Autoimmune/idiopathic thrombocytopenic purpura (ITP) is the destruction of platelets by

autoantibodies. Acute ITP is commonly seen in children following a viral infection. Chronic ITP typically occurs in adult females; it is normally idiopathic but may be associated with other autoimmune disorders, thyroid disease, malignancy or postviral infection.

> ■ KEY POINT
> The most frequent cause of a bleeding disorder is iatrogenic anticoagulation treatment.

Congenital disorders

Haemophilia A and B and von Willebrand disease make up over 95 per cent of inherited coagulation disorders (Dahlback, 2005; Peyvandi *et al.*, 2006).

Haemophilia A

- X-linked disorder resulting in factor VIII deficiency
- 30 per cent of cases occur as spontaneous mutations
- Disorder ranges from mild forms (5–30%) to severe forms (< 1%), depending on the amount of functional factor VIII
- Frequency of one in 5000–10 000 males; females are principally carriers
- In mild haemophilia, protracted bleeding is usually seen only after trauma
- In severe cases, spontaneous bleeding occurs into the muscles, joints, internal organs and brain
- Bleeding into joints (haemarthrosis) is the distinguishing feature of severe disease, causing loss of movement, fixed contractures and muscle wasting
- Treatment involves regular infusions of factor VIII concentrate from human plasma or recombinant DNA.

Haemophilia B (Christmas disease)

- Clinically indistinguishable from haemophilia A
- X-linked disorder causing factor IX insufficiency
- Disorder ranges from mild to severe
- At least 300 factor IX mutations have been identified; the majority are point mutations.

Von Willebrand disease

- The most common inherited bleeding disorder
- Due to a deficiency of vWF
- Lack of vWF prevents effective platelet adhesion and a secondary deficiency of factor VIII, as vWF is a carrier in the blood
- Clinically manifests as bleeding from the skin and mucous membranes
- There are three major subtypes:
  - Type 1: most common, autosomal dominant, deficiency of vWF
  - Type 2: several subtypes, qualitative defect in vWF
  - Type 3: very rare, autosomal recessive, clinically severe, virtual absence of vWF
- Severe forms are treated with vWF concentrate when bleeding episodes occur
- DDAVP is useful in type 1 as it increases the release of vWF and factor VIII from endothelial cells, but it is less useful in types 2 and 3.

> ■ KEY POINT
> Congenital bleeding disorders are rare; von Willebrand disease is the most common.

Coagulation factor deficiencies

- Rare defects, generally autosomal recessive
- Includes factors II (prothrombin), V, VII, X, XI and XIII.

Platelet function disorders

- Rare, usually manifest as mucocutaneous bleeding
- Include Glanzmann's thrombastenia (deficiency of a membrane receptor) and Bernard–Soulier syndrome (plasma platelet membrane defect).

● THROMBOPHILIA

Venous thromboembolism has a high prevalence among surgical and trauma patients. Thrombosis results from the interaction of several risk factors. These include environmental factors (e.g. surgery, immobility, trauma, oral contraceptive pill, hormone replacement therapy), medical conditions (e.g. cancer, pregnancy, infection, inflammatory states) and inherited or acquired thrombophilias (Buchanan *et al.*, 2003; Thomas, 2001).

> ■ KEY POINT
> Thrombosis in surgical and trauma patients is due to the interaction of several risk factors.

Thrombophilias produce a hypercoagulable state that predisposes to thrombosis due to an imbalance between pro- and anticoagulant factors. There are nine types of thrombophilia, which can occur in isolation or in combination:

> ■ KEY POINT
> Inherited or acquired thrombophilias predispose to thrombosis formation.

> ■ KEY POINT
> Thrombophilias can occur in isolation and in combination.

- *Anti-thrombin deficiency:*
    - Natural anticoagulant that inactivates thrombin, factors IXa, Xa, XIa and XIIa, and binds to exogenous and endogenous heparin
    - Rare autosomal dominant condition
    - Most serious of all inherited thrombophilias
    - Patients usually present with recurrent venous thromboembolism in the second or third decade. Arterial events also occur rarely
    - Mesenteric vessels are particularly prone to thrombosis
    - Patients should be treated with low-molecular-weight heparin (LMWH), as resistance to unfractionated heparin can occur
    - Lifelong anticoagulation is recommended after spontaneous or recurrent thromboses
- *Protein C deficiency:*
    - Vitamin K-dependent protein synthesised in the liver and that degrades procoagulant factors Va and VIIIa
    - Autosomal dominant disorder
    - Lifelong anticoagulation not usually needed
    - Care should be taken when initiating warfarin treatment due to the risk of warfarin necrosis
    - Prevalence in population of 0.4 per cent

- *Protein S deficiency:*
  - Cofactor for protein C inactivation of factors Va and VIIIa; can also directly inactivate factors Va and Xa
  - Autosomal dominant trait; prevalence 0.3–0.13 per cent
- *Dysfibrinogenaemias:*
  - Heterogeneous genetic disorder causing defective fibrinogen
  - Inherited as either autosomal recessive or dominant
  - Majority of molecular abnormalities are asymptomatic; 25 per cent cause mild haemorrhagic disorders and 20 per cent cause abnormal thrombosis
  - Routine laboratory testing is difficult – consider when common thrombophilias have been discounted but clinical presentation suggests an inherited disorder
- *Activated protein C resistance (factor V Leiden):*
  - Prevalence about 5 per cent; more common in white people
  - Due to a single point mutation in the factor V gene
  - Causes resistance to cleavage by protein C
  - Trait present in 10–50 per cent of individuals presenting with thromboembolic disease
  - Often found in conjunction with other thrombophilias, leading to a very high risk of thromboembolism
- *Prothrombin gene mutation:*
  - Single base substitution in the prothrombin gene
  - More prevalent in southern Europe
  - Considered a mild risk factor for thrombosis
- *Hyperhomocysteinaemia:*
  - Autosomal recessive disorder of homocysteine metabolism
  - Methionine metabolism produces the amino acid homocysteine
  - Homocysteine is metabolised by two pathways: one requires vitamin B6 and the enzyme cystathionine beta-synthase; the other requires vitamin B12, folic acid and the enzyme methionine synthase
  - Gene mutations in either pathway are exacerbated by vitamin B6, B12 or folic acid deficiency and cause high levels of homocysteine
  - Promotes thrombosis via multiple mechanisms – damage to endothelium, inhibition of thrombomodulin, protein C and prothrombin activation
- *Antiphospholipid syndrome:*
  - Most common hypercoagulable disorder
  - Acquired autoimmune condition of unknown cause
  - Diagnostic autoantibodies are lupus anticoagulant, anticardiolipin or anti-beta-2-glycoprotein I
  - Customarily divided into lupus anticoagulant syndrome and anticardiolipin syndrome (more common variant)
  - Causes inhibition of natural anticoagulants and the fibrinolytic system and activation of endothelial cells, monocytes, platelets and complement
  - Characterised by venous and arterial thrombosis and fetal loss
  - Affects up to 40 per cent of patients with systemic lupus erythematosus (SLE); can also present in isolation
  - Not all patients with antiphospholipid antibodies develop antiphospholipid syndrome, and therefore diagnosis is also based on clinical findings
  - Risk of recurrent thrombosis if antibody levels remain high
  - LMWH is recommended as warfarin fails in two-thirds of cases; if used, it is necessary to maintain an INR of 3–4

- *Elevated levels of procoagulant factors:*
  - Most common is increased levels of factor VIII
  - Genetic basis and mechanism causing thrombosis not known
  - Elevated levels of factors V, VII, IX, X and XI and fibrinogen also implicated.

SUMMARY

Shock is defined as impaired tissue oxygenation and is a clinical diagnosis. The leading cause of shock in surgical practice is hypovolaemia. The key aims of treatment are to restore the circulating volume, increase haemoglobin levels and stop the bleeding.

Red blood cell transfusions are given to treat tissue hypoxia. All red blood transfusions should be ABO-compatible and, in young women, also rhesus-compatible. A massive blood transfusion is the replacement of the total blood volume of a patient within 24 h. Coagulopathy, DIC and TRALI are severe complications of a massive transfusion. FFP, platelets and coagulation factors are needed for the treatment of particular bleeding disorders and in massive transfusions.

Injury to a blood vessel wall initiates immediate vasoconstriction followed by platelet plug formation. Fibrin clots reinforce the platelet plug, produced by the intrinsic and extrinsic coagulation cascades. Anticoagulation factors and the fibrinolytic system act in opposition to the coagulation cascade.

The most common cause of bleeding in a surgical patient is technical error. Coagulation disorders are usually acquired and are typically due to anticoagulation treatment. Congenital bleeding disorders are rare; the most common is von Willebrand disease.

QUESTIONS

1 What is the definition of shock? What are the five different classes of shock?
2 What is the initial management of hypovolaemic shock?
3 Explain the precautions that should be undertaken when giving blood.
4 What does the term 'massive blood transfusion' signify?
5 Describe the complications that can result from a massive blood transfusion.
6 Are there any alternatives to allogeneic blood transfusions? What are they and when would they be considered?
7 Give a brief outline of the physiological pathways involved in coagulation.
8 What are the most common acquired and congenital bleeding disorders?
9 What are the most frequent thrombophilias, and what is their impact on the surgical or trauma patient?

REFERENCES

Alpar EK, Killampalli VV (2004). Effects of hypertonic dextran in hypovolaemic shock: a prospective clinical trial. *Injury* **35**: 500–6.

Bishton M, Chopra R (2004). The role of granulocyte transfusions in neutropenic patients. *Br J Haematol* **127**: 501–8.

Buchanan GS, Rodgers GM, Ware Branch D (2003). The inherited thrombophilias: genetics, epidemiology, and laboratory evaluation. *Best Pract Res Clin Obstet Gynaecol* **17**: 397–411.

Bux J, Sachs UJ (2007). The pathogenesis of transfusion-related acute lung injury (TRALI). *Br J Haematol* **136**: 788–99.

Dahlback B (2005). Blood coagulation and its regulation by anticoagulant pathways: genetic pathogenesis of bleeding and thrombotic diseases. *J Intern Med* **257**: 209–23.

Franchini M, Lippi G, Manzato F (2006). Recent acquisitions in the pathophysiology, diagnosis and treatment of disseminated intravascular coagulation. *Thromb J* **4**: 4.

Goodnough LT, Shander A, Spence R (2003). Bloodless medicine: clinical care without allogeneic blood transfusion. *Transfusion* **43**: 668–76.

Hardy JF, de Moerloose P, Samama CM (2005). The coagulopathy of massive transfusion. *Vox Sang* **89**: 123–7.

Hebert PC, Wells G, Blajchman MA, *et al*. (1999). A multicenter, randomized, controlled clinical trial of transfusion requirements in critical care. Transfusion Requirements in Critical Care Investigators, Canadian Critical Care Trials Group. *N Engl J Med* **340**: 409–17.

Kim HW, Greenburg AG (2004). Artificial oxygen carriers as red blood cell substitutes: a selected review and current status. *Artif Organs* **28**: 813–28.

Krausz MM (2006). Initial resuscitation of hemorrhagic shock. *World J Emerg Surg* **1**: 14.

Madjdpour C, Heindl V, Spahn DR (2006). Risks, benefits, alternatives and indications of allogenic blood transfusions. *Minerva Anestesiol* **72**: 283–98.

Moore FA, McKinley BA, Moore EE (2004). The next generation in shock resuscitation. *Lancet* **363**: 1988–96.

O'Shaughnessy DF, Atterbury C, Bolton Maggs P, *et al*. (2004). Guidelines for the use of fresh-frozen plasma, cryoprecipitate and cryosupernatant. *Br J Haematol* **126**: 11–28.

Peyvandi F, Jayandharan G, Chandy M, *et al*. (2006). Genetic diagnosis of haemophilia and other inherited bleeding disorders. *Haemophilia* **12** (suppl. 3): 82–9.

Roberts K, Revell M, Youssef H, Bradbury AW, Adam DJ (2006). Hypotensive resuscitation in patients with ruptured abdominal aortic aneurysm. *Eur J Vasc Endovasc Surg* **31**: 339–44.

Spahn DR, Cerny V, Coats TJ, *et al*. (2007). Management of bleeding following major trauma: a European guideline. *Crit Care* **11**: R17.

Stainsby D, MacLennan S, Thomas D, Isaac J, Hamilton PJ (2006). Guidelines on the management of massive blood loss. *Br J Haematol* **135**: 634–41.

Thomas RH (2001). Hypercoagulability syndromes. *Arch Intern Med* **161**: 2433–9.

Worthley LI (2000). Shock: a review of pathophysiology and management. *Crit Care Resusc* **2**: 55–65.

Management of acute kidney injury in surgical patients

06

Andrew JP Lewington and Chas G Newstead

INTRODUCTION

The term 'acute kidney injury' (AKI) has been proposed by the Acute Kidney Injury Network (AKIN) to represent the entire spectrum of acute renal failure (Mehta *et al.*, 2007). Acute kidney injury affects 5–7 per cent of patients in hospital and has a high mortality, particularly when renal replacement therapy (RRT) is required. Even small rises in serum creatinine are associated with an increase in patient mortality (Praught and Shlipak, 2005). It is essential for all hospital disciplines to identify patients who are at risk of developing AKI and to understand the principles of prevention and treatment of the condition.

> ■ KEY POINT
> Acute kidney injury represents a spectrum of disease, and many surgical patients are at high risk.

> ■ KEY POINT
> Even small rises in creatinine in the in-patient setting are associated with an increase in mortality.

DEFINITION

Acute kidney injury can be considered as a reduction in the capacity of the kidney to maintain fluid, electrolyte and acid–base homeostasis occurring over a period of hours or days. The AKIN has proposed a new definition, along with easily measured staging criteria analogous to those used for chronic kidney disease (CKD). The diagnostic criteria must be used in the context of the clinical presentation and after adequate fluid resuscitation when applicable.

The AKIN diagnostic criteria for AKI are an abrupt (within 48 h) reduction in kidney function defined as an absolute increase in serum creatinine of $\geq 25\ \mu$mol/L (0.3 mg/dL) or an increase of 1.5-fold from baseline or a reduction in the urine output (documented oliguria of < 0.5 mL/kg/h for > 6 h).

CAUSES

It is helpful to subdivide the causes of AKI into three groups: pre-renal, intrinsic and post-renal (Table 6.1). The most common causes of AKI in the surgical patient are pre-renal, secondary

Table 6.1 Causes of acute kidney injury

Pre-renal	Intrinsic	Post-renal
Hypovolaemia	*Glomerular*	Calculus in single functioning kidney
Vomiting and diarrhoea	Glomerulonephritis	Bilateral renal calculi
Haemorrhage	*Tubular*	Retroperitoneal fibrosis
Decrease in effective circulating volume	Acute tubular necrosis	Prostatic hypertrophy
Cardiac failure	Rhabdomyolysis	Cervical carcinoma
Septic shock	Myeloma	Urethral stricture
Cirrhosis	*Interstitial*	Obstructed urinary catheter
Drugs	Interstitial nephritis	Intra-abdominal hypertension
ACE inhibitors		

ACE, angiotensin-converting enzyme.

to hypovolaemia, and intrinsic, secondary to ischaemic damage and acute tubular necrosis (ATN). Acute kidney injury secondary to pre-renal factors is usually reversible if the underlying cause is corrected; if not, the patient is at risk of developing intrinsic AKI. Post-renal causes of AKI can occur secondary to obstruction of any part of the urinary tract.

● DIAGNOSIS

It is essential to perform a thorough history and examination. A baseline set of laboratory investigations should be sent, along with more specific renal investigations depending on the clinical presentation. Early referral to a renal specialist should be considered in patients with AKI where the cause is not obvious from the clinical presentation and investigations, or where there is failure to respond promptly to appropriate management of the underlying medical condition.

> ■ KEY POINT
> Prompt diagnosis of the cause of AKI and its reversal where possible are critical.

Focused history
- *Previous history of CKD:* old notes, biochemistry laboratory, general practitioner
- *Comorbid conditions:* heart disease, peripheral vascular disease, diabetes mellitus, liver disease, myeloma
- *Poor fluid intake:* nausea, vomiting, reduced functional capacity
- *Excessive fluid losses:* fever, sweating, diuretics, diarrhoea, high stoma output, haemorrhage, burns
- *Drug history:* nephrotoxic drugs, radio-contrast media
- *Urinary tract symptoms:* prostatic disease, renal calculi.

Examination
- *Volume status:* core temperature, heart rate, jugular venous pressure (JVP), postural hypotension
- *Cardiovascular status:* peripheral perfusion, blood pressure, heart rate and rhythm
- *Palpable bladder:* prostatic hypertrophy, carcinoma of cervix

- *Bruits:* absent pulses, renovascular disease
- *Rash:* vasculitis, interstitial nephritis.

Investigations

- *Urine:* urinalysis (preferably not catheterised sample), spot urine Na^+, spot urine osmolality
- *Biochemistry:* urea and electrolytes (U&Es), bicarbonate, Ca^{2+}, PO_4^{3-}, liver function tests (LFTs), glucose, creatine kinase (CK), C-reactive protein (CRP)
- *Haematology:* full blood count (FBC), clotting screen
- *Microbiology:* urine microscopy and culture, blood culture (if septic)
- *Electrocardiogram* (ECG)
- *Chest X-ray* and/or kidney/ureter/bladder (KUB) X-ray (if obstructive cause suspected)
- *Renal tract ultrasound* (fails to demonstrate hydronephrosis in 5%).

● MANAGEMENT

Renal referral

Patients with pre-existing CKD, diabetes mellitus, liver failure or cardiac failure, and older people (> 65 years), are at higher risk of developing AKI following surgery. These patients need to be monitored closely postoperatively with a low threshold for seeking renal advice.

Prevention

Acute kidney injury following surgery is an important contributor to postoperative morbidity and mortality. The causes are often multifactorial, and identification of the high-risk patient and institution of preventive measures as shown in the first part of Figure 6.1 are valuable. There is no evidence base to support any specific pharmacological intervention (Zacharias *et al.,* 2005). Avoiding perioperative hypovolaemia is an essential component of patient management.

Fluid therapy

Hypovolaemia

In many cases AKI can be effectively treated and resolved by adequate volume replacement, treatment of the underlying medical condition (e.g. sepsis, haemorrhage) and avoidance of nephrotoxic medications. The choice of fluid replacement is guided by the nature of the fluid loss. Patients developing hypovolaemia secondary to haemorrhage require packed red blood cell (PRBC) transfusion if available. If PRBCs are not available, and in other cases of hypovolaemia, fluid replacement can be achieved through the rapid infusion of a balanced crystalloid solution such as Hartmann's solution (Na^+ 131 mmol/L, Cl^- 111 mmol/L) or Ringer's lactate (Na^+ 130 mmol/L, Cl^- 109 mmol/L) and a colloid solution such as hydroxyethyl starch or gelatine-based colloid with close clinical assessment. A central venous pressure (CVP) line and urinary catheter should be considered to aid the assessment of volume status. Fluid bonuses of 250 mL colloid or balanced crystalloid solution can be given with close attention to the CVP readings. If large volumes of colloid are administered, it is important to also administer an equal volume of balanced crystalloid solution in order to provide sufficient water for urine production and avoid a hyperoncotic state.

■ KEY POINT
Correction of hypovolaemia is the mainstay of treatment in the management of AKI.

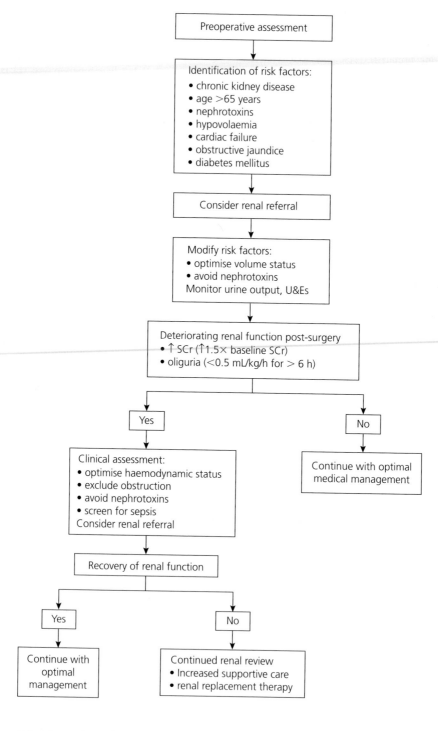

Figure 6.1 ● Prevention and management of acute kidney injury in the surgical patient.

SCr, serum creatinine; U&Es, urea and electrolytes.

There are caveats to these recommendations particularly relevant to patients who develop progressive oliguric AKI. Potassium-containing solutions (Hartmann's and Ringer's lactate) should be avoided in this scenario due to the risk of worsening hyperkalaemia; a crystalloid solution without potassium or a colloid should be used instead. It is also recommended on current evidence that high-molecular-weight hydroxyethyl starch should be used with caution in septic patients due to an increased risk of AKI.

Maintenance fluids

Once the patient is deemed to be euvolaemic, further fluid replacement can be prescribed as hourly fluid input = previous hour's output + 30 mL (this needs regular review). It is important to recognise that the daily sodium intake in health is 70–100 mmol/L. Following surgery the body's physiological response is to retain sodium and water through activation of the renin–angiotensin–aldosterone system and secretion of vasopressin. Therefore the inappropriate prescription of 0.9% sodium chloride (Na^+ 154 mmol/L, Cl^- 154 mmol/L) can potentially lead to a metabolic hyperchloraemic acidosis and significant fluid overload, which contributes to postoperative morbidity and mortality. If the patient is unable to resume oral intake of fluid, it is preferable to prescribe a combination of crystalloid solutions that provide the patient's daily electrolyte and fluid requirements, e.g. 0.45% sodium chloride/dextrose (Na^+ 75 mmol/L, Cl^- 75 mmol/L) or 0.18% sodium chloride/dextrose (Na^+ 30 mmol/L, Cl^- 30 mmol/L).

Pharmacological therapy

There is currently no evidence to support the routine use of loop diuretics (e.g. furosemide) or dopamine in the prevention or treatment of AKI (Kellum *et al.*, 2006). In certain situations, however, furosemide can be used to try to convert patients with oliguric AKI to non-oliguric AKI in order to facilitate the management of fluid and electrolyte disturbances. Dopamine should be avoided as it is associated with significant side effects, including cardiac arrhythmias and myocardial and intestinal ischaemia, which outweigh any renal treatment advantages. Patients with AKI may require a reduction in dose of medications that are usually excreted through the kidneys, such as antibiotics and fractionated heparin. Nephrotoxic medications such as aminoglycosides and non-steroidal anti-inflammatory drugs (NSAIDs) must be avoided in order to prevent further kidney injury.

Complications of acute kidney injury

Pulmonary oedema, acidosis and hyperkalaemia all require specific therapy.

Pulmonary oedema

- Sit the patient up and provide supplementary oxygen via a facemask. A non-rebreathing mask may be needed if there is severe pulmonary oedema. Give high-flow oxygen 60–100% as required.
- Buccal glyceryl trinitrate 2–5 mg works rapidly and can be repeated as frequently as required. If intolerable headache or hypotension develops, the effect rapidly resolves after removing the tablet from the mouth.
- Intravenous (IV) glyceryl trinitrate 50 mg in 50 mL 0.9% sodium chloride can be commenced at 2 mL/h and titrated up to 20 mL/h to maintain systolic blood pressure above 95 mmHg.
- Use IV furosemide, depending on the degree of renal failure. Give furosemide 250 mg (slow infusion over 1 h) if severe AKI.
- Use RRT and ventilation if the patient is in extremis.

■ KEY POINT
Pulmonary oedema, hyperkalaemia and acidosis may require urgent therapy.

Acidosis

- pH 7.2–7.4: very little evidence to support correction.
- pH < 7.2: isotonic sodium bicarbonate 1.26% solution can be used in stable patients not imminently requiring RRT. Bicarbonate therapy may worsen intracellular acidosis and deliver excessive sodium load. In the presence of hypocalcaemia, bicarbonate can provoke convulsions and should be used only when calcium is known and near normal.

Hyperkalaemia

Severe hyperkalaemia ($K^+ > 6.5$ mmol/L) or hyperkalaemia associated with ECG changes requires urgent treatment. The immediate principles of treatment include stabilisation of the myocardium and a reduction in plasma potassium concentration (increasing cellular uptake of potassium):

- IV 10 mL 10% calcium gluconate over 2–5 min (caution, as extravasation can cause tissue damage) stabilises the myocardium rapidly. There is no effect on serum potassium concentration. Further doses may be required until reduction in plasma potassium concentration is achieved. Onset of action: 2–4 min. Duration of action: 30–60 min.
- 10 units fast-acting insulin (Actrapid®) added to 50 mL of 50% dextrose infused IV over 20 min increases cellular potassium uptake. Blood glucose must be monitored closely. Onset of action: 15–30 min. Duration of action: 4–6 h.
- 10–20 mg salbutamol nebuliser stimulates cellular potassium uptake. Avoid in patients taking beta-blockers or with a history of cardiac arrhythmias. Onset of action: 30 min. Duration of action: 2–4 h.
- IV 1.26% sodium bicarbonate may be considered in patients not imminently requiring dialysis. Avoid in hypervolaemic patients due to the risk of precipitating pulmonary oedema.
- 15 g Calcium Resonium® orally three times daily (with lactulose to prevent constipation). Consider as a temporising measure if early recovery of renal function expected or dialysis is delayed. Onset of action: 2–3 h. Duration of action: 4–6 h.

If the cause of AKI is identified and can be treated promptly to restore renal function, then excretion of potassium will occur. If renal function fails to improve, then RRT will be necessary.

Renal replacement therapy

Renal replacement therapy may be required from the outset in patients with multiple organ system failure and may be initiated in patients who fail to respond to optimal medical management. The patient must be viewed as a whole and the AKI put in the context of their clinical condition and prognosis. The initiation of RRT is relatively straightforward if there is a recognised absolute indication to commence (Table 6.2). There is little consensus, however, as to when to initiate RRT in the absence of these criteria. The decision to commence treatment is dependent upon a number of different variables, including the physician's own beliefs, the clinical setting (AKI as part of multiorgan failure or as a single organ system failure) and the logistical capabilities of the institution. It has been proposed that early initiation of RRT may prevent the development of deleterious metabolic abnormalities and fluid overload but may unnecessarily expose the patient to the risks associated with the treatment, such as infection, haemorrhage and intradialytic hypotension.

■ KEY POINT

Renal replacement therapy is supervised by specialists but all doctors need to understand the indications for the treatment.

Table 6.2 Absolute indications for renal replacement therapy in patients with acute kidney injury

Indication	Characteristic
Hyperkalaemia	$K^+ > 6.5$ mmol/L with ECG changes (refractory to medical treatment)
Severe acidosis	pH < 7.15
Hypervolaemia	Pulmonary oedema resistant to diuretics
Uraemia	Urea > 35 mmol/L, pericarditis, encephalopathy

ECG, electrocardiogram.

Renal replacement therapy can be intermittent (intermittent haemodialysis, IHD) or continuous (continuous renal replacement therapy, CRRT). Continuous forms of RRT are preferred for patients who are haemodynamically unstable and who may require vasopressor support; therefore, CRRT is most commonly used in the intensive care unit setting in patients with multiorgan failure. Continuous renal replacement therapy may require anticoagulation, usually heparin, to allow the circuit to operate continuously. The practice of pre-dilution ultrafiltration lessens the need for heparin. Intermittent haemodialysis requires that the patient is more haemodynamically stable. It has the advantage over CRRT as it can be used without heparin anticoagulation if indicated due to its higher blood flows, which is an advantage in patients at risk of haemorrhage. Intermittent modes of RRT include haemodialysis (HD) and peritoneal dialysis (PD). More recently, hybrid therapies have been designed, including sustained low-efficiency dialysis (SLED) and extended daily dialysis (EDD). Peritoneal dialysis has been shown to be an effective therapy in paediatric patients developing AKI after cardiac surgery, but it is rarely used to treat adults with AKI. There is no evidence supporting the superiority of one modality of RRT over the other. The overall mortality from patients developing AKI is 50 per cent, but it ranges from 10 per cent to 80 per cent depending upon the severity of AKI and associated comorbidities. The majority of patients who survive AKI secondary to ATN recover renal function. It has been demonstrated, however, that 14 per cent of survivors develop end-stage kidney disease requiring long-term RRT.

Nutrition

Malnutrition has been identified as a predictor of in-hospital mortality for patients with AKI independent of complications and comorbidities. Acute kidney injury is associated with significant metabolic and immunological disturbances and the induction of a pro-inflammatory state that is exacerbated by malnutrition. As a general rule, patients with AKI should receive 20–35 kcal/kg/day and up to a maximum of 1.7 g amino acids/kg/day if hypercatabolic and receiving CRRT. Electrolytes must be monitored closely in order to avoid hypokalaemia and hypophosphataemia following the initiation of enteral nutrition (refeeding syndrome). Referral to a dietician for individual assessment is recommended, as nutrient requirements vary considerably depending on the course of the AKI, the underlying disease and the need for RRT.

● SPECIFIC SYNDROMES OF ACUTE KIDNEY INJURY

Contrast nephropathy

Acute kidney injury secondary to radiological contrast media is uncommon. It classically occurs within 72 h of receiving the contrast media and usually recovers over the following

5 days. Its incidence increases significantly in patients with risk factors and is associated with increased short- and long-term mortality. The kidney injury results from a combination of afferent arteriolar vasoconstriction and direct toxicity of the contrast media to the tubule epithelial cells. Prevention is important as there is no specific treatment (Stacul *et al.*, 2006). Management therefore involves the clinical assessment of the patient's volume status and potential risk factors (Figure 6.2). The patient should be adequately hydrated before the procedure and, if at risk of developing contrast nephropathy, should receive volume expansion with intravenous 0.9% sodium chloride (1 mL/kg/h) and iso-osmolar contrast. Presently there is no compelling evidence for the routine use of N-acetylcysteine (Kellum *et al.*, 2006). Renal function should be checked up to 48–72 h following the procedure if the patient is in a high-risk group in order to ensure stable renal function. Further exposure to contrast media should be delayed until full recovery of renal function, unless absolutely necessary.

> ■ KEY POINT
> Recognition of risk factors for AKI and use of preventive measures are mandatory when using radio-contrast agents and in the management of rhabdomyolysis.

Hepato-renal syndrome

Hepato-renal syndrome (HRS) occurs in patients with advanced cirrhotic liver disease, obstructive jaundice or acute liver failure and is a diagnosis that involves the exclusion of other causes of AKI. The pathophysiology of HRS is complex and incompletely understood. With progressive liver disease there is a rise in cardiac output and a fall in systemic vascular resistance (SVR). The decrease in SVR results from the splanchnic vasodilation that occurs in association with liver disease and has been proposed to be secondary to an increased secretion of a number of mediating factors, including glucagon, prostacyclin, nitric oxide and bacterial translocation. The reduced SVR in turn results in renal vasoconstriction and decreased renal blood flow (RBF) secondary to increased secretion of catecholamines, angiotensin, endothelin and antidiuretic hormone (ADH). Decreased RBF results in decreased renal perfusion and pre-renal AKI.

The onset of HRS is generally insidious but can be precipitated in a patient with advanced liver disease and ascites by a number of different insults, including gastrointestinal haemorrhage, sepsis, excessive diuresis and nephrotoxins. A low urinary sodium (< 10 mmol/L) is characteristic but not diagnostic of HRS. Management includes central venous monitoring and optimisation of the patient's volume status using colloid (20% salt-poor human albumin solution) while closely monitoring the urine output. Sepsis must be treated and intra-abdominal hypertension from tense ascites relieved if present. Large volume paracentesis has been demonstrated to result in a reduction in intravascular volume and renal dysfunction. The current recommendation based on the International Ascites Club guidelines is to infuse 6–8 g of albumin per 1 L of ascites fluid removed for paracentesis volumes greater than 5–6 L. There are some reports of success using terlipressin and human albumin solution to improve renal perfusion or the use of transjugular intrahepatic portosystemic shunt (TIPS) in patients with chronic liver disease. Patients with HRS secondary to liver cirrhosis have a mortality greater than 95 per cent. Renal replacement therapy is considered only if the patient is judged to have recoverable liver function or is a candidate for liver transplantation.

Rhabdomyolysis (crush syndrome)

Rhabdomyolysis results from skeletal muscle injury and cell lysis with the release of myoglobin and other muscle breakdown products (K^+, PO_4^{3-}, urate). Myoglobin is freely filtered by the

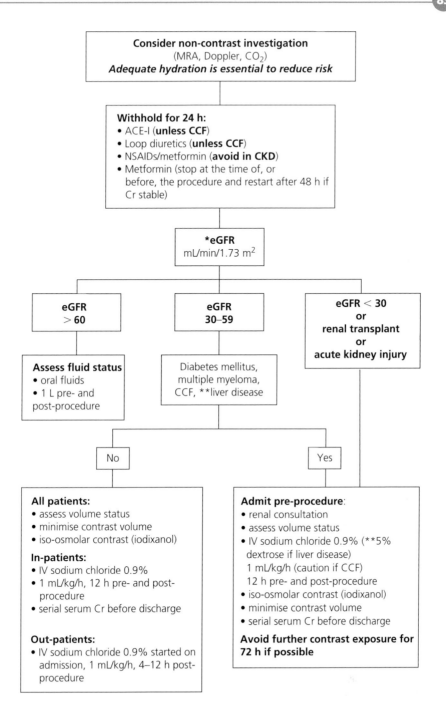

Figure 6.2 ● Contrast nephropathy protection guidelines.

ACE-I, angiotensin-converting enzyme inhibitor; CCF, congestive cardiac failure; CKD, chronic kidney disease; Cr, creatinine; eGFR, estimated glomerular filtration rate; MRA, magnetic resonance angiography; NSAID, non-steroidal anti-inflammatory drug.

*Online eGFR calculator available at www.renal.org.

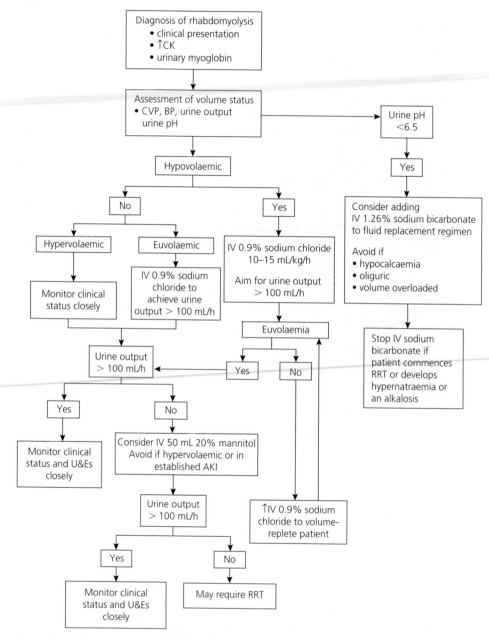

Figure 6.3 ● Prevention of rhabdomyolysis-induced acute kidney injury.

AKI, acute kidney injury; BP, blood pressure; CK, creatine kinase; CVP, central venous pressure; IV, intravenous; RRT, renal replacement therapy; U&Es, urea and electrolytes.

kidneys and is directly toxic to the tubular epithelial cells, particularly in the setting of hypovolaemia and acidosis. There are a number of causes, including trauma, burns, compartment syndrome and drugs (e.g. ecstasy, statins). Investigations supporting a diagnosis of rhabdomyolysis include increased CK, increased aspartate aminotransferase (AST) and urinary myoglobin. Additional electrolyte abnormalities include increased K^+, increased PO_4^{3-}, increased urate and decreased Ca^{2+} (binds to damaged muscle). Effective management requires correction of hypovolaemia in order to maintain renal perfusion pressure and dilute myoglobin and other toxins as outlined in Figure 6.3. Fluid resuscitation with 0.9% sodium chloride is preferred at a rate of 10–15 mL/kg/h. The effective circulating volume must be restored to maintain the urine flow rate of 100–150 mL/min. Although there is limited clinical evidence, it has been common practice to alkalinise the urine in order to prevent tubular precipitation of myoglobin. This can be achieved by the addition of sodium bicarbonate 1.26% to this regimen to maintain urinary pH above 6.5. Care must be taken to avoid causing hypernatraemia or precipitating a metabolic alkalosis and hypokalaemia.

Mannitol has traditionally been used to prevent AKI secondary to rhabdomyolysis because of its free-radical-scavenging activity and ability to promote renal vasodilation and osmotic diuresis. There is no evidence, however, that mannitol is superior to aggressive fluid resuscitation in preventing AKI in the setting of rhabdomyolysis. Mannitol can be harmful due to the risk of rapid intravascular volume expansion leading to pulmonary oedema and resulting in hyperoncotic kidney injury. Its use should therefore be restricted to the high dependency unit/intensive care unit environment and then only after careful evaluation of the patient's volume status. Hypocalcaemia should not be treated per se unless the patient is symptomatic or if intravenous calcium is required to treat hyperkalaemia, due to the risk of metastatic calcification and further tissue necrosis. Rebound hypercalcaemia can occur later following release of calcium from damaged muscle.

Obstruction

Urinary tract obstruction is identified in the majority of cases by ultrasound; however, the renal tract may fail to dilate in patients with obstruction secondary to retroperitoneal fibrosis or malignancy encasing the pelvis or ureter. Failure to identify obstruction may also occur when the patient is both obstructed and hypovolaemic. If obstruction is strongly suspected, then a computed tomography (CT) scan or cystoscopy with retrograde pyelography should be considered. Prompt relief of the obstruction must be achieved, as delay increases the risk of long-term kidney damage. Obstruction of a pyelonephrosis can result in rapid destruction of renal tissue.

Intra-abdominal hypertension

This can result in an abdominal compartment syndrome (ACS) characterised by cardiovascular, respiratory and renal dysfunction. There are a number of causes, including tight closure of a laparotomy wound (especially if there are dilated bowel loops), postoperative haemorrhage, tissue oedema secondary to sepsis or ischaemia, ascitic fluid and tumour load. The increased intra-abdominal pressure results in a decrease in renal blood flow secondary to a fall in cardiac output and increased renal venous pressure. There is also decreased glomerular filtration due to direct compression of the kidneys. The condition should be suspected from clinical examination and can be confirmed by measuring intra-abdominal pressure via a urinary catheter instilled with water and connected to a pressure transducer. Normal intra-abdominal pressure is less than 5 mmHg; intra-abdominal hypertension is defined as an intra-abdominal pressure greater than 12 mmHg or three measurements obtained 4–6 h apart. Abdominal compartment syndrome is defined as the presence of an intra-abdominal pressure of 20 mmHg or greater that is associated with a single or multiple organ system failure that was not present previously. The treatment of ACS is surgical decompression of the abdomen.

● SUMMARY

- Surgical patients with pre-existing risk factors are vulnerable to developing AKI postoperatively.
- It is important to identify patients at risk, as even small rises in creatinine are associated with an increase in mortality.
- The majority of cases of AKI can be effectively treated and resolved by adequate volume replacement, treatment of the underlying medical/surgical condition and avoidance of nephrotoxic insults.
- Early renal referral should be considered in patients developing AKI, as complications of AKI may require urgent treatment.

● QUESTIONS

1 Define acute kidney injury.
2 List four risk factors for patients developing acute kidney injury following surgery.
3 What is the daily sodium intake requirement? How much sodium chloride does 1 L of 0.9% sodium chloride contain?
4 What are the potential complications occurring in a patient with acute kidney injury?
5 List five non-dialysis strategies to manage pulmonary oedema in acute kidney injury.
6 What is the immediate management of a patient with hyperkalaemia secondary to AKI with associated ECG changes?
7 List four potential precipitants of hepato-renal syndrome.
8 List four electrolyte abnormalities that occur with rhabdomyolysis.

● REFERENCES

Kellum J, Leblanc M, Venkataraman R (2006). Renal failure (acute). *Clin Evid* (15): 1191–212.

Mehta RL, Kellum JA, Shah SV, *et al.* (2007). Acute Kidney Injury Network (AKIN): report of an initiative to improve outcomes in acute kidney injury. *Crit Care* **11**: R31.

Praught ML, Shlipak MG (2005). Are small changes in serum creatinine an important risk factor? *Curr Opin Nephrol Hypertens* **14**: 265–70.

Stacul F, Adam A, Becker CR, *et al.* (2006). Strategies to reduce the risk of contrast-induced nephropathy. *Am J Cardiol* **98**: 59–77K.

Zacharias M, Gilmore IC, Herbison GP, Sivalingam P, Walker RJ (2005). Interventions for protecting renal function in the perioperative period. *Cochrane Database Syst Rev* (3): CD003590.

Respiratory failure and acid–base balance

Julie O'Riordan and Laura Harvey

INTRODUCTION

The primary function of the respiratory system is the exchange of oxygen (O_2) and carbon dioxide (CO_2) between the body and the environment. Respiratory failure – defined as an arterial oxygen tension (PaO_2) of less than 8 kPa while breathing air or an arterial carbon dioxide tension ($PaCO_2$) of greater than 6.7 kPa – occurs when this gas exchange is unable to meet the metabolic requirements of the body. It is a common postoperative complication.

RESPIRATION – AN OVERVIEW

Breathing is controlled by the brainstem. After a latent period of several seconds, increased firing of the inspiratory neurons results in stimulation of the respiratory muscles. Contraction of the diaphragm, the intercostal muscles and the dilator muscles of the upper airway results in increased intrathoracic volume, decreased intrapleural pressure and opening of the upper airway. Consequently, air is drawn in through the nose, where it is warmed and humidified, and then flows through the pharynx, larynx, trachea and bronchi to the terminal bronchioles. From here the air travels to and from the alveoli by diffusion.

In the alveoli, the gas diffuses across the alveolar epithelium, basement membrane, capillary endothelium, plasma and red cell membrane before combining with haemoglobin. Carbon dioxide diffuses in the opposite direction.

As inspiration continues, stretch receptors in the lung and chest wall provide a negative feedback to the inspiratory neurons, which cease firing, allowing expiration to occur passively.

Mechanics of respiration

The lungs can be divided into various volumes, which can be measured to assess lung function. These volumes vary with age, sex and body weight:

- Tidal volume (TV)
- Inspiratory reserve volume (IRV)
- Expiratory reserve volume (ERV)
- Residual volume (RV)
- Total lung capacity (TLC)
- Functional residual capacity (FRC)

- Inspiratory capacity (IC)
- Vital capacity (VC).

Figure 7.1 shows a spirometer trace of lung volumes and Table 7.1 shows typical values.

When the system is at rest (i.e. at the end of a normal expiration), there is a balance between the tendency of the elastic lungs to collapse and the semi-rigid thorax to expand. This is known as the FRC. This is not a fixed volume, and it varies with normal respiration, gravity and numerous other factors (Figure 7.2). The FRC is important because of its relationship with the closing capacity. The closing capacity is the volume of the lung at which small airways begin to collapse during expiration. Normally closing capacity is less than FRC and therefore not relevant clinically. However, as FRC decreases, FRC can become less than closing capacity, resulting in areas of lung collapse (atelectasis) during normal tidal breathing and, consequently, hypoxia.

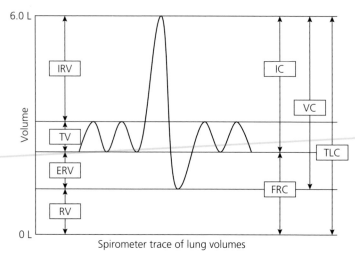

Spirometer trace of lung volumes

Figure 7.1 ● Spirometry.

Table 7.1 Typical spirometry values

Volume	Males (mL)	Females (mL)	Definition
Total lung capacity (TLC)	6000	4200	Volume of gas in lungs after maximal inspiration
Tidal volume (TV)	500	500	Amount of gas inspired/expired during normal quiet breathing
Inspiratory reserve volume (IRV)	3300	1900	Extra volume that can be inspired with maximal inspiration
Expiratory reserve volume (ERV)	1000	700	Amount of gas that can be forcefully expelled at end of normal tidal expiration
Residual volume (RV)	1200	1100	Gas remaining in lungs after maximal expiration

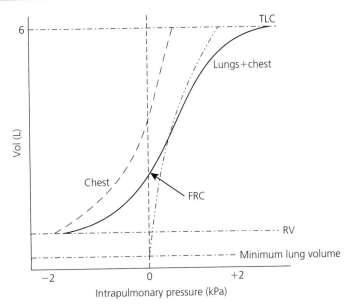

Figure 7.2 ● Functional residual capacity (FRC).

RV, residual volume; TLC, total lung capacity.

Compliance

The lungs and chest wall both expand in response to a change in transpulmonary pressure. Compliance (expressed in mL/cmH$_2$O) is a measure of the ease with which they expand in response to a given change in pressure and can be derived from the pressure–volume curve of a normal isolated lung undergoing inflation.

Compliance is usually maximal at FRC but is approximately linear over most of the range of lung volumes during normal breathing. At the extremes of lung volumes, however, compliance is reduced. At low volumes greater pressures are required to expand collapsed areas of lung, while at high volumes the elastic fibres are stretched to their limit. Compliance is also decreased at extremes of age and by many lung diseases.

The lung demonstrates hysteresis – that is, the pressure–volume curves for inspiration and expiration are not identical, meaning the compliance differs between inspiration and expiration (Figure 7.3). This is due mainly to the extra work required to overcome the elastic recoil of the tissues and the airway resistance during inspiration.

Distribution of ventilation and perfusion

Under normal physiological conditions, ventilation ($\dot{V}$) and perfusion ($\dot{Q}$) are near-perfectly matched, with a ratio ($\dot{V}/\dot{Q}$) of about 1. Ventilation and perfusion are both greatest in the most dependent part of the lung.

Local fine-tuning also occurs within the lung as the pulmonary arteries are capable of reflex vasoconstriction in response to alveolar hypoxia (hypoxic pulmonary vasoconstriction, HPV). This means that the blood is diverted away from the areas that are being poorly ventilated.

Disease processes can lead to changes in the $\dot{V}/\dot{Q}$ ratio. If ventilation exceeds perfusion, then $\dot{V}/\dot{Q}$ is greater than 1; conversely, if perfusion exceeds alveolar ventilation, then $\dot{V}/\dot{Q}$ is less than 1.

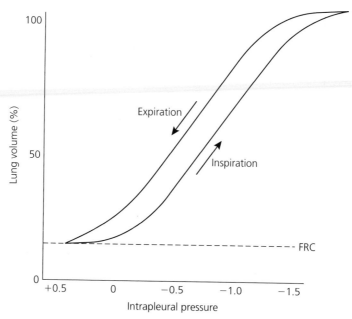

Figure 7.3 ● Lung hysteresis.

FRC, functional residual capacity.

Gas exchange

Oxygen cascade

The transport of oxygen relies on a partial pressure gradient known as the oxygen cascade. The partial pressure of oxygen (PO_2) in the atmosphere is 21 kPa; this falls to 0.5 kPa in the mitochondria where it is utilised. This drop in PO_2 is caused by a variety of factors, including the humidification of inspired gases by the upper airway, dilution in the alveoli by expired gases, incomplete diffusion across the alveolar membrane, and dilution in the arteries by shunted blood.

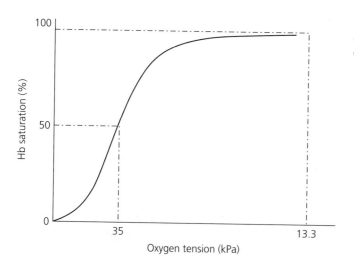

Figure 7.4 ●
Oxyhaemoglobin
dissociation curve.

Oxygen transport

Most (97%) of the oxygen in the blood is transported bound to haemoglobin (Hb) in a readily reversible bond. Each molecule of Hb can bind up to four molecules of oxygen. As one oxygen molecule binds to the Hb, there is a conformational change in the Hb molecule, encouraging further binding of more oxygen molecules, which results in the sigmoid shape of the oxy-haemoglobin dissociation curve (Figure 7.4).

The shape of the curve has several advantages. The upper flat portion means that even if alveolar PO_2 falls slightly, the loading of O_2 on to Hb will be little affected. The steep part of the curve means that the tissues can withdraw large amounts of oxygen for only a small drop in capillary PaO_2.

The position of the curve is defined by the oxygen tension when the haemoglobin saturation is 50 per cent (P50) under standard conditions. P50 is normally about 3.5–3.9 kPa.

The Bohr effect is a shift of the oxyhaemoglobin dissociation curve to the right due to increasing H^+ concentration. Acidosis shifts the curve to the right, while alkalosis (decrease in H^+ concentration) shifts it to the left.

2,3-Diphosphoglycerate (2,3-DPG) is produced by glycolysis and influences ion changes in the red cell. An increase in 2,3-DPG moves the oxyhaemoglobin dissociation curve to the right.

An increase in PCO_2 moves the curve to the right, and a decrease moves it to the left. Pyrexia shifts the curve to the right and hypothermia moves it to the left.

A small amount of oxygen (0.023 mL/100 mL blood/kPa) is carried dissolved in the blood. Oxygen content (CaO_2) of blood can be calculated as follows:

$$CaO_2 \text{ (mL/100 mL blood)} = [(1.34 \times Hb \text{ in g/dL}) \times (SaO_2/100)] + 0.023 \, PaO_2$$

where SaO_2 is the percentage saturation of Hb with oxygen, and 1.34 is the *direct* measurement of the oxygen-carrying capacity of Hb (theoretical = 1.39).

Oxygen delivery to the tissues (DO_2) is

$$CaO_2 \times CO.$$

The primary goal of the respiratory system is to deliver adequate oxygen to the tissues in order to meet their metabolic requirements.

Carbon dioxide

Carbon dioxide diffuses down its concentration gradient from the mitochondria to the capillaries. Transfer is rapid due to its high solubility. Carbon dioxide is carried in the blood in three forms: as bicarbonate ions (70%), combined with proteins as carbamino compounds (22%) and dissolved (8%).

● RESPIRATORY FAILURE

Respiratory failure can occur from an abnormality in any component of the respiratory system. It can be classified as hypoxaemic or hypercapnic.

Hypoxaemic (type 1) respiratory failure is the most common form. It is characterised by a PaO_2 of less than 8 kPa while breathing air with a normal $PaCO_2$. Type 1 respiratory failure is caused by a $\dot{V}/\dot{Q}$ mismatch and is associated with most acute lung diseases (e.g. pneumonia, pulmonary oedema, acute asthma). Pathophysiological causes include the following:

- *Low inspired oxygen (FiO_2)*: e.g. at high altitude, inadvertent administration of hypoxic gas.
- *Hypoventilation*: usually occurs from depression of the central nervous system by drugs (e.g. morphine, sedatives) or neuromuscular diseases affecting respiratory muscles.

- $\dot{V}/\dot{Q}$ mismatch: *the most common cause of hypoxaemia.* Areas with a $\dot{V}/\dot{Q}$ greater than 1 waste ventilation but do not affect gas exchange unless quite severe. A $\dot{V}/\dot{Q}$ of less than 1 may occur either from a decrease in ventilation secondary to airway or interstitial lung disease (e.g. pneumonia) or from overperfusion in the presence of normal ventilation. Administration of 100% oxygen will eliminate the low $\dot{V}/\dot{Q}$ units, thus leading to correction of hypoxaemia.
- *Shunt:* pulmonary capillary blood enters the arterial circulation having bypassed ventilated areas of lung. This poorly oxygenated blood then mixes with blood from the lung and has the effect of decreasing the PaO_2. An important feature of shunt is that it cannot be overcome by giving the patient 100% oxygen. It is observed primarily in pneumonia, atelectasis and severe pulmonary oedema.

Hypercapnic (type 2) respiratory failure is characterised by a $PaCO_2$ greater than 6.7 kPa. It indicates inadequate alveolar ventilation. It is usually associated with hypoxia in patients who are breathing room air. Common causes include drug overdose, neuromuscular disorders and severe chronic lung conditions.

Many cases of respiratory failure, such as severe pneumonia and pulmonary oedema, have a mixture of $\dot{V}/\dot{Q}$ mismatch and shunt. High-flow oxygen should always be given, as there will be some improvement in oxygenation even if it is not corrected fully.

> ■ KEY POINT
> Respiratory failure is a common postoperative complication.

Acute versus chronic respiratory failure

Acute hypercapnic respiratory failure occurs over minutes and hours, with an acute and therefore uncompensated rise in $PaCO_2$. Arterial blood gases (ABGs) will show a low pH (< 7.3), a normal bicarbonate (22–28 mmol/L) and a normal base excess (−2 to +2).

Chronic respiratory failure occurs over many days or years, allowing time for the renal system to compensate for the high $PaCO_2$ by retaining bicarbonate; therefore ABGs show an elevated $PaCO_2$, with a normal pH and a raised bicarbonate (> 28 mmol/L). Clinical markers of longstanding hypoxia include polycythaemia and cor pulmonale.

A common presentation is acute respiratory failure in a patient with underlying lung disease. This acute-on-chronic picture classically produces ABGs with a pH that is lower than normal but with an elevated bicarbonate.

> ■ KEY POINT
> Hypoxia can occur with or without hypercapnia. It can be acute, chronic or acute-on-chronic.

Signs of acute respiratory failure

The patient with acute respiratory failure may not appear distressed, despite being critically ill. Other signs include the following:

- Tachypnoea – the most sensitive sign
- Cyanosis
- Inability to speak or to say full sentences
- Signs of airway obstruction, e.g. tracheal tug, pursed lips, intercostal indrawing, wheeze, stridor, paradoxical respiration (abdomen and thorax move in opposite directions)
- Decreased conscious level, confusion
- Signs of CO_2 retention, e.g. warm peripheries (vasodilation), bounding pulses, flapping tremor, tachycardia, arrhythmias
- Respiratory arrest.

> ■ KEY POINT
> Onset can be insidious; tachypnoea is an early and sensitive sign.

Monitoring

- Pulse oximetry
- Respiratory rate
- ABGs.

Investigations

- ABGs
- Chest X-ray
- Electrocardiogram (ECG) – ?cardiac cause
- Spirometry – usually not suitable in acute setting
- Sputum culture.

Management

- Oxygen therapy to correct hypoxaemia
- Treat specific precipitating event, e.g. antibiotics for pneumonia, nebulisers for asthma/chronic obstructive pulmonary disease (COPD), diuretics for pulmonary oedema, consider naloxone if hypoventilation secondary to opiate overdose, anticoagulation for pulmonary embolism
- Physiotherapy
- Airway control, if required (respiratory failure most common indication for intubation)
- Respiratory support – non-invasive ventilation (NIV), intubation and ventilation on intensive care unit (ICU).

Myth: all patients with COPD retain CO_2; therefore, you should avoid high levels of O_2.
Truth: very few patients rely on a hypoxic drive to stimulate their breathing. Hypoxia is more of a threat to life, and therefore *all* patients should be given high-flow oxygen initially, with subsequent regular monitoring of ABGs.

> ■ KEY POINT
> Oxygen therapy is the main priority.

RESPIRATORY SUPPORT

Indications for respiratory support in a patient who has a reasonable chance of recovery are as follows:

- Continues to deteriorate despite treatment, e.g. rising respiratory rate
- Tiring
- Extreme hypoxia
- Rising $PaCO_2$
- Decreased consciousness level.

Intubation and ventilation

Conventional invasive positive-pressure ventilation (IPPV) has long been the routine method of providing respiratory support. Its efficacy is well accepted and it can undoubtedly be life-saving. However, IPPV requires the patient to be intubated and initially sedated on an ICU (Garfield, 2001). The benefits of IPPV include the following:

- Secure, protected airway
- Aspiration of secretions
- Ventilator setting can be adjusted to alter tidal volume and therefore alter $PaCO_2$ levels
- Removes the work of breathing and therefore reduces the body's oxygen consumption
- Can administer high concentrations (up to 100%) of oxygen
- Can apply positive end expiratory pressure (PEEP; see below).

Intubation and ventilation are, however, associated with the following complications:

- Insertion of endotracheal tube (ETT) – cardiovascular instability during intubation, failure to intubate, misplacement of tube, trauma to airway
- Presence of ETT – ventilator-associated pneumonia, impairment of ciliary function, inability to talk/eat/drink
- Disconnection or mechanical failure
- Need for sedation – cardiovascular instability, delayed weaning, reduced cough
- Barotrauma – overdistension, pneumothorax, subcutaneous emphysema, potential long-term lung damage
- Cardiovascular complications – IPPV impedes venous return, resulting in a decrease in cardiac output
- Gastrointestinal complications – many patients develop abdominal distension associated with ileus
- Salt and water retention – IPPV, especially with PEEP, causes increased secretion of antidiuretic hormone
- Critical illness neuropathy (Garfield, 2001).

Non-invasive ventilation

Non-invasive ventilation is increasingly being used in the treatment of respiratory failure, as it reduces the (potential) complications associated with endotracheal intubation. A meta-analysis of randomised controlled clinical trials comparing NIV with standard (intubation and ventilation) medical therapy in acute respiratory failure showed substantial reductions in mortality and subsequent need for invasive ventilation, especially in the COPD subgroup. Success depends on early initiation of treatment, preferably with an arterial pH above 7.25 (Ram *et al.*, 2004).

> ■ KEY POINT
> Non-invasive ventilation has been shown to be effective in preventing intubation and invasive ventilation.

The equipment consists of a ventilator, tubing and an interface, of which there are several types available. Full facemasks have been shown to be the most effective, especially in reducing $PaCO_2$. The nasal mask is the most tolerable but requires the cooperation of the patient to keep their mouth closed. Both types of mask have problems with pressure effects and ulceration of the nasal bridge. Alternatives include the nasal pillow, which is a bung that fits inside the nose, and a hood, which is well tolerated and allows the patient to communicate.

Non-invasive ventilation machines are often portable. They provide high gas flow by entraining air and therefore are unable to deliver very high levels of oxygen. Devices can be volume-controlled (to deliver a set tidal volume) or pressure-controlled (to deliver a set pressure change, such that the tidal volume depends on the compliance of the respiratory system).

The simplest form of NIV is continuous positive airway pressure (CPAP). This is the application of a preset positive pressure (usually 5–10 cmH$_2$O) throughout the respiratory cycle to a patient who is breathing spontaneously. The pressure recruits alveoli that have a tendency to collapse, and shifts tidal volume to the steeper part of the pressure–volume curve, thereby reducing the work of breathing.

Another popular form is biphasic positive airways pressure (BiPAP). The ventilator time cycles between two set pressure levels – a high-level P_{insp} usually set between 10 cmH$_2$O and 20 cmH$_2$O and a PEEP usually set at 5 cmH$_2$O. Patients are able to breathe spontaneously at both levels while the airway pressure is adjusted to maintain the preset levels. It can also fully ventilate a patient who is not making any spontaneous breaths. The compliance of the lung determines the volume change produced in cycling between the two pressures. PEEP acts in the same way as CPAP.

Absolute contraindications to NIV include the following:

- Respiratory arrest
- Severe cardiovascular instability
- Reduced consciousness level
- Inability to protect the airway
- Patient uncooperative/refusal
- Oral/airway surgery.

Relative contraindications to NIV include the following:

- Difficulty forming a seal with mask, e.g. facial trauma/deformity
- Air-swallowing a problem, e.g. after oesophagectomy – increased risk of anastomotic breakdown
- Frequent interruption of NIV required, e.g. copious secretions (Garfield, 2001).

Minor complications of NIV are common and include air leaks, discomfort from mask, nasal bridge ulceration and facial erythema. Major complications such as aspiration, cardiovascular instability and pneumothorax are rare.

RESPIRATORY FAILURE IN THE POSTOPERATIVE PERIOD

Respiratory failure is a recognised complication of the postoperative period. With an ageing population, the incidence of patients with significant respiratory problems presenting for surgery is increasing.

Patients at risk
Patient risk factors include the following:

- Pre-existing lung disease
- Smoking
- Obesity, history of obstructive sleep apnoea
- Sepsis/trauma – associated with acute lung injury (ALI) and acute respiratory distress syndrome (ARDS).

Surgical factors include the following:

- Anaesthesia – interferes with most aspects of respiratory physiology
- Intra-abdominal or thoracic surgery
- Prolonged laparoscopic surgery – splinting of diaphragm by gas can cause atelectasis
- Blood transfusion – transfusion-related acute lung injury (TRALI).

Smoking and the surgical patient
Smokers are six times more likely than non-smokers to develop postoperative complications (Moppett and Curran, 2001). Smoking has the following major effects on respiratory physiology:

- Reduced oxygen carriage in blood: Hb has 250 times the affinity for the carbon monoxide produced than for O_2, and therefore the amount of Hb available for O_2 transport is decreased.
- A smoker is already close to the point on the dissociation curve where any further decrease in PaO_2 will lead to rapid desaturation.
- Pulse oximeters cannot differentiate between carboxyhaemoglobin (COHb) and oxyhaemoglobin (HbO_2) and will therefore overestimate O_2 saturation.
- Smokers have irritable airways, making them prone to laryngospasm and breath-holding on induction of anaesthesia, which can become life-threatening.

Minimising the risk of respiratory complications

Much can be done before the operation in order to minimise the risk of respiratory postoperative complications. For patients with chronic lung disease, it is important to ensure that they are as well as they can be before surgery.

The preoperative assessment should involve the following:

- Identify patients at risk (see above).
- Take a history to establish extent of limitation, e.g. how far can the patient walk on the flat/uphill? Can they manage a flight of steps?
- If moderate to severe limitation of exercise tolerance, patients will require:
  - chest X-ray;
  - ABGs (on room air);
  - pulmonary function tests.
- Patients who are stable and have had tests within the past year do not need them repeating.
- Arrange physiotherapy for the patient both pre- and postoperatively.
- If the patient has had recent exacerbations of their condition, it is wise to postpone surgery where possible.
- Smokers should be encouraged to stop smoking, both to reduce their chance of complications postoperatively and for their general health. As it can take up to 6 months for a reduction in risk after stopping smoking (Table 7.2), encouragement is best given when the patient is seen in clinic.

■ KEY POINT

Patients at risk can be identified preoperatively.

For patients deemed to be at risk, regional anaesthesia (e.g. epidural, spinal) should be considered, as this has been shown to reduce the incidence of postoperative respiratory complications (Nishimori et al., 2006).

Table 7.2 Benefits of stopping smoking

Time frame	Effect
12–24 h	Clearance of carbon monoxide
2–10 days	Improvements in upper airway reactivity
1 month	Possible increased risk of postoperative complications
5–6 months	Reduction in postoperative complications
Years	Reduction in lung cancer, COPD, IHD, CVA

COPD, chronic obstructive pulmonary disease; CVA, cerebrovascular accident; IHD, ischaemic heart disease.
From Moppett and Curran (2001, p. 124), with permission from Oxford University Press.

● ACID–BASE BALANCE AND BLOOD GAS ANALYSIS

The concentration of hydrogen ions is one of the most tightly controlled systems in the body. The pH is the negative $\log_{10}$ of the hydrogen ion (H^+) concentration. The normal value at 37 °C is 7.34–7.42.

Normal pH is controlled by three basic mechanisms:

- Respiratory control of the partial pressure of carbon dioxide in arterial blood ($PaCO_2$) by the respiratory centre, which regulates alveolar ventilation. The higher the concentration of H^+, the more CO_2 is expired from the lungs. This is a rapid compensatory system.
- Renal excretion of bicarbonate and metabolic acids. This is a relatively slow mechanism taking hours or days.
- Buffering by bicarbonate, sulphate and haemoglobin. This minimises very rapid, acute changes.

The traditional approach to acid–base control centres on the Henderson–Hasselbalch equation. This describes the carbonic acid buffer system. Carbon dioxide reacts with water to form carbonic acid, which dissociates to form bicarbonate and H^+:

$$CO_2 + H_2O = H_2CO_3 = H^+ + HCO_3^-$$

If

$$[H^+][HCO_3^+]/[H_2CO_3] = k \text{ (constant)}$$

then by rearranging and taking the logs of each side:

$$pH = pKa + \log[HCO_3]/0.03 \times PaCO_2$$

and so pH can be defined as the ratio of bicarbonate to carbon dioxide. Therefore, alterations in acid–base result from either changes in CO_2 (respiratory) or changes in HCO_3 (metabolic). Compensatory mechanisms exist in order to maintain this ratio.

Standard base excess or deficit quantifies the amount of acid in mmol/L that must be added or subtracted from the blood sample in order to regain a normal pH at a $PaCO_2$ of 40 mmHg. So, the more negative the base excess, the more acidic is the blood sample.

Blood gas analysers directly measure pH, $PaCO_2$ and partial pressure of oxygen (PaO_2). Bicarbonate is calculated from a modified Henderson–Hasselbalch equation, while base excess is derived from computerised nomograms.

Acidosis and alkalosis

Blood pH is normally maintained at 7.36–7.44. A blood or plasma pH below this range is an acidaemia. Acidosis is a condition in which $[H^+]$ is raised or would be raised in the absence of compensatory mechanisms. Acidosis leads to acidaemia, but often the terms are used interchangeably. The same is true for alkalosis and alkalaemia.

Respiratory acidosis

Respiratory acidosis occurs when there is an increase in $PaCO_2$ above the normal range as a result of inadequate alveolar ventilation, which may be due to respiratory failure, drugs (particularly opiates) or central nervous system (CNS) pathology. Renal compensation occurs by increasing H^+ excretion and retaining bicarbonate, but this takes several days to occur.

Respiratory alkalosis

Respiratory alkalosis is caused by a decrease in $PaCO_2$, which is due to alveolar hyperventilation. It is important to look at the PaO_2, as the hyperventilation may be in response to hypoxia and underlying lung pathology. Other causes include pain, anxiety and CNS disease. Renal compensation causes a decrease in bicarbonate and takes days to occur.

Metabolic acidosis

The primary change is a decrease in bicarbonate caused by a primary metabolic abnormality. To compensate, there is an increase in alveolar ventilation in an attempt to decrease $PaCO_2$ and return the pH towards normal. Patients become very tachypnoeic and can often reduce the $PaCO_2$ to extremely low levels.

The causes of metabolic acidosis are many and can be divided into those that cause a high anion gap and those that cause a normal anion gap.

In blood, the sum of cations is equal to the sum of anions.

$$Na^+ + K^+ + \text{unmeasured cations} = Cl^- + HCO_3^- + \text{unmeasured anions}$$
$$\text{Anion gap} = (Na^+ + K^+) - (Cl^- + HCO_3^-) = 12\text{–}18 \text{ mmol/L}$$

A high anion gap acidosis is caused by the presence of unmeasured anions such as lactate, ketoacids, ethanol, salicylates or organic acids. Lactic acidosis is caused by inadequate tissue oxygen delivery, and renal failure produces an increase in organic acids, so both of these are common causes of high anion gap metabolic acidosis.

Normal anion gap acidosis is caused by hyperchloraemia and loss of bicarbonate or accumulation of H^+. Causes include gastrointestinal losses, ureteric fistulae and giving large volumes of intravenous normal saline.

Metabolic alkalosis

Caused by an increase in bicarbonate, metabolic alkalosis is often related to the use of diuretics. Other causes include loss of acid from the upper gastrointestinal tract, and administration of bicarbonate or its precursors (e.g. citrate, lactate).

Respiratory compensation for this is by increasing $PaCO_2$, but this is limited as the chemoreceptors will also try to compensate for an elevated $PaCO_2$, which overrides the response to the metabolic alkalosis. Generally the kidney itself will compensate well by excreting more bicarbonate.

Plan for interpreting blood gases

It is important to interpret results with knowledge of the patient's clinical condition in mind.

- Look at the pH for the primary–acid base disorder.
- Look at $PaCO_2$: an abnormality indicates a respiratory cause for the disorder.
- Look at the base excess (BE) and/or the standard bicarbonate for the metabolic acid–base status. There may be evidence of compensation or of a mixed respiratory and metabolic component.
- Calculate the anion gap.
- Look at the PaO_2.

Example 1

pH: 7.22
$PaCO_2$: 4.0 kPa
PaO_2: 12.8 kPa
HCO_3^-: 11.8
BE: –13.7

In this example there is a metabolic acidosis, as indicated by the low pH, the negative base excess and the low bicarbonate. Some respiratory compensation has occurred, as indicated by the low $PaCO_2$, although the pH has not reached normal.

Example 2

> pH: 7.35
> Pa_{CO_2}: 9.44 kPa
> Pa_{O_2}: 7.3 kPa
> HCO_3^-: 39.8
> BE: +9.4
> O_2 sat: 87%

This shows respiratory acidosis (raised Pa_{CO_2}) compensated by a metabolic alkalosis (high bicarbonate and positive BE), with the pH in the lower part of the normal range. This is the typical picture seen in patients with COPD with renal compensation. It indicates that the hypercarbia is chronic and not acute in nature, since renal compensation takes at least days to occur.

● SUMMARY

Respiratory failure is a common postoperative complication. Understanding respiratory physiology is very helpful in understanding respiratory failure. There are two types of respiratory failure – hypoxaemic (type 1) and hypercapnic (type 2) – which are caused by different problems. Onset can be insidious, with tachypnoea being an early and sensitive sign.

Oxygen therapy is the main priority in treating respiratory failure.

Patients at risk of respiratory failure can be identified preoperatively and should be optimised before surgery in order to minimise postoperative complications.

● QUESTIONS

1 What is FRC?
2 How is carbon dioxide carried in the blood?
3 Would acute pulmonary oedema usually cause type 1 or type 2 respiratory failure?
4 What is shunt? Can it be corrected with 100% oxygen?
5 What is CPAP? How does it work?
6 Would non-invasive ventilation be helpful in a patient with type 2 respiratory failure who is confused and agitated? Why?

● REFERENCES

Garfield MJ (2001). Non-invasive ventilation. *Br J Anaesth CEPD Rev* **1**: 142–5.

Moppett I, Curran J (2001). Smoking and the surgical patient. *Br J Anaesth CEPD Rev* 1: 122–4.

Nishimori M, Ballantyne JC, Low JHS (2006). Epidural pain relief versus systemic opioid-based pain relief for abdominal aortic surgery. *Cochrane Database Syst Rev* (3):CD005059.

Ram FSF, Picot J, Lightowler J, Wedzicha JA (2004). Non-invasive positive pressure ventilation for treatment of respiratory failure due to exacerbations of chronic obstructive pulmonary disease. *Cochrane Database Syst Rev* (3):CD004104.

● FURTHER READING

Pinnock C, Lin T, Smith T (2003). *Fundamentals of Anaesthesia*, 2nd edn. London: Greenwich Medical Media.

West JB (2005). *Respiratory Physiology: The Essentials*, 7th edn. Philadelphia, PA. Lippincott Williams & Wilkins.

Wound healing and the metabolic response to surgery

Timothy R Wilson, Qassim F Baker and A Al Zein

INTRODUCTION

Wound healing and the metabolic response to surgery are inevitable physiological consequences of operating. Understanding these processes can help the surgeon to pre-empt and detect problems in the postoperative recovery of patients. Postoperative complications have a significant effect on the patient's wellbeing and the burden of cost to the health service.

THE WOUND HEALING PROCESS

All wounds heal with the same three-step process, as outlined below and in Figures 8.1–8.3. The three steps are not entirely sequential and overlap to some degree.

Inflammatory response phase (Figure 8.1)

Wound healing starts with clot formation. Platelets adhere to the wound edges and release several important cytokines including platelet-derived growth factor (PDGF) and endothelial growth factor (EGF). These attract macrophages and neutrophils, which release further cytokines, amplifying the process. Serotonin (released from platelets) and histamine (released from mast cells) increase vascular permeability and allow neutrophils and macrophages into the wound. Within a few hours, the wound is occupied by an amorphous collection of white and red blood cells, plasma, coagulation proteins, fibrin and fibronectin. This mass supports the wound until collagen can be laid down. Macrophages play an essential role in wound healing by phagocytosis of bacteria and dead tissues and by secreting growth factors.

Proliferation phase (Figure 8.2)

Macrophages and platelets release transforming growth factors alpha and beta (TGF-α, TGF-β). TGF-β encourages fibroblasts to migrate to the edge of the wound and begin laying down immature collagen. TGF-α along with EGF causes proliferation and migration of epithelial cells to cover the surface of the wound. New blood vessel formation (angiogenesis) is triggered by low oxygen tension in the wound edges. These new capillary loops give the typical granular appearance of open wounds and give rise to the term 'granulation tissue'.

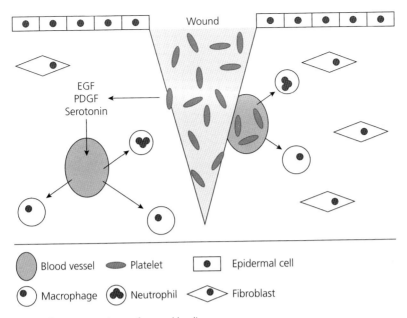

Wound

EGF
PDGF
Serotonin

Blood vessel	Platelet	Epidermal cell
Macrophage	Neutrophil	Fibroblast

Figure 8.1 ● Inflammatory phase of wound healing.

EGF, endothelial growth factor; PDGF, platelet-derived growth factor.

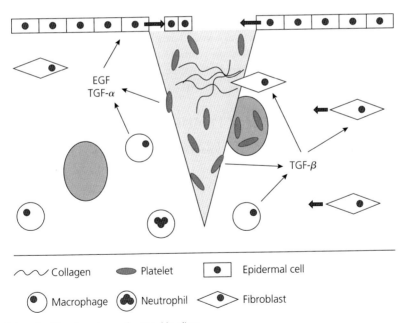

EGF
TGF-α

TGF-β

Collagen	Platelet	Epidermal cell
Macrophage	Neutrophil	Fibroblast

Figure 8.2 ● Proliferative phase of wound healing.

EGF, endothelial growth factor; TGF-α, transforming growth factor alpha; TGF-β, transforming growth factor beta.

Remodelling phase (Figure 8.3)

Immature collagen is broken down by collagenases. This is replaced by mature collagen, which is also secreted by fibroblasts. This form of collagen is aligned along the skin tension lines

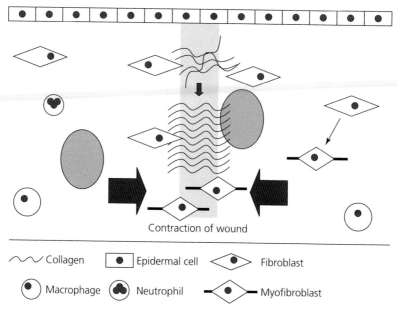

Contraction of wound

~~~ Collagen   ● Epidermal cell   ◇● Fibroblast

◉ Macrophage   ◉ Neutrophil   —◇●— Myofibroblast

Figure 8.3 ● Remodelling phase of wound healing.

(Langer's lines) and has increased tensile strength formed by the cross-linkage between the mature collagen fibrils. It takes about 3 months for the wound to achieve satisfactory tensile strength. However, collagen turnover in the wound can last for more than a year. The tensile strength of the fully healed wound will never return to normal. After more than 7 days, some of the fibroblasts differentiate to myofibroblasts. These cells are responsible for contraction in the wound.

● OPTIONS FOR WOUND CLOSURE

Three broad options are available for the closure of wounds: primary union, delayed primary suture and secondary union.

Primary union (first intention)

Primary union refers to full and immediate closure of wounds by sutures, metal clips, Steristrips® or tissue glue. It is the method of choice for any clean, neatly incised surgical wound.

Mid-line laparotomy wounds are normally closed in one layer (mass closure) adhering to Jenkins' rule, which states that the length of suture required should be four times the length of the wound. Bites should be taken 1 cm from the edge of the wound and 1 cm apart. Other abdominal wounds are usually closed in layers.

Delayed primary suture

In cases where the wound may be infected (e.g. following a laparotomy for purulent peritonitis), the deeper layers may be closed but the skin and subcutaneous layers left open to allow any residual infection to drain. If, after a few days, the wound is clean, the patient can be taken back to theatre to close the skin. Alternatively, the infected wound can initially be closed loosely with subcuticular prolene, which can be tightened to close the wound on the ward when the infection is cleared.

Secondary union (second intention)

Where wounds are known to be infected (e.g. following drainage of an abscess), they may be left open to heal. Granulation tissue fills up the cavity and with wound contracture the cavity will diminish in size substantially. These wounds often need regular packing by a district nurse and may take many weeks to heal.

● IMPAIRMENT OF WOUND HEALING

Factors that contribute to poor wound healing may be systemic or local.

Systemic factors

- *Age:* immune function declines with age; consequently, the inflammatory phase of wound healing is impaired with older age. Collagen synthesis is also reduced. Older people are also more likely to have coexisting cardiorespiratory disease.
- *Vascular disease:* impaired cardiac output and diseased peripheral arteries result in reduced delivery of nutrients and oxygen to the wound.
- *Pulmonary disease and smoking:* pulmonary disease and smoking impair oxygen exchange and subsequent delivery to the wound. Oxygen is important for angiogenesis and helps with resisting infection.
- *Poor nutrition:* the three main nutritional elements for wound healing are:
  - protein, which is necessary for all aspects of wound healing, but especially for laying down collagen;
  - zinc, which helps with enzyme activity;
  - vitamin C, which is essential for collagen formation.
  Other important elements include vitamins A and B12, folate, iron, selenium and magnesium.
- *Immunosuppression:* results in an impaired immune response to healing.
- *Steroids:* directly influence wound healing by dampening the inflammatory response, and also impair collagen synthesis and epidermal proliferation. Their deleterious effect on immune function also increases the risk of wound infection.
- *Diabetes mellitus:* wound healing in diabetes can be impaired for a number of reasons, including impaired immunity, increased risk of infection and impaired blood supply from microvascular disease.
- *Jaundice:* associated with impaired wound healing and increased risk of wound infection.
- *Malignancy:* in the presence of malignancy, tissue healing can be disrupted through poor nutrition or through an impaired immune response.

Local factors

- *Site of wound:* wounds on sites with an abundant blood supply (e.g. the face) heal better than those with less good supply (e.g. pre-tibial area of the leg). The presence of localised arterial disease (e.g. following amputation for ischaemia) is also important. With bowel anastomoses, local blood supply is a vital component for healing. Left-sided colonic anastomoses are associated with high rates of breakdown in comparison with right colonic or small bowel anastomoses due to a less dependable blood supply.
- *Infection:* the presence of infection frequently results in superficial dehiscence and slow healing of wounds. This is discussed further below.
- *Foreign body:* the presence of a foreign body may act as a nidus for infection, resulting in chronic non-healing wounds. This is a rare but recognised complication of using non-absorbable synthetic mesh for hernia repair. Such infections rarely settle until all the foreign material has been removed.

- *Tension:* increased tension across wounds increases the risk of dehiscence. Laparotomy wounds are more prone to dehiscence if intra-abdominal pressure is abnormally high. Tension is particularly important for the healing of bowel anastomoses.
- *Surgical technique:* it is important to recognise that wound edges swell due to oedema as part of the physiological response to healing. Sutures should not be placed too tight, since this may result in local wound ischaemia and necrosis. This is particularly important when closing the abdominal muscles, where tension may be exacerbated further by intra-abdominal pressure increasing the risk of dehiscence or incisional hernia.
- *Previous radiotherapy:* radiotherapy may impair the local blood supply to healing tissues. Infection and poor healing are often seen in perineal wounds following abdominoperineal resections for cancer after pelvic radiotherapy.

EARLY COMPLICATIONS OF WOUND HEALING

Primary bleeding

Primary bleeding occurs within 24 h of surgery and is due to inadequate haemostasis. This may result in external bleeding or haematoma formation. The risk is increased in patients on anticoagulants or antiplatelet drugs. For most operations, anticoagulants (warfarin) and clopidogrel should be stopped before surgery. Initial treatment involves direct pressure where possible, using a local pressure bandage. If bleeding is from the skin edge, then a non-absorbable suture may be placed to under-run the bleeding under local anaesthetic. If bleeding is ongoing or if the haematoma is extensive and causing pain, then surgical exploration may be necessary. This is particularly important in surgical wounds of the neck (e.g. thyroidectomy), as progressive haematoma and resultant laryngeal oedema may lead to stridor and airway obstruction. In theatre, the haematoma should be evacuated, the cavity washed with normal saline, and a search for the cause instigated. In the majority of cases no active bleeding point is recognised at the time of exploration.

> ■ KEY POINT
>
> If bleeding is ongoing or if the haematoma is extensive and causing pain, then surgical exploration may be necessary, particularly in surgical wounds of the neck, as progressive haematoma and resultant laryngeal oedema may lead to stridor and airway obstruction.

Wound seroma

Seromas (accumulation of serum) are common following breast and axillary surgery and other operations where there is extensive dissection in the subcutaneous plane. Seromas usually present several days following surgery. If small and asymptomatic, they can be left alone. Larger symptomatic collections may need aspiration, which can be performed satisfactorily in the clinic setting with a 22 gauge (green) needle. Repeated aspiration is often necessary, but it is inadvisable in patients who have undergone surgery involving mesh or other implants, because of the risk of introducing infection.

Wound infection

True wound infection occurs within 30 days of surgery and can be defined by the presence of pus or by signs of local inflammation in the presence of microorganisms. The bacterial count is typically in the order of 1 000 000 organisms per 1 g of tissue. Wound infection is one of the major contributors to delayed healing and protracted hospital stay. It has been estimated that

Table 8.1 Classification of wound contamination

Classification	Definition	Examples	Wound infection
Clean	No contamination or breach of mucosa	Thyroid, breast	2%
Clean–contaminated	Breach of mucosa with potential for minimal contamination	Biliary or upper gastrointestinal surgery	5–10%
Contaminated	Breach of mucosa with significant contamination	Elective colorectal surgery	10–20%
Dirty	Frank contamination or infection	Perforated appendix	40%

wound infections may affect up to 10 per cent of surgical patients and cost the NHS about £1 billion a year.

Risk factors

The risk of wound infection is related directly to the degree of contamination to which the patient is exposed at operation. Table 8.1 shows how this degree of contamination is classified. Infection after clean operations is due to exogenous organisms entering the wound during surgery or due to organisms from the patient's own skin. The most commonly encountered pathogen is *Staphylococcus aureus*, which accounts for 50 per cent of all wound infections. Infection of contaminated wounds is invariably due to the patient's own endogenous flora from the site of operation. In the upper gastrointestinal tract and biliary tree this predominantly comprises Gram-negative organisms, while in the lower tract anaerobic organisms predominate.

Other salient risk factors for wound infection mirror those that contribute to poor wound healing (see above). General factors include obesity, diabetes, immunosuppression and steroids, malnutrition and jaundice. Local factors relate to the degree of contamination, haematoma formation and surgical technique. During the operation, tissues should be handled with care to avoid unnecessary bleeding or ischaemia. Although adequate haemostasis is important, excessive use of diathermy should be avoided as this may predispose to infection.

Prevention of infection

Prevention of wound infection begins before any surgery is performed. Patients should be admitted for as short a time as possible before surgery as lengthy hospital stays before theatre increase the risk of infection. In operations involving prosthetic implants, it may be necessary to screen for and eradicate problematic endogenous organisms such as meticillin-resistant *Staphylococcus aureus* (MRSA). Blood sugars should be controlled tightly in all diabetic patients before and after surgery. If the patient needs to be shaved, then this should be performed immediately before surgery, as preoperative shaving has been shown to increase wound infections through minor injury to the skin.

Prophylactic antibiotics should be used where contamination is expected, where prosthetic implants or mesh is to be used, and when the patient is at high risk of infection (e.g. immunosuppression, prosthetic heart valves, valvular heart disease). Appropriate prophylactic antibiotics should be given during induction of anaesthesia so that tissue levels are sufficiently high before surgery begins. Once the incision is made, vessels at the wound edge will undergo vasospasm and tissue penetration of antibiotic at the wound edge may be poorer.

Management of wound infection

Simple wound infections comprise abscess (pus) or cellulitis, or both. Treatment primarily involves drainage of any infected fluid or pus. This can usually be accomplished on the ward by removing some or all of the sutures and gently probing the wound with sterile forceps or a bacteriology swab to facilitate drainage. If the patient is unable to tolerate drainage, if the collection is large or if necrotic tissue is found, then formal drainage with or without debridement under anaesthetic is necessary. Fluid or tissue should be sent for culture. Once the wound is drained, antibiotics are rarely necessary unless cellulitis is marked, the patient is systemically unwell, prosthetic material or mesh is present, or the patient is at risk of infection (e.g. valvular heart disease). Antibiotics should be tailored to the likely organism. *Staphylococcus aureus* is the likely pathogen responsible for infections after clean surgery, in which case flucloxacillin is usually satisfactory. After contaminated surgery, Gram-negative and anaerobic organisms should be covered. Previous microbiological specimens may be helpful with regard to the decision-making process in more complex situations.

Complicated forms of wound and soft tissue infection require further discussion.

Necrotising fasciitis

This is a serious soft tissue infection of the fascial plane characterised by thrombosis of cutaneous vessels resulting in development of gangrene in the skin and subcutaneous tissue, whilst leaving the muscle relatively spared. It is associated with systemic sepsis and high mortality. Necrotising fasciitis can be caused by a variety of organisms including *Streptococcus, Staphylococcus, Bacteroides, Enterococcus, Escherichia coli, Clostridium* and anaerobes. Two distinct groups of infection are recognised:

- *Haemolytic streptococcal gangrene:* this form of fasciitis is caused by haemolytic streptococci. Although people with lowered immunity are at increased risk, young fit individuals are also susceptible. The infection is acquired through the skin, usually through minor, unnoticed trauma, but surgical wounds may also give rise to this condition. All areas of the body may be susceptible, although limbs are more commonly affected. Patients are systematically unwell with fever and have localised pain, swelling and redness. Blistering may develop within 24–48 h. This is followed by gangrene, which appears initially as bluish-tinged blotches. Discharge is not a feature of streptococcal infection. As the infection evolves, the patient becomes profoundly septic; mortality affects one in three affected patients.

- *Synergistic gangrene:* this is caused by a combination of bacteria, typically Gram-negative and anaerobic organisms. These organisms may invade through the skin or may arise in the urinary track or anorectum. Affected individuals usually have a degree of medical comorbidity, particularly diabetes, chronic alcoholism and immunosuppression. The lower limb is particularly susceptible in people with arterial disease, as is the scrotal skin (Fournier's gangrene). However, this infection may also complicate surgical wounds. In comparison with streptococcal fasciitis, the presentation of synergistic gangrene is often less acute, but the skin changes are similar, with oedema, redness and ensuing necrosis. In addition, a thin 'dishwater' discharge often occurs. In some cases infection may spread to involve tissue deep to the fascial layer. Worsening systemic sepsis is also part of the clinical presentation, and mortality may be as high as 40 per cent.

Fournier's gangrene is used to describe necrotising fasciitis of the scrotal skin and perineum (Figure 8.4). This is usually the result of synergistic gangrene, although streptococcal infection may also be responsible.

Diagnosis of necrotising fasciitis is predominantly made on clinical grounds with a high index of suspicion. Plain radiographs may show evidence of soft tissue gas. Computed tomography (CT) or magnetic resonance imaging (MRI) reveals fascial thickening, but neither is

Figure 8.4 • Fournier's gangrene of the scrotum developing after drainage of a perianal abscess. Note thickening and cellulitis of the scrotum, with two small necrotic patches.

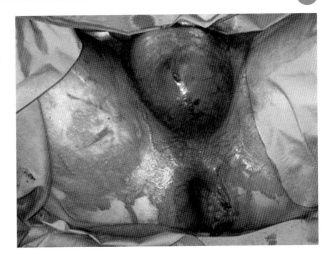

wholly specific or sensitive and may delay urgent treatment. Some clinicians advocate the finger test in which a 2-cm incision is made down to deep fascia. If the subcutaneous tissues can be easily separated from the fascia with gentle finger dissection, then the test is positive. Thin watery discharge and absent bleeding are also suspicious findings. When available, histological diagnosis can be confirmed from a frozen section.

The management of necrotising fasciitis is three-fold, comprising vigorous systemic resuscitation, broad-spectrum antibiotics and radical surgical debridement. If the causative organism is unknown, penicillin, third-generation cephalosporin and metronidazole should cover most of the likely pathogens. Piperacillin with tazobactam, and gentamicin, are also commonly used as part of an antibiotic regime. Surgery consists of debriding all affected skin and subcutaneous fat back to healthy tissue (Figure 8.5). Once healthy tissue is reached, dissection should continue beyond this margin until subcutaneous tissue cannot be separated from the underlying fascia with ease. No compromise should be made, no matter how extensive the resection. Where a limb is affected, amputation may be the preferred option. Following excision, the

Figure 8.5 • Extensive resection of necrotising fasciitis of the abdominal wall complicating a laparotomy wound.

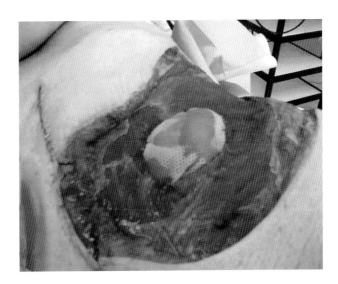

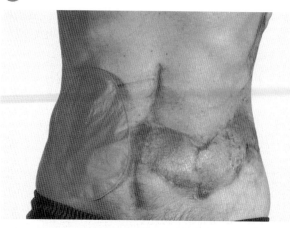

Figure 8.6 ● End result of reconstructive surgery to repair the abdominal wall defect seen in Figure 8.5.

wound should be dressed and re-inspected under anaesthetic after 24 h, as further debridement may be required. Inspections should be repeated as necessary, until the surgeon can be sure that the infection is eradicated. Reconstructive surgery is frequently required in those patients who survive such extensive debridement (Figure 8.6).

Gas gangrene

This infection, caused by *Clostridium welchii* and other *Clostridium* species, is rarely seen. The organisms invariably affect wounds with a compromised blood supply, as they favour an anaerobic environment. Consequently, arteriopathic patients and other patients with general debilitation are at increased risk. Unlike necrotising fasciitis, the infection results in muscle necrosis. Patients are usually profoundly septic. Skin changes, including oedema, purple discolouration and thin purulent discharge, are late signs. The organisms may produce gas, resulting in signs of crepitus or radiological soft tissue gas. Treatment involves high-dose benzylpenicillin and radical surgical debridement. At surgery, the affected muscles appear black, are non-contractile and do not bleed on cutting. The use of hyperbaric oxygen as part of treatment has also been advocated by some.

Tetanus

Tetanus may potentially cause problems in traumatic wounds. The responsible organism *Clostridium tetani* secretes a neurotoxin that inhibits cholinesterase at the motor end plate, resulting in local acetylcholine excess and sustained tonic muscle spasm. Tetanus infection can be prevented by active immunization with tetanus toxoid. This is given initially as three vaccinations, with subsequent booster vaccinations required every 10 years. The tetanus vaccination status should be obtained from any patient with contaminated traumatic wounds. Figure 8.7 details the procedure to be followed with regard to tetanus immunisation in these patients. Established infection should be treated with surgical debridement and antibiotics. If tetany is established, the patient may require paralysis with respiratory support.

Wound dehiscence

Early failure of the abdominal muscle repair combined with non-healing of the skin can result in complete wound dehiscence ('burst abdomen'). In addition to all of the risk factors for wound healing listed above, patients are also at risk from increased intra-abdominal pressure due to postoperative vomiting, paralytic ileus, chest infection or abdominal compartment syndrome. Wound dehiscence typically occurs 5–8 days after surgery and may be heralded by serosanguinous discharge from the wound. In the case of complete dehiscence, patients should

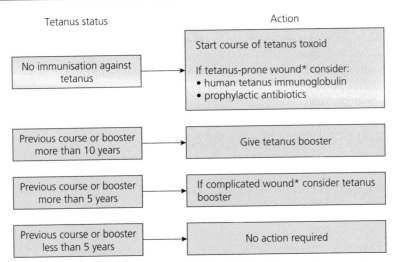

Figure 8.7 ● Schedule of tetanus toxoid and immunoglobulin administration for traumatic wounds.

*Tetanus-prone wound: deep, puncture, infected, contaminated, devitalised, bites.

ideally be examined under anaesthetic. The abdominal contents should be inspected to look for any underlying cause. After washout, the muscle layer should be carefully resutured using a non-absorbable suture. If the muscle layer does not come together without excessive tension, then consideration should be given to laparostomy or closure with mesh. Partial dehiscence (where the bowel is visible, but not eviscerated) may be managed conservatively where patients are unfit or not suitable for further surgery. Mortality following dehiscence is high, reflecting the poor physiological state of the patients involved.

● LATE COMPLICATIONS OF WOUND HEALING

Incisional hernia

Incisional hernia is a late complication of wound healing, resulting from failure of the deeper muscle layers to unite where the skin heals. The above risk factors for poor wound healing and poor surgical technique are the main contributing factors. Incisional hernias are usually wide-necked and therefore are at low risk of strangulation. Consequently, in high-risk patients, it may be appropriate to manage them conservatively, with a surgical corset where necessary. Surgical repair should be offered in symptomatic patients and in those whose hernias are increasing in size and difficult to control. Recurrence is higher in obese patients and, where possible, such patients should be advised to lose weight before surgery. Surgical repair increasingly involves the use of mesh to assist in closing defects, which are frequently associated with weak muscles and poor-quality tissue. Laparoscopic repairs are increasing in popularity following the introduction of specially coated meshes that do not adhere to bowel and can be placed across the abdominal defect from inside the peritoneal cavity.

Malignant change

Dysplasia and squamous cell cancer may develop in chronic wounds that are subjected to long-standing inflammation. The best-known example is the eponymous Marjolin's ulcer, which arises in chronic venous ulceration.

Hypertrophic and keloid scarring

Hypertrophic and keloid scars are caused by excessive scar tissue production. In hypertrophic scars this excess is confined by the wound edges, but in keloid scars it extends beyond the boundaries of the wound. Keloid scarring is due to an abnormality in collagen production. People with dark skin are more commonly affected. The scars tend to complicate wounds on the upper chest, head and neck.

● ADJUNCTS TO WOUND HEALING

Wound dressings

An ideal dressing should possess the following properties:

- Maintain a moist environment
- Remove excess exudate
- Provide a barrier to infection and protect the wound
- Allow gaseous exchange
- Require infrequent removal
- Be non-adherent
- Be non-allergenic.

There is a bewildering array of dressings available for wounds. It is important to bear in mind that no one dressing is suitable for all types of wound. Table 8.2 outlines the common types of dressings available, their properties, and the wounds for which they are suited. The nature of some chronic wounds may change with time, and the type of dressings used should be altered accordingly.

Antibiotics

Chronic wounds are frequently colonised by bacteria, and routine culture of wounds may lead to the identification of innocent organisms. Antibiotics should be reserved for evidence of infection as manifested by pus, cellulitis or systemic symptoms. The indiscriminate use of antibiotics in non-infected colonised wounds does not expedite healing and is likely to cause pathogenic resistance. Where deep-seated pus and necrotic tissue are present, surgery may also be necessary to eradicate infection.

> ■ KEY POINT
> The indiscriminate use of antibiotics in non-infected colonised wounds does not expedite healing and is likely to cause pathogenic resistance.

Topical negative pressure therapy

Topical negative pressure (TNP) therapy involves the application of negative pressure to the wound edge to help facilitate healing. The use of negative pressure is thought to decrease tissue oedema, resulting in capillary dilation and increased blood flow to the wound. The pressure may also affect growth factor release and cellular proliferation. In addition, pathogens and other inhibitors of healing are removed from the wound. As well as facilitating healing, TNP therapy is an effective method of dealing with large amounts of wound exudates.

Figure 8.8 demonstrates how TNP therapy works. Foam dressings are inserted into the wound cavity. Where multiple cavities are present, the cavities may be joined by internal or external foam bridges, which distribute negative pressure throughout the wound. A suction

Table 8.2 Overview of types of wound dressing

Dressing type	Examples	Properties	Uses
Low adherent	Jelonet Mepitel	Low adherence Allow exudates to pass Maintain moist wound	Fragile skin Open granulation
Semipermeable	Opsite Tegaderm	Impermeable to fluid and bacteria Permeable to air and water vapour Maintain moist wound Allow visual checks May be left for several days	Shallow wounds Low exudates only
Hydrocolloids	Granuflex Aquacel	Gel formed on wound contact Absorbs exudate Maintains moist wound Impermeable to air/water vapour	Moderate to high exudates Rehydration dry eschar
Hydrogels	Intrasite GranuGel	Desloughing action Allow some hydration wound Can absorb some exudate May lead to maceration	Sloughy or necrotic wounds Low to moderate exudate *Not* for dry gangrene
Alginates	Kaltostat Sorbsan	Highly absorptive Sticks to low-exudate wounds	High exudate wounds *Not* for low exudates
Foam	Allevyn	Good cushioning/protection Absorbs exudate May be left for several days	Shallow or cavity wounds with some exudate
Antimicrobial	Inodene Aquacel Silver	Can reduce bacterial load	Chronic infected wounds

tube connects the foam packing to a vacuum device that generates negative pressure, typically in the region of 125 mmHg. An occlusive dressing is then applied to maintain the vacuum with an airtight seal.

Topical negative pressure therapy may be used in acute and chronic wounds, but it is contraindicated in the following situations:

- Necrotic tissue or eschar
- Exposed organs or blood vessels
- Unexplored fistulae
- Malignancy in the wound.

Some patients may experience pain and discomfort during the therapy, which may be ameliorated by reducing the negative pressure or periodicity of the suction. Although portable devices are available, patient mobility is impaired with the use of these devices.

Topical negative pressure machines are rented on a daily basis; consequently, the therapy is expensive. The cost may be offset by significant reductions in healing times. Nevertheless, a 2007 *Drug and Therapeutics Bulletin* review concluded that there is currently insufficient evidence regarding the efficacy of TNP therapy for the majority of wounds and called for more robust clinical trials to be performed.

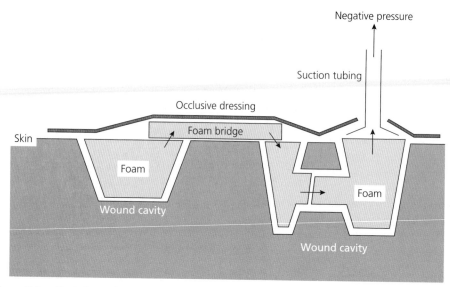

Figure 8.8 ● Topical negative pressure wound therapy.

Laparostomy

Laparostomy (leaving the abdomen open) is a useful adjunct to managing some abdominal wounds where the abdominal wall cannot be closed, where closure may result in intra-abdominal compartment syndrome (Box 8.1) or when a re-look laparotomy is planned.

Simply covering the intestine with saline-soaked gauze is not recommended due to resulting trauma and the possibility of fistulae developing. Where it is anticipated that the abdomen will be primarily closed at a later stage, some form of temporary covering should be used. A cheap, commonly used covering is an empty sterile saline bag (Bogota bag), which can be sutured to the fascial sheath. Synthetic mesh can also be used in this manner and has the advantage of allowing ascites to drain. Alternatively a non-adherent dressing can be placed over the abdominal contents, usually combined with suction to maintain adherence and reduced wound effluent. Specialist dressings designed to be used with commercial TNP systems are available, but dressings can also be improvised using suction drains and non-adherent dressings (e.g. Opsite®).

If the fascia and skin cannot be brought together, then a permanent covering should be considered. If synthetic mesh is used in this situation, then consideration should be given to an absorbable mesh, which will dissipate as the wound granulates. Non-absorbable mesh runs the risk of resulting in a chronically infected, non-healing wound. Skin grafts can be placed over granulating wounds to facilitative early skin coverage. If the fascia cannot be closed but the skin comes together easily, then an alternative strategy is to close the skin and create a deliberate incisional hernia.

Hyperbaric oxygen therapy

Hyperbaric oxygen therapy has been used to assist with wound healing for diabetic foot ulcers, pressure sores and refractory osteomyelitis. Patients are exposed to 100% oxygen at pressures greater than one atmosphere to increase the amount of oxygen delivered to the tissues. This therapy can only be delivered in hyperbaric chambers and is therefore not widely available.

Box 8.1 Abdominal compartment syndrome

Abdominal compartment syndrome (ACS) refers to abnormally increased pressure inside the abdominal cavity, which results in physiological impairment. The abdominal musculature acts like the fascial compartments of the limbs, and any intra-abdominal swelling therefore results in increased intra-abdominal pressure. Normal intra-abdominal pressure is around 5–7 mmHg. Intra-abdominal hypertension is said to occur when intra-abdominal pressure exceeds 12 mmHg. The extent of resulting physiological disruption increases as intra-abdominal pressure rises. Renal perfusion is impaired, resulting in reduced urine output, which may precipitate acute renal failure. Pressure on the diaphragm results in reduced tidal volume, which can lead to difficulties in ventilation and to the development of respiratory complications and respiratory failure. Venous return is also impaired, resulting in reduced cardiac output. Reductions in splanchnic blood flow may impair the gut barrier function, which is implicated in the development of the systemic inflammatory response syndrome and sepsis. Initially the body is able to compensate for this physiological disruption, but as intra-abdominal pressures exceed 20 mmHg the body is less able to do so. Abdominal compartment syndrome is defined as an intra-abdominal pressure of 20 mmHg or more in the presence of one or more newly dysfunctioning or failing organs.

Abdominal compartment syndrome may complicate abdominal surgery or may be seen in patients presenting with an acute abdomen. Any pathology resulting in increased abdominal swelling may be implicated. Common causes include the following:

- Postoperative oedema
- Resection of abdominal wall with primary closure
- Blunt or penetrating trauma
- Intra-abdominal bleeding
- Pancreatitis
- Distended bowel (obstruction, pseudo-obstruction or ileus).

The prevalence of ACS is about 3–5 per cent in the intensive care setting and is as high as 15 per cent following abdominal trauma.

Intra-abdominal pressure can be assessed by measuring intravesical (or, less commonly, intragastric) pressure. The empty catheterised bladder is instilled with 25 mL of normal saline. A pressure transducer can then be attached to a green needle inserted into the catheter's specimen port.

Management of ACS depends on the underlying cause and the degree of physiological disruption. Where distended bowel is implicated, a nasogastric or flatus tube may be sufficient to compress the bowel and reduce excess abdominal pressure. Ascites may be tapped percutaneously if required. In patients presenting with an acute abdomen and concurrent ACS, surgery should be expedited where indicated. In postoperative patients, it may be possible to manage ACS conservatively. Fluid boluses and inotropes may be used to optimise perfusion, and adequate ventilation can be maintained with respiratory support. However, when pressures exceed 25 mmHg, laparostomy is usually necessary to decompress the abdomen. If it is anticipated that ACS will occur postoperatively, then consideration should be given to initial laparostomy rather than forced primary closure of the abdomen.

Skin grafts and flaps

Skin grafts and flap procedures are a highly useful adjunct to wound healing, but this subject is beyond the scope of this chapter.

● THE METABOLIC RESPONSE TO SURGERY

Wound healing is one part of a larger generalised metabolic response to surgical trauma. It is important for surgeons to be familiar with the causes and consequences of these metabolic changes. Minimising the effects of this response can reduce postoperative complications and expedite patient recovery. This forms the basis for enhanced recovery programmes, which are gaining in popularity. It should also be recognised that an excessive metabolic response may result in the systemic inflammatory response syndrome (SIRS). Where the metabolic response is massive (e.g. in response to major trauma or burns), multiorgan failure can ensue.

> ■ KEY POINT
> Minimising the effects of the metabolic response to surgical trauma can reduce postoperative complications and expedite patient recovery. This forms the basis for enhanced recovery programmes.

Initiating factors

The metabolic response has a number of initiating factors. The main factors involved and their mediating pathways are summarised in Table 8.3.

Controlling systems

Many physiological systems are responsible for mediating the metabolic response. A brief summary of the salient systems is provided below.

Sympathetic nervous system

Stimulation of sympathetic nerves results in the release of adrenaline and noradrenaline, which act on alpha and beta adrenoceptors with the following effects:

Table 8.3 Initiators of the metabolic response to surgery

Initiators	Sympathetic nerves	Cytokines	ACTH	AVP	Aldosterone
Pain	+		+	+	
Tissue injury		+			(+)
Infection	+	+			
Hypovolaemia				+	+
Starvation			+		
Hypoxia and acidosis	+		+	+	
Temperature			+	+	
Anxiety	+		+	+	

ACTH, adrenocorticotrophic hormone; AVP, vasopressin.

- *Cardiovascular effects:* reduced blood flow to skin and viscera (α); increased blood flow to brain, heart and skeletal muscle (β_2); increase in heart rate and contractility (β_1)
- *Visceral effects:* inhibition of intestinal and bladder motility; increased sphincter tone and bronchodilation (β_1)
- *Metabolic effects:* release of glucagon; inhibition of insulin; glycolysis; gluconeogenesis; lipolysis; ketogenesis.

The cytokine acute-phase response

Cytokines are released from granulocytes, mononuclear cells, fibroblasts and endothelial cells in response to infection, trauma, toxins or haemorrhage. Important cytokines include interleukin 1 (IL-1), interleukin 6 (IL-6) and tumour necrosis factor (TNF), which initiate the acute-phase response and stimulate release of adrenocorticotrophic hormone (ACTH) from the pituitary. IL-1 and TNF cause systemic symptoms, including fever, malaise, headache and myalgia. Additional effects of the acute-phase response are activation of the complement and coagulation cascades, up-regulating the liver production of acute-phase proteins and initiating the vascular endothelial response.

The vascular endothelial response

The vascular endothelial response is mediated largely by platelet activating factor (PAF), which is released from the endothelium in response to cytokines (TNF, IL-1). This results in platelet aggregation and an increase in vascular permeability. Prostaglandins are also important mediators of increased vascular permeability and vasodilation.

Glucocorticoids

Adrenocorticotrophic hormone is released from the pituitary in response to direct stimuli (see Table 8.3) and also from the actions of cytokines, vasopressin and catecholamines. Release of ACTH results in release of glucocorticoids from the adrenal glands, leading to protein catabolism, gluconeogenesis and inhibition of insulin. The glucocorticoid response normally lasts for 24 h but may continue for days after major trauma or burns.

> ■ KEY POINT
> The glucocorticoid response normally lasts for 24 h but may continue for days after major trauma or burns.

Aldosterone

Aldosterone may be released in response to hypovolaemia, hyponatraemia, hyperkalaemia and ACTH. Aldosterone release results in resorption of water and sodium by the kidney.

Vasopressin

Vasopressin (AVP), also known as antidiuretic hormone (ADH), is released from the posterior pituitary in response to hypovolaemia or increasing osmolality. It causes solute-free water resorption.

Other hormones

Other hormone responses include an increase in glucagon and growth hormone and a decrease in insulin and thyroxine.

Clinical effects

The clinical effects of the metabolic response to surgery can be summarised as follows:

- Hypovolaemia (third space loss and increased vascular permeability)
- Low urine output (reduced excretion of sodium and water)
- Catabolic metabolism:
  - Increased energy expenditure
  - Increased circulating glucose
  - Muscle breakdown
  - Weight loss
  - Negative nitrogen balance
- Changes in serum biochemistry:
  - Hypoalbuminaemia
  - Hyperkalaemia (tissue damage and reduced excretion)
  - Hyponatraemia (solute-free water resorption)
  - Increase in acute-phase proteins (e.g. C-reactive protein, CRP)
- Impaired immunity:
  - Impaired immune cell function
  - Breakdown of gut barrier function and risk of bacterial translocation
- Increased cardiac index
- Activation of clotting cascade.

● ENHANCED RECOVERY PROGRAMMES FOR SURGERY

Advances in surgical and anaesthetic techniques along with a better understanding of the metabolic response to surgery have enabled the development of fast-track recovery programmes for surgery. The goals of such programmes are to optimise the preoperative physiological and nutritional status of the patient and to minimise the metabolic response sustained by the patient during and after surgery. The aim is to expedite patient recovery, reduce morbidity and increase wellbeing. A brief overview of the common elements included in such programmes follows.

Preoperative optimisation

- Physiological optimisation to minimise hypovolaemia, hypoxia and acidosis. (In colorectal surgery, full preparation of the bowel is discouraged since it may result in significant preoperative hypovolaemia.)
- Preoperative nutritional support should be given to malnourished patients.
- Where feeding cannot be implemented immediately after surgery, a preoperative carbohydrate-rich beverage may be given a few hours before surgery to help reduce the metabolic consequences of perioperative starvation.
- Adequate preoperative counselling should be given to reduce perioperative anxiety, which can stimulate sympathetic and adrenal responses.

Carefully controlled surgery

- The patient should be kept in physiological equilibrium where possible:
  - Warming blankets should be used to maintain normothermia.
  - Patients should not be over-hydrated during surgery. Transoesophageal Doppler monitoring can be used to guide fluid administration.
- Analgesia should be given pre-emptively before surgery, with epidural commonly employed for abdominal procedures.

- Careful anaesthetic techniques should be used to minimise postoperative nausea and vomiting, which allows for early postoperative feeding.
- Meticulous attention to surgery technique should be employed to minimise unnecessary tissue damage.
- The use of laparoscopic techniques should be considered to minimise the tissue trauma created by access.

Postoperative management

- Postoperative oxygen supplementation can be employed to reduce hypoxia and may also help with tissue healing.
- Good postoperative pain relief is essential in order to minimise metabolic triggers and to reduce respiratory and cardiovascular complications.
- Postoperative feeding should begin at the earliest opportunity:
  - Nasogastric tubes should be avoided in order to allow early feeding and to reduce respiratory complications.
  - Medication should be given routinely to control postoperative nausea.
- Bed rest should be minimised in order to reduce muscle wasting and to prevent deep vein thrombosis.

SUMMARY

- A proper understanding of the processes of wound healing and the metabolic response to surgery is essential.
- In treating contaminated wounds, there should be no hesitation in leaving the wound open with a view to delayed primary suture or allowing the wound to granulate.
- There is no ideal wound dressing that possesses all the required properties.
- Vacuum-assisted closure (VAC) therapy may assist in the healing of chronic wounds.
- Leaving the abdomen open (laparostomy) may be needed in order to avoid tight closure and development of abdominal compartment syndrome, or if a 'second look' is necessary.

QUESTIONS

1 What are the most urgent wound complications that you might expect following thyroidectomy?
2 How would you manage seromas following mastectomy?
3 What are the predisposing factors for burst abdomen?
4 What are the options for surgical wound closure?
5 What general factors can interfere with wound healing?
6 What are the predisposing factors for gas gangrene?
7 Explain the properties of ideal wound dressing.
8 Define enhanced recovery programmes for surgery.
9 What are the common causes of abdominal compartment syndrome?

FURTHER READING

Deodhar AK, Rana RE (1997). Surgical physiology of wound healing: a review. *Postgrad Med J* **43**: 52–6.
Drug and Therapeutics Bulletin (2007). Topical negative pressure for chronic wounds. *Drug Ther Bull* **45**: 57–61.
Jones V, Grey JE, Harding KG (2006). Wound dressings. *Br Med J* **332**: 777–80.
Tahir Khan M (1997). Metabolic response to trauma. *Surgery* **15**: 129–32.
Wilmore DW, Kehlet H (2001). Recent advances: management of patients in fast track surgery. *Br Med J* **322**: 473–6.

09 Systemic inflammatory response syndrome and sepsis

Ramanathan Kandasamy, Ahmed Al-Bahrani and Munther I Aldoori

● INTRODUCTION

The systemic inflammatory response syndrome (SIRS) is defined as the presence of two or more objective signs, such as an increase in heart rate, temperature and respiratory rate (Table 9.1). The SIRS is associated with a variety of stimuli, including infection, multiple trauma, inflammation, severe burns, pancreatitis, major surgery, cardiopulmonary bypass and shock. The SIRS may progress to sepsis, severe sepsis, septic shock and multiorgan dysfunction syndrome (MODS). It is important to understand certain definitions in order to understand the subject better (Table 9.2). Effective treatment of organ failure is essential, because of the cumulative burden of organ failure, leading to death. The average risk of death increases by 15–20 per cent with failure of each additional organ. A median of two-organ failure in severe sepsis is associated with a mortality rate of 30–40 per cent. In this chapter we review some of the concepts of the pathology of sepsis and the current management options available.

> ■ KEY POINT
> SIRS is associated with a variety of stimuli, e.g. infection, multiple trauma, inflammation, severe burns, pancreatitis, major surgery, cardiopulmonary bypass and shock.

● PATHOPHYSIOLOGY OF SEPSIS AND MULTIORGAN DYSFUNCTION SYNDROME

Infective and non-infective stimuli such as trauma and pancreatitis lead to SIRS and the release of pro-inflammatory cytokines such as tumour necrosis factor (TNF), interleukin 1 (IL-1) and interleukin 6 (IL-6), with the aim of destroying damaged tissues and promoting repair. Anti-inflammatory mediators such as interleukin 10 (IL-10) are subsequently released to regulate the inflammatory response and restore homeostasis. Although inflammation is an essential host response, excessive levels of pro-inflammatory cytokines lead to systemic endothelial damage, while high levels of anti-inflammatory mediators can result in immune suppression. Inflammatory cytokines cause increased synthesis of nitric oxide (NO), which is a potent vasodilator leading to decreased systemic vascular resistance, characteristic of shock.

Tumour necrosis factor contributes to the disruption of the tight junction between endothelial cells, resulting in increased permeability to plasma protein and fluid, which leads to generalised tissue oedema. Interleukin 6 alters hepatocyte protein synthesis, inducing acute-phase protein synthesis, and also down-regulates the production of albumin and anticoagulant pro-

Table 9.1 Definition of systemic inflammatory response syndrome (SIRS)

Two or more of the following clinical signs of systemic response to endothelial inflammation:

Temperature > 38 °C or < 36 °C

Heart rate > 90 beats/min

Tachypnoea (respiratory rate > 20 breaths/min) or hyperventilation ($Paco_2$ < 4.25 kPa)

White blood cell count > 12×10^9/L or < 4×10^9/L, or the presence of more than 10% immature neutrophils

In the setting or strong suspicion of a known cause of endothelial inflammation, such as:

Infection (bacteria, viruses, fungi, parasites, yeasts, other organisms)

Pancreatitis

Ischaemia

Multiple trauma and tissue injury

Haemorrhagic shock

Immune-mediated organ injury

Absence of any other known cause for such clinical abnormalities

$Paco_2$, arterial carbon dioxide tension.
Based on Bone *et al.* (1992).

Table 9.2 Definitions for sepsis

Term	Definition
Infection	Inflammatory response to microorganisms or invasion of normally sterile tissues
Sepsis	Confirmed or suspected source of infection plus ≥ 2 SIRS criteria
Severe sepsis	Sepsis with evidence of ≥ 1 organ dysfunction
Septic shock	Sepsis-induced hypotension (systolic blood pressure < 90 mmHg or a reduction of ^{3}40 mmHg from baseline) despite adequate fluid resuscitation
Multiorgan dysfunction syndrome (MODS)	Presence of altered organ function in an acutely ill patient such that homeostasis cannot be maintained without intervention

SIRS, systemic inflammatory response syndrome.
Based on Bone *et al.* (1992).

teins such as protein C. Simultaneous activation of cytokines and decreased production of anticoagulant proteins contributes to disseminated intravascular coagulation (DIC).

● MANAGEMENT OF SEPSIS

The primary aim when treating the critically ill septic patient is the prevention of organ failure. All risk factors should be identified and corrected in order to prevent the development of MODS. Measures such as early goal-directed therapy, use of activated protein C (APC), appropriate use of antibiotics, identification and eradication of infection, enteral feeding and neutralisation of inflammatory mediators may be used to prevent organ failure. In addition, however, general support of cardiovascular, respiratory, endocrine and renal function is very important in the treatment of sepsis.

> ■ KEY POINT
> The primary aim when treating the critically ill septic patient is the prevention of organ failure.

Early goal-directed therapy

The evolution of organ failure from SIRS involves many pathological changes, including circulatory abnormalities, tissue hypoxia and microvascular changes. Early optimisation of oxygen delivery and circulation may prevent organ failure in patients at risk. Rivers *et al.* (2001) demonstrated that early goal-directed therapy guided by central venous oxygen saturation ($ScvO_2$) decreased in-hospital mortality from 46.5 per cent to 30.5 per cent when comparing the standard and the treatment group (Figure 9.1).

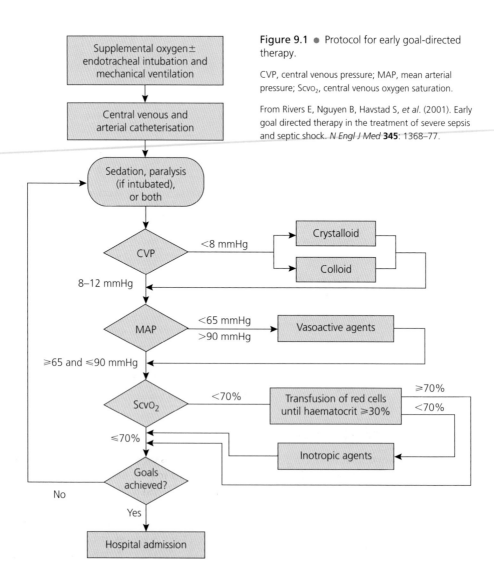

Figure 9.1 ● Protocol for early goal-directed therapy.

CVP, central venous pressure; MAP, mean arterial pressure; $ScvO_2$, central venous oxygen saturation.

From Rivers E, Nguyen B, Havstad S, *et al.* (2001). Early goal directed therapy in the treatment of severe sepsis and septic shock. *N Engl J Med* **345**: 1368–77.

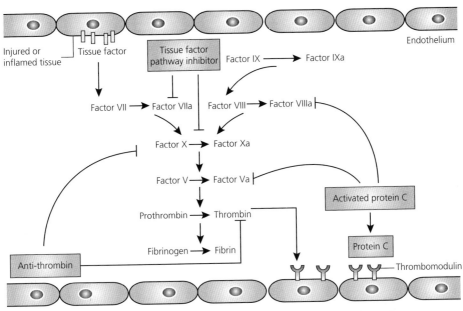

Figure 9.2 ● Coagulation cascade and the three major anticoagulant pathways in sepsis.

From Marshall JC (2004). Sepsis: current status, future prospects. *Curr Opin Crit Care* **10**: 250–64.

The benefits of early goal-directed therapy are mainly due to prevention of sudden cardio-vascular collapse, which may subsequently decrease the need for vasopressor and mechanical ventilation. The practice of blood transfusion to achieve a haematocrit of 30 per cent in patients with an $ScvO_2$ of 70 per cent or less is controversial. Monitoring of $ScvO_2$ requires the use of a special catheter and central venous cannulation.

Activated protein C

Disseminated intravascular coagulation in sepsis can impair oxygen delivery and aggravate tissue injury. The coagulation cascade has emerged as a promising target in preventing multi-organ failure due to sepsis. Recombinant APC is the first agent to be used clinically to alter the coagulation cascade (Figure 9.2).

Activated protein C limits thrombin formation by inactivating factors Va and VIIIa and thereby providing negative feedback regulation of coagulation. APC is also an important modulator of the systemic response to infection and has anti-thrombotic and pro-fibrinolytic activities. APC causes a rapid decline in thrombotic markers such as D-dimers, IL-6 and thrombin/anti-thrombin levels and a more rapid increase in protein C and anti-thrombin levels. APC also restores endogenous fibrinolytic potential.

Identification and eradication of infection

All patients presenting with sepsis syndrome should be evaluated for possible sources of infection and source control measures, including drainage of abscess, wound debridement and removal of infected devices (e.g. central venous catheter). Appropriate specimens for culture and sensitivity testing should be obtained before empirical antibiotic therapy is started.

Enteral nutrition

Early jejunal feeding may help to maintain the normal bacterial flora and the barrier function of the intestine. This minimises bacterial and endotoxin translocation into the systemic circulation. Patients also develop an immunosuppressed state characterised by reduced cell-mediated immunity. The addition of glutamine to the enteral or parenteral feeding improves T-cell function, enhances bactericidal function of the neutrophils and preserves the intestinal morphology.

Specialised immuno-nutrition formulations are available for enteral feeding to modify the inflammatory response; however, they do not act uniquely on the immune system. Glutamine, ornithine α-ketoglutarate, arginine, nucleotides and omega-3 fatty acids are used alone or in combination. The evidence base in humans for various additional substrates is variable.

General support of organ function

Cardiovascular system

Early goal-directed therapy aims to prevent sudden deterioration of the cardiovascular system, improve oxygen delivery and prevent tissue hypoxia. After adequate volume resuscitation, this is achieved with the help of vasopressor agents such as noradrenaline or adrenaline; however, this is associated with increased tissue oxygen demand, and decreased renal and mesenteric blood flow.

Vasopressin, a potent vasoconstrictor, has an established role in systemic arterial pressure maintenance. In septic shock, a relative vasopressin deficiency along with enhanced sensitivity exists. Vasopressin acts on the VIa receptors in the vascular smooth muscle and produces organ-specific vascular effects, including vasodilation of the cerebral, coronary and pulmonary vessels, and vasoconstriction of the skeletal and skin blood vessels. Vasopressin also decreases the noradrenaline requirement significantly.

Respiratory system

Respiratory failure in septic shock frequently leads to acute respiratory distress syndrome (ARDS), which requires mechanical ventilation. Despite advances in mechanical ventilation strategies, the mortality is around 36 per cent (which has decreased from 50 per cent over the past decade). Acute respiratory distress syndrome is diagnosed by acute onset of severe respiratory distress with bilateral pulmonary infiltrates consistent with pulmonary oedema. This bilateral non-cardiogenic pulmonary oedema leads to varying degrees of refractory hypoxemia. A PaO_2/FiO_2 ratio of 200 or less is defined as ARDS. The aetiology is usually pulmonary or extrapulmonary in origin. The causes are shown in Table 9.3. Sepsis-associated ARDS carries the highest mortality. The pathogenesis of ARDS involves endothelial dysfunction and loss of epithelial integrity, resulting in alveolar oedema and damage to type II pneumocytes, which

Table 9.3 Causes of acute respiratory distress syndrome

Pulmonary	Extrapulmonary
Aspiration	Sepsis
Pneumonia	Shock
Near-drowning	Trauma
Smoke inhalation	Pancreatitis
Burns	Fat embolism
Pulmonary contusion	Multiple blood transfusion
	Cardiopulmonary bypass

causes surfactant deficiency. Atelectasis results in increased shunt, leading to refractory hypoxaemia. Management of ARDS includes mechanical ventilation, fluid management and supportive treatment of the aetiology.

Mechanical ventilation

Patients with ARDS require intermittent positive-pressure ventilation (IPPV) with positive end expiratory pressure (PEEP). The ARDS Network trial demonstrated a 22 per cent decrease in mortality with 6 mL/kg compared with 12 mL/kg tidal volume ventilation and with a PEEP of 8–12 cmH$_2$O. With low tidal volume ventilation, the respiratory rate may go up to 35 breaths/min in order to clear the carbon dioxide. This can contribute to high levels of intrinsic PEEP, minimising the alveolar recruitment/derecruitment process.

Prone-position ventilation

In the supine position, atelectasis in the dependent region of lungs in ARDS creates large intrapulmonary shunt and hypoxaemia. Prone-position ventilation (PPV) is thought to recruit and ventilate the atelectatic dorsal lung units, thus improving ventilation perfusion and gas exchange.

Newer ventilatory strategies

High-frequency oscillatory ventilation (HFOV) oscillates the lung around a constant mean airway pressure, which allows maintenance of alveolar recruitment while providing low end expiratory and peak pressures.

Novel strategies

Granulocyte–macrophage colony-stimulating factor (GS-CSF) deficiency leads to impaired homeostasis of pulmonary surfactant and the development of an alveolar proteinosis-like disease. GM-CSF restores impaired function of granulocytes and macrophages and haematopoiesis.

Endocrine system

Functional adrenal insufficiency and tight glycaemic control are two important aspects in the management of septic patients. Patients with severe sepsis may develop relative adrenal insufficiency or SIRS-induced glucocorticoid receptor resistance. Studies suggest that, in severe septic patients, hydrocortisone 50 mg every 6 h is beneficial.

Hyperglycaemia and insulin resistance are common in critically ill patients, increasing the risk of complications such as severe infection, critical illness polyneuropathy and multiorgan failure. Van den Berghe et al. (2001) demonstrated that the maintenance of blood glucose between 4.4 mmol/L and 6.1 mmol/L reduced the morbidity and mortality in critically ill patients.

Renal replacement therapy

Acute renal failure is a complication of septic shock that can precipitate life-threatening complications such as hyperkalaemia, acidosis and fluid overload. Haemofiltration is the main form of continuous renal replacement therapy (CRRT) used to support renal function in acute renal failure. Critically ill patients do not tolerate the higher flow rates required in haemodialysis and develop hypotension. Septic patients tolerate haemofiltration better with hypotension. The concept of direct removal of pro- and anti-inflammatory mediators from the circulation may interrupt the inflammatory cascade and hence attenuate the septic shock.

● SUMMARY

The treatment of sepsis has changed significantly over the past few years; however, adopting these newer practices can be a real challenge to physicians. In the UK, all intensive care units are adopting these practices in the form of 'sepsis care bundle' and 'ventilatory care bundle'. The 'bundle' is defined as a group of interventions related to a disease process that, when implemented together, results in a better outcome than when implemented individually. Before initiating a new high-cost therapy, basic measures such as effective resuscitation can make a significant difference in the outcome of the patient.

● QUESTIONS

1 What is sepsis?
2 What is septic shock?
3 What is MODS?
4 What is the role of early-goal-directed therapy in septic shock?
5 What is ARDS?
6 What are the causes of ARDS?
7 What is the pathogenesis of ARDS?
8 What do you understand by the term 'PEEP'?
9 What is the treatment for ARDS?
10 What is activated protein C?
11 What is the mechanism of action of activated protein C?

● REFERENCES

Bone RC, Balk RA, Cerra FB, *et al.* (1992). Definitions for sepsis and organ failure and guidelines for the use of innovative therapies in sepsis: the ACCP/SCCM Consensus Conference Committee – American College of Chest Physicians/Society of Critical Care Medicine. *Chest* **101**: 1644–55.

Marshall JC (2004). Sepsis: current status, future prospects. *Curr Opin Crit Care* **10**: 250–64.

Rivers E, Nguyen B, Havstad S, *et al.* (2001). Early goal directed therapy in the treatment of severe sepsis and septic shock. *N Engl J Med* **345**: 1368–77.

Van den Berghe G, Wouters P, Weekers F, *et al.* (2001). Intensive insulin therapy in critically ill patients. *N Engl J Med* **345**: 1359–67.

● FURTHER READING

Finney SJ, Evans TW (2001). Mechanical ventilation in acute respiratory distress syndrome. *Curr Opin Anaesthesiol* **14**: 165–71.

Intensive Care National Audit and Research Centre. www.icnarc.org.

Kandasamy R (2006). Current concepts in the management of MODS. *Ind J Trauma Crit Care* **7**: 478–86.

Marshall JC (2001). Inflammation, coagulopathy and the pathogenesis of multiple organ dysfunction syndrome. *Crit Care Med* **29**: S99–106.

Richard DG (2003). Specialised nutrition support in critically ill patients. *Curr Opin Crit Care* **9**: 249–59.

Management of intestinal fistulae and enteral and parenteral nutrition

10

William Ainslie, Kishore Sasapu and Munther I Aldoori

INTRODUCTION

A fistula is an abnormal communication between two epithelial surfaces. Intestinal fistulae are an infrequent phenomenon, but they are distressing to the patient, are associated with significant morbidity and mortality (up to 33 per cent in recent reports) and result in prolonged periods of hospitalisation.

CLASSIFICATION OF FISTULAE

Fistulae may be simple – a short, direct tract between the two epithelial surfaces – or complex – with long, often multiple tracts, which may feed into an abscess cavity. Arbitrarily, 500 mL of fluid output a day is the volume above which a fistula is deemed to be a high-output fistula and below which it is deemed to be a low-output fistula. The causes are listed Table 10.1.

MANAGEMENT OF FISTULAE

The aims of fistula management are to treat any associated sepsis, replace fluid and electrolyte losses, and optimise conditions to allow spontaneous or surgical closure. Treatment of fistulae may be time-consuming, complex and often frustrating, but the principles of management can be summarised simply into five categories that can be recalled with the acronym SNAPP:

- *Sepsis:* management of sepsis, including associated issues of fluid and electrolyte balance
- *Nutrition:* provision of adequate nutrition for patients who are malnourished and catabolic
- *Anatomy:* delineation of the level and course of the fistula
- *Protection:* care of the of the skin and wound edges as enteric contents damage skin
- *Planning:* thorough and careful planning of any definitive procedure.

> ■ KEY POINT
> The aims of fistula management are to treat any associated sepsis, replace fluid and electrolyte losses, and optimise conditions to allow spontaneous or surgical closure.

Table 10.1 Causes of fistulae

Category	Example	Incidence (%)
Postoperative	Inadvertent enterotomy, anastomotic leakage	75–85
Spontaneous, secondary to underlying pathology	Crohn's disease, malignancy, diverticular disease, radiation, tuberculosis, pancreatitis	15–25

Management of sepsis, fluid and electrolyte balance

Sepsis

Sepsis is the leading cause of mortality as it may result in multiple organ failure and often necessitates admission to intensive care or a high dependency setting. Sepsis drives catabolism, which contributes to impaired healing of wounds. Treatment includes oxygen administration, fluid resuscitation and antibiotics. Computed tomography (CT) scanning is required to identify sources of sepsis and, if feasible, accessible collections should be drained percutaneously. If this is not possible and the patient has an uncontrolled fistula with peritonitis or an abscess that is inaccessible to percutaneous drainage, then surgical options to control the situation, such as laparotomy and drain insertion, resection of the affected segment and exteriorisation of bowel ends, or enteric diversion with a proximal loop stoma, may be required. If there are multiple fistulae, a laparostomy may be necessary in order to achieve control of the situation.

Fluid and electrolyte balance

Enteric fluid is rich in sodium and potassium. These electrolytes have to be replaced aggressively. To achieve this effectively, fluid balance must be recorded rigorously and losses promptly replaced with sodium-based fluids such as 0.9% saline or Hartmann's solution. Drugs such as proton pump inhibitors are effective in reducing gastric acid secretion, while octreotide injections or somatostatin infusions may reduce losses and aid fluid balance management. However, there is no good evidence of an improved rate of spontaneous healing of fistulae with octreotide or somatostatin.

Nutrition

Malnutrition is rife due to reduced nutritional intake, increased losses of protein-rich fluid and catabolism. Options available for providing nutrition treatment include the following:

- *Parenteral nutrition:* for intestinal failure and to manage high-output fistulae
- *Enteral feeding with low-output fistulae:* associated with a lower incidence of septic complications. The use of glutamine in critically ill patients is associated with a lower incidence of mucosal atrophy
- *Enteral feeding beyond the fistula into healthy bowel:* fistuloclysis.

Anatomy

It is advisable to discuss the situation and imaging requirements with a radiologist in order to agree on which investigations to perform and to optimise the yield of information achieved from these. Imaging is required to identify the level and cause of the fistula and to exclude distal obstruction. The latter is essential if there is to be any hope of spontaneous closure and to prevent recurrence and leaks after a definitive procedure, should the fistula fail to close spontaneously. Typical imaging studies include CT or a fistulogram, with or without oral and retrograde contrast studies.

Protecting the skin and wound edges

Small-bowel effluent contains activated enzymes and is harmful to surrounding tissue. Stoma nurses are an invaluable asset, and the need for their early involvement and input throughout the patient's management cannot be overstated. They are able to come up with many ingenious solutions to problems associated with the collection of effluent, which helps in both the accurate measurement of fluid balance and the protection of the skin.

> ■ KEY POINT
> Small-bowel effluent contains activated enzymes and is harmful to surrounding tissue.

Planning the procedure

About a third of fistulae close spontaneously, but fistulae that persist beyond 2 months are unlikely to heal spontaneously and require resection. Definitive surgery can be planned once the above steps have been completed, and the patient is free from sepsis and adequately nourished.

Surgery should be avoided before 6 months (unless a source of sepsis cannot be drained otherwise), in order to allow the peritoneal cavity to be re-established. This is often indicated by prolapse of the fistula. Principles of surgery are as follows:

- Enter peritoneal cavity at point away from fistula.
- Mobilise the bowel.
- Resect the fistula(e): there is a high incidence of recurrence if not resected.
- Perform anastomosis.
- Close abdomen in order to reduce risk of further fistulation. Avoid use of prosthetic mesh directly over the anastomosis.

It is important to remember that prolonged periods of illness and hospitalisation require psychological support of both the patient and their relatives. For this, consider the involvement of specialist nurses or psychologists. Also, throughout the process, advice and assistance can be obtained from regional centres that specialise in intestinal failure.

> ■ KEY POINT
> Prolonged periods of illness and hospitalisation require psychological support of both the patient and their relatives.

● STOMAS

A stoma is a surgically created opening of the bowel or urinary tract on to the abdominal wall. Stomas may be classified in the following ways:

- *Type*: an *end stoma* with only one intestinal lumen is brought out when the bowel is transected (such as an end ileostomy after a subtotal colectomy or an end colostomy after a Hartmann's procedure). A *loop stoma* contains both the afferent and efferent loops brought out together. It is used to divert enteric contents (e.g. to protect an anastomosis after a low anterior resection or as part of treatment for Crohn's disease of the perineum). Some surgeons place a temporary bar underneath this to support it while it heals.
- *Nature*: stomas may be *temporary* (created with an intention to reverse it in the future) or *permanent*.
- *Site*: jejunostomy, ileostomy, colostomy, ileal conduit.

Common indications for stoma creation

- No distal bowel to re-establish intestinal continuity (abdominoperineal resection of rectum)
- To avoid an anastomosis in acute setting (end ileostomy after a subtotal colectomy, colostomy with a Hartmann's procedure, resection of ischaemic bowel after thromboembolic event)
- To protect a distal anastomosis (after low anterior resection of rectum)
- To divert the faecal stream for treatment of a distal pathology (perianal sepsis, radiotherapy for anal canal tumours, distal obstruction in a patient too unfit for definitive surgery)
- To divert the urinary stream (ileal conduit after cystectomy).

Rules of stoma formation

- Always discuss stoma formation before surgery where this will or may be likely.
- Always mark potential sites preoperatively with an indelible marker – avoid skin creases, bony prominences and waist bands/belts, and place it where it can be seen and accessed by the patient. Stoma nurses are particularly good at selecting stoma sites.
- Insert a marker suture in the skin at the start of the procedure – this avoids the 'indelible' mark being wiped off during the procedure by the combined action of skin preparation fluid and blood.
- Create an opening about the width of two fingers through the abdominal wall and the rectus muscle. The bowel should sit snugly but not tightly within the tract and should be free from tension. Ensure the bowel is well perfused.
- Open the bowel and create the stoma after all other wounds have been closed and covered.
- Ileostomies should have a spout to minimise contact between the alkaline effluent (with activated enzymes) and skin. Colostomies can be flush.

Complications of stomas

Complications can be categorised as early and late. Early complications include the following:

- *Retraction:* either partial or complete, due to inadequate mobilisation of bowel. Partial retraction can cause local infection, fistula formation or, with a loop stoma, overflow of effluent into the distal limb. Sometimes this may be treated conservatively, but it may require resiting of the stoma. Complete retraction causes peritonitis, which requires reoperation.
- *Ischaemia:* due to inadequate perfusion. This requires reoperation, resection of the affected segment and creation of a new stoma. It can result from the following:
  - Excessive tension (inadequate mobilisation)
  - External pressure as bowel passes through abdominal wall
  - vasopressors.
- *Fluid and electrolyte losses:* as with fistulae, ileostomy output can be very high (up to 6 L/day). Management includes strict fluid balance, adequate replacement and use of antidiarrhoeal agents.

Late complications of stomas include the following:

- *Parastomal hernia:* predisposing factors include obesity, increased intra-abdominal pressure and a wide opening in the fascia. These are mostly asymptomatic, but they can interfere with appliances and can strangulate. They can be repaired with a mesh or relocated.
- *Stenosis:* result of ischaemia or a tight opening in fascia. Rarely due to Crohn's disease. Can be treated by dilation but may require revision.
- *Prolapse:* most commonly affects loop colostomies. Predisposing factors are as for parastomal hernias and also include excessive mobility of the bowel or the presence of a redundant loop. Treatment includes excision of the redundant portion if the stoma is permanent, or reversal of the stoma if it is temporary. Loop transverse colostomies are best avoided as they are notorious for this problem (consider a loop ileostomy instead).

- *Haemorrhage:* can occur at the stoma margin from friable granulation tissue. Always consider a proximal cause of the haemorrhage.
- *Diversion colitis:* chronic inflammation in the distal defunctioned bowel. Usually this is asymptomatic, but it may cause discharge of blood and mucus per rectum. The cause is considered to be due to lack of contact of the mucosa with short-chain fatty acids.
- *Fistulae:* may occur late from Crohn's disease.
- *Skin irritation:* caused by contact with effluent, particularly from an ileostomy. Predisposing factors include an inadequate spout on an ileostomy and poorly fitting appliances. Patients can also develop sensitivity to adhesives and appliances. Rarer causes include Crohn's disease and pyoderma gangrenosum. The stoma nurse is invaluable in the management of these problems.

Unusual stomas

- *Appendicostomy:* to administer antegrade colonic enemas ('ACE' procedure) for slow-transit constipation.
- *Caecostomy:* used rarely for decompression in pseudo-obstruction. Now supplanted by loop stomas or a formal right hemicolectomy.

Reversal of stomas

- Ensure the patient is fit for the procedure. Most hospitals now offer some form of pre-admission anaesthetic assessment.
- Check the distal bowel to ensure there is no evidence of a stricture or a leak. This can be performed with radiological contrast and endoscopic studies.
- Loop stomas (e.g. loop ileostomy) may be reversed by local mobilisation and re-anastomosis without resorting to laparotomy.
- End stomas can be reversed laparoscopically or at laparotomy.
- There is a small but significant risk of leak and of mortality associated with reversal. Always ensure that the patient is aware of this and is prepared to take the risk.

● NUTRITION

An adequate nutritional state is of the utmost importance for a patient to withstand the impact of surgical trauma. Despite this, malnutrition is much more common in surgical patients than has previously been appreciated, even though its relevance to outcome is well established. Contemporary estimates suggest that up to 39 per cent of surgical patients are malnourished. Although many cases are due to the nature of the disease process itself, many are down to inadequate consideration of, and delivery of, nutrition. Detrimental effects of malnutrition include increased infectious morbidity, impaired immunological function, prolonged ventilator dependence, decreased wound healing, prolonged hospital stay and increased mortality. It is therefore necessary to have the necessary tools to diagnose, assess and intervene in cases of malnutrition.

> ■ KEY POINT
> Up to 39 per cent of surgical patients are malnourished.

Definition of malnutrition

Malnutrition occurs when the supply of nutrients is inadequate or poorly balanced, or there is impaired absorption and utilisation of these nutrients. A global deficiency of carbohydrate, proteins and fats is termed 'protein energy malnutrition', while a deficiency of vitamins or minerals is termed 'micronutrient malnutrition'.

Table 10.2 Causes of malnutrition

Cause		Examples
Decreased intake	Fasting	Preoperative patient
	Inability to swallow/eat	Oesophageal pathology, stroke, dementia, malignancy
Malabsorption	Impaired digestion	Pancreatic insufficiency
	Impaired absorption	Crohn's disease, intestinal resection
	Excessive losses	Enterocutaneous fistula, diarrhoea
Increased requirements	Metabolic response to injury	Surgery, trauma, burns, sepsis

Causes of malnutrition

See Table 10.2.

Consequences of malnutrition

Identification and treatment of malnutrition are essential, as malnutrition leads to prolonged recovery from illness, increased length of hospital stay and delayed return to work. Mechanisms through which these occur include the following:

- *Impairment of immune response:* predisposition to infection
- *Impairment of wound healing:* can increase the likelihood of surgical wound dehiscence, anastomotic breakdown, fistulae, wound infection and fracture malunion
- *Reduction in muscle strength:* the patient becomes easily fatigued and finds it difficult to breathe or cough effectively. Patient may require prolonged ventilation. This also affects the patient's ability to mobilise and self-care, which necessitates additional physiotherapy and nursing care
- *Water and electrolyte disturbances:* retention of whole-body sodium and water, with peripheral and pulmonary oedema. This further affects ventilation and mobility. There is also depletion in whole-body potassium, magnesium and phosphate, which are essential for protein synthesis. There is a risk of refeeding syndrome
- *Vitamin and micronutrient deficiencies:* although rare, these deficiencies can result in refeeding syndrome or deficiency syndromes such as scurvy and Wernicke–Korsakoff syndrome
- *Impairment of psychosocial function:* malnutrition results in apathy, depression and self-neglect
- *Impairment of immune response:* predisposition to infection.

Screening and diagnosis of malnutrition

Early identification of patients requiring nutritional support is necessary. Following recent guidance from the National Institute for Health and Clinical Excellence (NICE), every institution needs to have pathways in place to assess all patients and to recognise those who require nutritional support. Body mass index ($BMI = weight/height^2$) is used to identify patients who are under- and overweight, but it does not give an indication of current nutritional status or the necessity for nutritional support. An isolated biochemical marker such as serum albumin is not useful, as this is a negative acute-phase protein and normally reduces with surgical stress. Changes in weight in the intensive care setting are largely due to changes in total body water and so do not reflect nutritional status. Tools such as the Malnutrition Universal Screening Tool (MUST) are more useful, as the score generated by this combines an estimation of BMI, recent weight loss and the effect of the pathological process on the nutritional intake of the patient.

METHODS OF FEEDING – ENTERAL VERSUS PARENTERAL FEEDING

Having decided that a patient requires nutritional support, a further decision is required about how to supply that support. Enteral feeding is the preferred choice whenever possible, using either oral supplements or formulated enteral feeds via feeding tubes. For these, the patient must have a functioning gut. In patients with a non-functioning or inaccessible gut, who need parenteral nutrition, every attempt needs to be made to move on to enteral feeding as soon as possible. Enteral feeding is associated with fewer septic complications, a reduction in gut mucosal atrophy with an improvement of gut barrier function through the direct contact of nutrients (in particular, glutamine), and a lower risk of hepatic steatosis.

Enteral feeding

Indications and contraindications for enteral feeding
See Table 10.3.

Access for enteral tube feeding
The choice depends on the expected period of feeding, the clinical condition and the anatomy:

- *Nasogastric tubes:* easily passed on the ward for short-term feeding of patients with functioning gut but poor appetite and reduced ability to maintain oral intake. Fine-bore tubes are preferable but are more prone to blockage.
- *Nasojejunal tubes:* used for post-pyloric feeding in patients with impairment of gastric emptying but distal functioning gut in situations such as pancreatitis and pyloric stenosis. Best positioned endoscopically or radiologically.
- *Gastrostomy:* provides more permanent access for long-term enteral feeding. A percutaneous gastrostomy is placed either endoscopically (percutaneous endoscopic gastrostomy, PEG) or radiologically (radiologically inserted gastrostomy, RIG). A jejunal extension is available for patients with gastroparesis or significant reflux. Surgically inserted gastrostomies are reserved for patients in whom endoscopic or radiological placement has failed or is not possible.
- *Feeding jejunostomy:* usually placed surgically at laparotomy or, increasingly, laparoscopically.

Management of enteral feeding tubes
- Ensure proper positioning before commencing feed (pH testing, chest X-ray).
- The patient should be propped up when feeding in order to minimise aspiration.
- Start infusion with small (30 mL) hourly volumes and increase in increments of 20–30 mL every

Table 10.3 Indications and contraindications for enteral feeding

Indications	Contraindications
Unconscious	Basal skull fracture
Swallowing disorder	Non-functioning gut: intestinal obstruction, ileus
Debility, anorexia	Perforation
Upper gastrointestinal surgery	
Increased nutritional requirements with poor appetite	

Table 10.4 Complications of enteral tube feeding

Type	Complication
Insertion	Nasogastric: nasal damage, pharyngeal/oesophageal pouch perforation, bronchial intubation PEG/PEJ: bleeding, leakage, intestinal/colonic perforation
Displacement	Tube falls out, bronchial administration of feed
Reflux	Oesophagitis, aspiration
Feed intolerance	Nausea, bloating, pain, diarrhoea
Contamination	Bacterial
Metabolic	Refeeding syndrome, hyperglycaemia, fluid overload, electrolyte disturbance

PEG, percutaneous endoscopic gastrostomy; PEJ, percutaneous endoscopic jejunostomy.

4 h until target volume (75–100 mL) is reached. Allow a rest period of 4–8 h once feeding is established. Most patients require 25–30 kcal/kg/day.

- Flush tubes routinely before and after feeds in order to prevent clogging.

Complications of enteral tube feeding
See Table 10.4.

Parenteral nutrition

Parenteral nutrition refers to the administration of nutrients by the intravenous route. It is administered via a dedicated central or peripheral line and is used where there is a failure of gut function and the consequent intestinal failure has persisted for and is likely to do so for 5 days. Parenteral nutrition is invasive, expensive and associated with multiple potential complications. Careful consideration is therefore required when deciding to use it.

> ■ KEY POINT
> Parenteral nutrition is invasive, expensive and associated with multiple potential complications.

Indications and contraindications for parenteral feeding

Total parenteral nutrition (TPN) is required by patients who have a non-functioning gut and are not expected to resume oral intake for more than 5 days (Table 10.5).

Table 10.5 Indications and contraindications for parenteral feeding

Indications	Contraindications
Non-functioning gut: obstruction ileus, peritonitis	Functioning gut
Enterocutaneous fistula	
Short bowel syndrome	
Malabsorption	
Burns, severe trauma	

Access for parenteral feeding

- *Peripheral access:* full intravenous feeding can be given through a peripheral small catheter, changed every 48 h, or a long line to major veins via a peripheral vein. Normal intravenous nutrition solutions are not tolerated well by peripheral veins, resulting in early thrombophlebitis. More dilute solutions are used but, as a consequence, require larger volumes to provide the required number of calories as central TPN.
- *Central venous catheters:* catheters are placed in the internal jugular or subclavian veins using an aseptic Seldinger technique under ultrasound guidance. Internal jugular venous access has a lower risk of pneumothorax than subclavian access but is less suited to ambulatory patients. Tunnelled catheters need fluoroscopic guidance and are indicated for long-term nutrition (> 30 days).

Management of central venous catheters and feeding

- Ensure proper positioning before commencing feed (chest X-ray).
- Strict asepsis is essential when the catheter is handled and the catheter and infusions are changed. Many institutions employ staff who are trained specifically in, and dedicated to, central line handling.
- Use a dedicated central line if possible. If this is not practical, one lumen of a multi-lumen catheter should be devoted solely to feeding.
- Review biochemical parameters, fluid balance and nutritional requirements daily.
- Insulin may be required due to hyperglycaemia. However, consider a reduction in glucose content, as forced glucose utilisation may increase CO_2 production and promote lipogenesis.

Estimation of nutritional requirements

- Most surgical patients require 25–30 kcal/kg/day.
- Fats provide 9.3 kcal/g of energy, glucose 4.1 kcal/g and protein 4.1 kcal/g.
- Energy is supplied through the administration of carbohydrates (70%) and lipids (30%).

An excessive dependence on glucose as the energy source in critically ill patients can result in poor utilization due to insulin resistance. The CO_2 released during glucose metabolism increases the ventilatory effort to clear CO_2 in the critically ill patient and can result in respiratory failure. The excess glucose is converted in the liver to fatty acids by liponeogenesis. Relying solely on glucose may lead to deficiency of essential fatty acids. Therefore in the critically ill patient more than 50 per cent of energy needs should be from lipids.

A normal adult requires at least 50 g of protein per day (0.8 g/kg/24 h). Although the nitrogen content of individual amino acids varies, overall 6.25 g of protein produces 1 g of nitrogen. During periods of starvation it is muscle that provides the main labile pool of amino acid precursors for hepatic gluconeogenesis to meet cerebral energy requirements (about 100 g of glucose per day). For each gram of nitrogen that is excreted as a result of amino acid oxidation, 6.25 g of protein is lost, which is equivalent to 30–35 g in weight of skeletal muscle. A maintenance diet should supply a patient with approximately 0.15 g/kg/day of nitrogen and up to 0.2–0.3 g/kg/day for the depleted patient. The calorie-to-nitrogen ratio should be around 150 kcal to 1 g of nitrogen.

- Essential amino acid-enriched solutions are often used for renal failure patients and branched chain amino acids may be used in hepatic failure.
- Immune modulation regimes like glutamine have been used in the critically ill.

The respiratory quotient (RQ = CO_2 production divided by O_2 consumption) can be used to monitor adequacy of the support. An RQ of more than 1 suggests overfeeding and lipogenesis,

Table 10.6 Complications of parenteral feeding

Type	Complication
Catheter-related	Pneumothorax/haemothorax
	Vascular injury/arterial puncture
	Misplacement in contralateral subclavian or jugular veins, right atrium
	Thrombosis
	Air embolus
Contamination	Sepsis
Metabolic	Refeeding syndrome, hyperglycaemia, fluid overload, electrolyte disturbance, vitamin and mineral deficiencies, hepatic steatosis

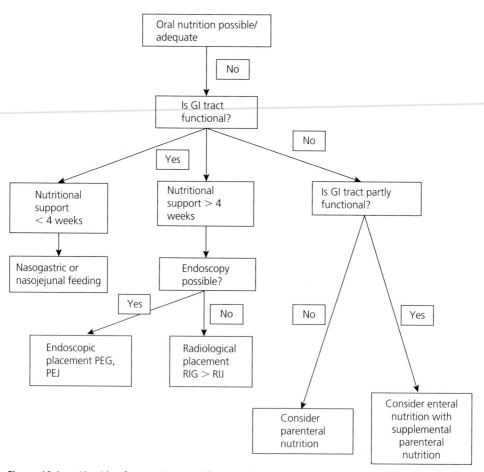

Figure 10.1 ● Algorithm for assessing need for enteral or parenteral nutrition.

GI, gastrointestinal; PEG, percutaneous endoscopic gastrostomy; PEJ, percutaneous endoscopic jejunostomy; RIG, radiologically inserted gastrostomy; RIJ, radiologically inserted jejunostomy.

while an RQ of 1 indicates pure carbohydrate utilization. Pure fat utilization produces an RQ of 0.7 and the value suggests underfeeding. Mixed substrate utilization, the desired goal, is suggested when the RQ is between 0.8 and 0.9.

Estimation of fluid and electrolyte requirements

- Fluid requirements are 30–35 mL/kg + 150 mL per 1 °C rise in temperature.
- All gastrointestinal losses should be measured and replaced with 0.9% normal saline with 20 mmol potassium added per 1 L.
- Sodium = 2 mmol/kg.
- Potassium = 1 mmol/kg.
- Chloride = 1 mmol/kg.
- Phosphate = 0.7 mmol/kg.
- Other electrolyte and micronutrient requirements should be assessed depending on the duration of support.

Trace elements

- *Zinc:* Daily requirement is 15 mg. The human body contains 1.5–3 g, predominantly in bones teeth and soft tissues. It is bound to albumin and globulin in circulation. It is a cofactor in more than 10 enzymes involved in protein and nucleic acid synthesis, and is required for tissue healing and immune function. Zinc deficiency manifests as apathy, depression, diarrhoea, skin rash and alopecia.
- *Selenium:* Daily requirement is 50–200 µg. It is absorbed from the duodenum and transported in the circulation bound to low and very low-density lipoproteins. It is used to synthesise selenoaminoacids, which are required for the synthesis of the antioxidant enzyme glutathione peroxidase and is also necessary for prostaglandin metabolism. Selenium levels fall rapidly in acutely ill surgical patients. Severe deficiency may give rise to cardiomyopathy, which may be reversible.
- *Copper:* Daily requirement is 203 mg. The body contains 150 mg. It is a cofactor in many enzymes such as cytochrome and super oxide dismutase. Copper is transported bound to albumin and incorporated into ceruloplasmin in the liver. Ceruloplasmin oxidises the ferrous to ferric ion to allow its transport by ferritin. Deficiency may result in hypochromic anaemia and defects in collagen synthesis.
- *Iron:* Daily requirement is 10–18 mg. The body contains up to 5 g, 65 per cent in haemoglobin, 30 per cent in the reticuloendothelial system as ferritin and 10 per cent in myoglobulin. It is transported in the circulation by transferrin or haemosiderin. It is a key component of enzymes and proteins involved in energy transfer and oxygen transport.

Complications of parenteral feeding

See Table 10.6.

Refeeding syndrome

Refeeding syndrome can occur on commencing enteral or parenteral nutrition. Too rapid or unbalanced nutrition support can create increased demands for electrolytes and micronutrients, resulting in micronutrient deficiencies and fluid electrolyte imbalance. Catabolism results in loss of intracellular electrolytes and phosphate. On reintroducing carbohydrate, there is an increase in insulin levels, which result in increased uptake of phosphate by the cells and shift of sodium and water out of the cells. This results in hypophosphataemia, hypokalaemia, hypomagnesaemia and occasionally hypocalcaemia. Initial symptoms may be vague but rhabdomyolysis, respiratory failure, cardiac failure, dysrhythmias, coma and sudden death can ensue.

Treatment involves infusion of 50 mmol of phosphate over 24 h and further monitoring of phosphate levels are required. Enteral and parenteral feeds should be commenced at half rate and only gradually increased if over the next 4 days there is no biochemical evidence of refeeding syndrome.

Multidisciplinary nutrition teams

Due to the complexity and specialist nature of nutrition, many hospitals now use a specialist multidisciplinary team consisting of dieticians, pharmacists, specialist nurses, gastroenterologists and surgeons to review the issues and advise on nutrition for patients who require additional nutritional support.

Algorithm for assessing need for enteral or parenteral nutrition

See Figure 10.1

● SUMMARY

A fistula is an abnormal communication between two epithelial surfaces. Fistulae are infrequent but are associated with significant morbidity and mortality. The aims of fistula management are to treat any associated sepsis, replace fluid and electrolyte losses, and optimise conditions to allow spontaneous or surgical closure.

A stoma is a surgically created opening of the bowel or urinary tract on to the abdominal wall. It may be temporary or permanent and is utilised when intestinal continuity cannot be re-established or when there would be significant risk of leakage of an anastomosis. Alternatively, it can be used to divert the faecal stream as part of a treatment plan for distal pathology. It should be borne in mind that they are not without complications and reversal can be associated with morbidity and mortality. A stoma nurse should always be involved in the management of stomas to aid patients with the many practical and psychological issues that accompany them.

Malnutrition is rife among surgical patients and requires aggressive identification and management. Whenever feasible, enteral nutrition is the preferred choice with parenteral nutrition reserved for situations when the gastrointestinal tract is non-functioning or not accessible. A multidisciplinary team is now a pre-requisite to review the issues and advise on nutrition for patients who require additional nutritional support.

● QUESTIONS

1 What is the definition of a fistula?
2 Outline the principles of management of a fistula (remember SNAPP).
3 If a fistula fails to heal spontaneously, when and how should it be repaired?
4 What is the definition of a stoma?
5 When would you create a stoma?
6 What complications can occur with a stoma?
7 What is malnutrition?
8 How would you identify a patient who is malnourished or who is at risk of malnutrition?
9 When would you recommend enteral nutrition?
10 When would you recommend parenteral nutrition?
11 What is refeeding syndrome and how would you avoid it?
12 How would you work out a patient's requirements for a prescription for TPN?

● FURTHER READING

Brent A (2006). Information websites for patients with stomas. *Ann R Coll Surg Eng* **88**: 82–3.

Department of Surgical Education, Orlando Regional Medical Center (2005). Octreotide in the prevention and management of gastrointestinal and pancreatic fistulas. www.surgicalcriticalcare.net/guidelines/octreotide.pdf.

Hearing SD (2004). Refeeding syndrome. *Br Med J* **328**: 908–9.

Lloyd DAJ, Gabe SM, Windsor ACJ (2006). Nutrition and management of enterocutaneous fistula. *Br J Surg* **93**: 1045–55.

Malnutrition Advisory Group (2004). Malnutrition Universal Screening Tool. www.bapen.org.uk/pdfs/must/must_full.pdf.

Saunders RN, Hemingway D (2005). Intestinal stomas. *Surgery* **23**: 369–72.

11 Management of surgical jaundice

Amer Aldouri, Hassan Malik and Peter Lodge

● INTRODUCTION

Jaundice is a condition characterised by yellow discoloration of the skin, sclera and mucous membranes due to excessive deposition of bilirubin. The discoloration is detected clinically once the serum bilirubin level rises above 50 μmol/L.

Yellow discoloration of the sclera and oral mucous membranes may be detected during examination of patients complaining of jaundice or symptoms such as abdominal pain, weight loss or fever. To differentiate between jaundice and other conditions that cause yellow discoloration of skin (e.g. excessive consumption of vegetables high in beta-carotene or medication such as rifampicin), the sclera and oral mucous membranes should be inspected in natural light, since only jaundice causes such discoloration.

Guidelines from the American Gastroenterological Association stress that it is nearly always possible to differentiate between conjugated and unconjugated hyperbilirubinaemia on clinical grounds alone: conjugated hyperbilirubinaemia is associated with dark urine and pale faeces, while unconjugated hyperbilirubinaemia tends not to be (Frank, 1989).

Blood biochemistry confirms the presence of jaundice by revealing elevated serum bilirubin and helps to differentiate predominantly conjugated (direct) hyperbilirubinaemia from predominantly unconjugated (indirect) hyperbilirubinaemia on the basis of their behaviour in the van den Bergh (diazo) reaction.

Unconjugated hyperbilirubinaemia may arise from:

- increased bilirubin production (haemolysis, reabsorption of large haematoma);
- decreased hepatic uptake or conjugation as in Gilbert's syndrome (a common genetic defect in the UDP-glucuronyl transferase gene, where patients report yellow discoloration of their skin during stress, e.g. exercise or fasting, with spontaneous resolution).

Conjugated hyperbilirubinaemia usually arises when the liver has lost at least 50 per cent of its excretory capacity as a consequence of hepatocellular damage (hepatic jaundice) or obstruction of biliary ductal system (obstructive jaundice). The latter could arise from several causes (Table 11.1).

In this chapter we discuss the management of patients with obstructive jaundice, which is traditionally most relevant to the general surgeon.

Table 11.1 Causes of obstructive jaundice

Common	Infrequent	Rare
Choledocholithiasis	Ampullary carcinoma	Benign strictures – iatrogenic (e.g. following cholecystectomy), trauma
Carcinoma of the head of pancreas	Chronic pancreatitis	Recurrent cholangitis
Malignant porta hepatis lymph nodes	Hepatic metastatic tumours	Mirrizi's syndrome
		Sclerosing cholangitis
		Cholangiocarcinoma
		Biliary atresia
		Choledochal cysts
		Parasitic infection

Table 11.2 History-taking in patients with conjugated jaundice

Pain	Severe pain suggests obstructive jaundice (malignancy or gallstone); upper abdominal discomfort is usually associated with hepatitis
Weight loss	Suggests obstructive jaundice (malignancy)
Pruritus	Suggests obstructive jaundice (malignancy or gallstone)
Medications	Common medications associated with cholestatic jaundice include chlorpromazine, ciprofloxacin, phenytoin, erythromycin, cloxacillin, amoxicillin–clavulanic acid, cimetidine, oestrogen, enalapril and captopril
Transfusions/injections	Suggests hepatitis
Contacts	Contact with jaundiced patient suggests hepatitis
Alcohol intake	Suggests liver cirrhosis

● DIAGNOSIS

It is essential to differentiate between hepatic and obstructive jaundice in order to initiate appropriate management. History (Table 11.2), physical examination and blood biochemistry are reliable tools that help to distinguish between these two causes of conjugated hyperbilirubinaemia (Figure 11.1).

Hepatic jaundice may be associated with:

- history of excessive alcohol consumption or presenting acutely with low-grade fever, abdominal pain and flu-like symptoms (acute hepatitis);
- stigmata of liver disease encountered during physical examination (palmer erythema, Dupuytren's contracture, chest wall spider angioma, gynaecomastia);
- signs of portal hypertension (mental changes, flapping tremor, caput medusa, ascites, splenomegaly).

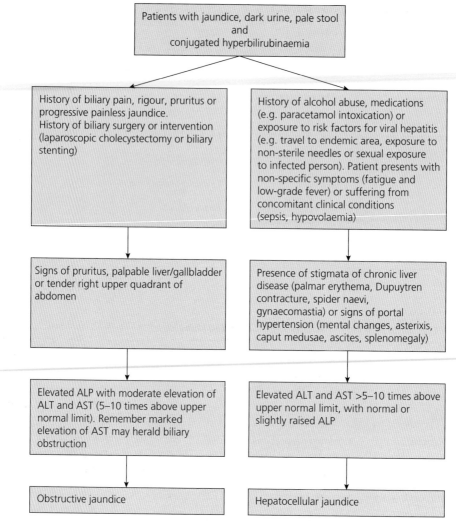

Figure 11.1 ● Suggested diagnostic algorithm for patient presenting with conjugated hyperbilirubinaemia.

ALP, alkaline phosphatase; ALT, alanine aminotransferase; AST, aspartate aminotransferase.

It is often the pattern of liver enzyme alteration on blood biochemistry, however, that helps to distinguish hepatic from obstructive jaundice.

Full assessment involves identification of the predominant pattern of liver enzyme abnormalities, the magnitude of the enzyme alterations, and the nature and rate of enzyme alteration:

● Slightly elevated conjugated serum bilirubin (< 35 μmol/L), with markedly elevated aspartate aminotransferase (AST) and alanine aminotransferase (ALT) levels, and a mild abnormality of alkaline phosphatase (ALP) and γ-glutamyl transpeptidase (GGT), are suggestive of hepatocellular jaundice, as injury to hepatocytes results in elevation of both AST and ALT.

- Altered liver enzymes with a predominantly elevated ALP and a mild raise in ALT are suggestive of obstructive jaundice.

It is important to remember that an atypical obstructive enzyme pattern could be due to a cholestatic drug reaction (including commonly used drugs, e.g. angiotensin-converting enzyme inhibitors or oestrogens) and may also occur in autoimmune cholestatic diseases (primary biliary cirrhosis, primary sclerosing cholangitis).

IMAGING FOR PATIENTS WITH SUSPECTED OBSTRUCTIVE JAUNDICE

Imaging is a mandatory step in the management of obstructive jaundice. Imaging:

- confirms the presence of obstructive jaundice;
- determines the level and the cause of obstruction;
- may be necessary in order to stage the disease if the cause is malignancy.

A transabdominal ultrasound scan is the first imaging test usually performed in patients in whom the clinical and biochemical tests suggest obstructive jaundice. This scan is an inexpensive, non-invasive and widely available test, but it is operator-dependent and is affected by the patient's body habitus.

Transabdominal ultrasound scanning can detect common bile duct (CBD) dilation greater than 7 mm (> 10 mm in patients who have undergone cholecystectomy) with an accuracy of 95 per cent. The reliability of transabdominal ultrasound in detecting CBD stones varies between 23 per cent and 80 per cent; however, the findings of dilated CBD and small stones in the gallbladder are highly suggestive of CBD stones.

Transabdominal ultrasound scanning is reliable in detecting hepatic lesions, with a sensitivity of 94 per cent for lesions larger than 20 mm and of 56 per cent for lesions smaller than 10 mm.

In clinical practice we request ultrasound scanning to confirm the diagnosis of obstructive jaundice (dilated biliary tree) and to detect gallstones. If ultrasound scanning does not reveal bile duct dilation, then the diagnosis of obstructive jaundice is unlikely, except in the following cases:

- Early ultrasound test, when the pressure inside the CBD is not high enough to cause dilation
- Failure of the ducts to dilate, e.g. in primary sclerosing cholangitis (PSC) or cirrhosis
- Intermittent obstruction (CBD stone, ampullary tumour).

In order to exclude these exceptional situations, further imaging tests can be carried out, such as magnetic resonance cholangiopancreatography (MRCP), spiral computed tomography (CT) scanning, endoscopic ultrasound (EUS), endoscopic retrograde cholangiopancreatography (ERCP), percutaneous transhepatic cholangiography (PTC) and hydroxy-imino-diacetic acid (HIDA) scanning.

Magnetic resonance cholangiopancreatography

This non-invasive test is usually combined with magnetic resonance imaging (MRI) to detect tumour masses. It can detect 95 per cent of CBD stones with a specificity of 89 per cent. It demonstrates benign and malignant biliary, hepatic and pancreatic lesions.

Spiral computed tomography

In cases where the diagnosis of CBD stones is unlikely (when ultrasound does not reveal gallstones or the patient suffers from backache, anorexia or weight loss), spiral CT is the next imaging test used to visualise the pancreas, as pancreatic cancer is the second most common cause of obstructive jaundice after CBD stones.

Spiral CT with thin-slice images of 1.25 mm (pancreatic protocol) can detect 90 per cent of pancreatic lesions larger than 20 mm (60 per cent for smaller lesions). Fine-needle aspiration cytology (FNAC) can be obtained under CT guidance. Spiral CT has 95 per cent accuracy in determining:

- superior mesenteric artery encasement;
- extensive superior mesenteric and portal vein involvement;
- extensive lymph node infiltration;
- liver metastases.

Endoscopic ultrasound

In cases of lower CBD obstruction with no obvious cause on spiral CT, EUS is useful. Endoscopic ultrasound may detect and stage small pancreatic lesions and peri-ampullary tumours, and it provides a safe route for biopsy.

Endoscopic retrograde cholangiopancreatography

The gold standard in CBD imaging remains ERCP. This identifies the presence, level and nature of biliary obstruction. It also offers therapeutic options. With sphincterotomy, ERCP achieves up to 95 per cent clearance of CBD stones; in the remaining 5 per cent ERCP allows insertion of a nasobiliary tube or stent in order to decompress the CBD and prevent stone impaction of the distal CBD. Correction of coagulopathy and the use of prophylactic antibiotics are necessary.

> ■ KEY POINT
> The gold standard in CBD imaging remains ERCP.

Endoscopic retrograde cholangiopancreatography is associated with mortality of 1 per cent (Christensen *et al.*, 2004) and a 10 per cent risk of complications (Choudari *et al.*, 2000), including:

- pancreatitis (5% in diagnostic ERCP, 10% in therapeutic ERCP);
- haemorrhage (5%);
- cholangitis (1%);
- retroperitoneal duodenal perforation (1.3%).

The authors believe that ERCP is an option when therapeutic measures are required, as in the case of acute cholangitis or worsening and severe obstructive jaundice.

Percutaneous transhepatic cholangiography

Percutaneous transhepatic cholangiography is another investigation that provides direct cholangiography, but it is associated with a 4 per cent risk of haemorrhage, bile leak and cholangitis. It is of use as a therapeutic manoeuvre for relief of jaundice in high biliary obstruction and is preferred to ERCP in some centres. Both ERCP and PTC can be used to provide access for direct visualisation by cholangioscopy, but this is not currently available except in specialised centres.

Hydroxy-imino-diacetic acid scanning

This is a radioisotope scan in which technetium-labelled HIDA is excreted in the bile after intravenous injection. Generally, HIDA scanning is used to demonstrate patency of the biliary

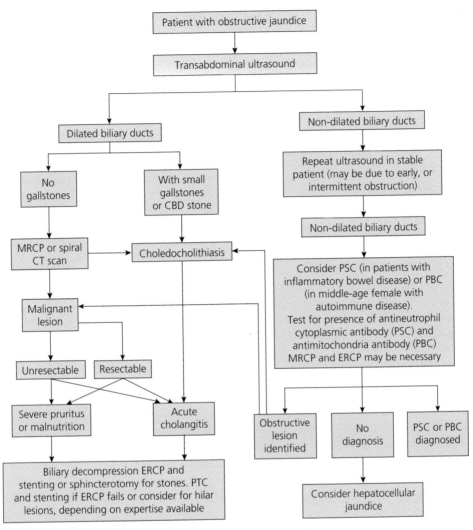

Figure 11.2 ● Imaging algorithm for patients with obstructive jaundice.

CBD, common bile duct; CT, computed tomography; ERCP, endoscopic retrograde cholangiopancreatography; MRCP, magnetic resonance cholangiopancreatography; PBC, primary biliary cirrhosis; PSC, primary sclerosing cholangitis; PTC, percutaneous transhepatic cholangiography.

tree or biliary anastomosis. In investigating a patient with obstructive jaundice, HIDA scanning can be helpful to demonstrate the obstruction, providing that the bilirubin level is less than 100 µmol/L. In severe jaundice the isotope is not excreted in the bile.

To summarise, in clinical practice the first-line imaging test in investigating a patient with obstructive jaundice is ultrasound, with second-line imaging tests being MRCP with MRI, spiral CT scan, ERCP, PTC, EUS and HIDA scanning (Figure 11.2). Although in our practice we prefer MRCP, the choice of second-line imaging modality is often determined by the local expertise available in each centre. Cholangioscopy provides an unparalleled level of visualisation and is likely to be more readily available in the future.

MANAGEMENT OF CHOLEDOCHOLITHIASIS

If ultrasound reveals CBD dilation with small gallstones in the gallbladder or identifies stones in CBD, then the diagnosis of choledocholithiasis is made. The need for further imaging tests will depend on four factors:

- Presence of sepsis (rigors and swinging fever indicates acute cholangitis)
- Severity of obstructive jaundice (serum bilirubin level > 90 μmol/L)
- Presence of progressive obstructive jaundice
- High-risk patient for laparoscopic cholecystectomy.

If one of these factors is present, then urgent biliary decompression (ERCP with endoscopic sphincterotomy and stone removal or biliary stent) should be performed following patient resuscitation, antibiotic administration and correction of coagulopathy by intravenous administration of vitamin K.

Choledocholithiasis is the most common cause of obstructive jaundice. These stones usually originate in the gallbladder and migrate to the CBD (secondary choledocholithiasis). Primary choledocholithiasis originates in the bile duct in association with impaired bile duct motility, ampullary stenosis and peri-ampullary diverticulum. Studies suggest that 73 per cent of choledocholithiasis pass spontaneously to the duodenum; however, patients with obstructive jaundice or cholangitis are less likely to pass stones spontaneously.

> ■ KEY POINT
> Choledocholithiasis is the most common cause of obstructive jaundice.

Csendes and colleagues (1996) demonstrated that 58 per cent of people with asymptomatic choledocholithiasis had a positive bile culture, and those with cholangitis mainly cultured aerobic Gram-negative bacilli (*Escherichia coli, Klebsiella, Pseudomonas*), enterococci and anaerobes. Proliferation of these microorganisms in an obstructed biliary system makes it a potentially life-threatening condition, as the increasing hydrostatic pressure in the biliary tree leads to cholangiovenous reflux of bacteria and its toxic products to the venous circulation, resulting in the stimulation of an immune response that is responsible for multiple organ dysfunction.

Initial resuscitation of a patient with acute cholangitis includes:

- adequate oxygen delivery;
- fluid replacement, with monitoring of urine output and central venous pressure;
- administration of the appropriate antibiotics.

Piperacillin has been shown to be as effective as the combination of ampicillin and aminoglycoside (tobramycin) in improving the outcome of 70 per cent of patients with acute cholangitis (Thompson *et al.*, 1990). The addition of the β-lactamase inhibitor tazobactam increases the spectrum of piperacillin activity.

Other investigators have demonstrated that intravenous ciprofloxacin alone is as effective as triple therapy (ampicillin, ceftazidime, metronidazole) and resulted in improvement of outcomes in 85 per cent of the 46 patients treated with ciprofloxacin (Sung *et al.*, 1995).

Biliary decompression is essential in order to control the sepsis and to treat the cause of the jaundice. Endoscopic retrograde cholangiopancreatography with endoscopic sphincterotomy has been shown to be associated with lower mortality and fewer complications compared with emergency surgical decompression. Lai and colleagues (1992) randomised 82 patients with severe acute cholangitis due to choledocholithiasis into endoscopic biliary drainage (41 patients) or surgical decompression of the biliary tract (41 patients), followed by definitive treatment. The mortality among those who underwent endoscopic decompression was 10 per cent compared with 32 per cent in those treated with surgical drainage. Complications were significantly lower among the endoscopic group (34 per cent) than the surgical group (66 per cent). Based on this evidence, ERCP with endoscopic sphincterotomy is the treatment of choice in patents with acute cholangitis.

> ■ KEY POINT
> ERCP with endoscopic sphincterotomy is the treatment of choice in patients with acute cholangitis.

If ERCP is unsuccessful, unavailable or not feasible (e.g. in patients who have had previous gastric surgery with duodenal exclusion or disconnection), then PTC should be performed.

Then definitive treatment (cholecystectomy for secondary choledocholithiasis; choledocho-jejunostomy for primary choledocholithiasis) should be performed in fit patients.

Patients with choledocholithiasis who have no signs of sepsis or severe or progressive jaundice, and who are suitable for laparoscopic cholecystectomy, should be listed for laparoscopic cholecystectomy with either preoperative ERCP or intraoperative cholangiography. Preoperative ERCP has the advantage of clearing the CBD in 95 per cent of cases and decompression of the CBD with stent insertion in the remaining 5 per cent; however, it is associated with mortality of 1 per cent and morbidity of 10 per cent. Alternatively, perioperative cholangiography may reveal choledocholithiasis, which can be removed by laparoscopic trans-cystic CBD exploration with success rates of up to 70 per cent; in unsuccessful cases, laparoscopic choledochotomy can be performed (if the CBD diameter is > 10 mm). Conversion to open choledochotomy should be considered if the laparoscopic choledochotomy was unsuccessful and in the presence of multiple or large impacted CBD stones. Open choledochotomy is also indicated when ERCP is unsuccessful, unavailable or not feasible. There is ongoing debate regarding the best management for choledocholithiasis; however, the choice between preoperative ERCP or intraoperative cholangiography with laparoscopic exploration of CBD depends on local facilities and expertise.

● MANAGEMENT OF JAUNDICED PATIENTS WITH PANCREATIC CANCER

If ultrasound fails to demonstrate gallstones, or there is a suspicion that a concomitant obstructive lesion coexists with gallstones (a patient with progressive jaundice and vague epigastric pain, weight loss or anorexia), then further detailed imaging should be carried out in order to exclude a malignant lesion and to assess the resectability if such a lesion is identified. The second most common cause of obstructive jaundice is pancreatic cancer, which is best detected and staged using spiral CT. Magnetic resonance cholangiopancreatography with MRI of the pancreas is also useful in detecting and assessing the resectability of pancreatic tumours, but again this depends on local expertise. If spiral CT or MRI findings are inconclusive, then EUS is helpful in detecting small lesions. Furthermore, EUS allows FNAC or biopsy for tissue diagnosis. Preoperative tissue diagnosis may help to avoid resection of benign lesions, which are encountered in 10 per cent of cases, but negative cytology does not exclude malignancy, due to the sclerotic nature of pancreatic adenocarcinoma. Although spiral CT has 95 per cent accuracy in detecting unresectable lesions, studies demonstrate that nearly a third of resectable lesions on spiral CT are found to be unresectable at the time of resection. This emphasises the need for staging laparoscopy, which can be useful in detecting peritoneal carcinomatosis, ascites, liver metastases and lymph node infiltration before resection. Centres favouring open operative palliative procedures continue to question the impact of laparoscopic staging, but laparoscopic palliative manoeuvres such as gastroenterostomy and biliary diversion procedures are increasingly being done in specialised units.

> ■ KEY POINT
> The second most common cause of obstructive jaundice is pancreatic cancer.

If preoperative assessment reveals a resectable lesion (20% of all pancreatic cancer cases), then:

- the patient should be evaluated for cardiovascular and pulmonary fitness, with a view to major resection;
- dehydration should be corrected, with monitoring of urine output and central venous pressure;
- any coagulation abnormality should be corrected preoperatively with vitamin K.

Preoperative biliary decompression remains controversial: there is little evidence that relief of jaundice is helpful except in severe cases, and both ERCP and PTC introduce a risk of biliary sepsis. Many authors reserve biliary decompression for patients with acute cholangitis or deteriorating renal function.

Surgery for carcinoma of the head of the pancreas involves a pancreaticoduodenectomy, Whipple's operation (Figure 11.3).

The need for vascular resection is a relative contraindication to surgery, but there is increasing experience with portal vein resection and reconstruction with autologous vein.

There appears to be no benefit in carrying out more than a regional lymphadenectomy.

In a study, adjuvant chemoradiotherapy (after resection) in pancreatic adenocarcinoma based on 5-fluorouracil, adriamycin and mitomycin C showed better median survival (20 months v. 11 months) compared with the surgery group (Gastrointestinal Tumor Study Group, 1987).

In patients with unresectable pancreatic cancer (80% of all pancreatic cancer), obstructive jaundice may require biliary decompression if sepsis, pruritus or progressive malnutrition interferes with the quality of life:

- ERCP and stenting is the treatment of choice for patients with lower CBD obstruction.
- PTC with stenting is preserved for unsuccessful cases and patients with higher biliary lesions.

For patients with advanced malignancy and longer life expectancy (> 6 months), surgical biliary drainage by Roux-en-Y choledochojejunostomy is indicated and provides longer biliary

Figure 11.3 ● Whipple's operation.

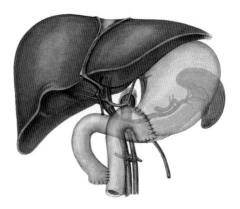

patency. Studies have demonstrated that both stenting and surgical bypass are equally effective in the relief of obstruction. Although stenting is associated with lower short-term morbidity and a shorter initial hospital stay, long-term biliary patency is higher in patients who undergo surgical bypass. Patients found to have unresectable tumour on laparotomy should have chole-dochojejunostomy and gastrojejunostomy performed, as evidence suggests that 20 per cent of patients will develop gastric outlet obstruction.

● MANAGEMENT OF JAUNDICED PATIENTS WITH CHOLANGIOCARCINOMA

Cholangiocarcinoma is an uncommon cause of obstructive jaundice, with an incidence of 1.7 per 100 000 population in Western countries. In two-thirds of cases it arises at the hilar confluence of the hepatic ducts (Klatskin tumour), while in nearly a third of cases it arises in the lower CBD; 6 per cent arise from the intrahepatic ducts.

Cholangiocarcinoma should be suspected in the following:

- Patients known to have PSC (up to 36% develop cholangiocarcinoma)
- Patients known to have choledochal cyst (up to 30% develop cholangiocarcinoma)
- Patients who have had a previous biliary-enteric drainage
- Patients living in South-East Asia (*Opisthorchis viverrini, Clonorchis sinensis*).

Imaging is usually by MRCP with MRI in combination with magnetic resonance angiography (MRA), as this allows assessment of both the biliary stricture and the involvement of the hepatic artery and portal vein. Magnetic resonance cholangiopancreatography has been shown to be superior to ERCP as a diagnostic procedure for cholangiocarcinoma (Yeh *et al.*, 2000). If MRCP is not available, then spiral CT is useful.

Tissue diagnosis is not usually obtained before surgery, because of the dangers of liver biopsy in the presence of dilated ducts and the risk of tumour spillage.

Preoperative biliary decompression by ERCP or PTC drainage remains controversial, because of the risk of introducing biliary sepsis, but jaundice is a major risk factor for perioperative mortality following major liver resection.

Assessment of resectability depends on:

- involvement of the hepatic ducts and hepatic vasculature;
- extent of lymph node infiltration;
- the individual hepatic reserve.

In patients with a potentially resectable tumour:

- Evaluation of cardiovascular and pulmonary function should be performed in order to assess the patient's fitness for such major resection.
- The patient should receive nutritional support.
- Correction of any coagulopathy is mandatory.

Hilar cholangiocarcinoma (Klatskin tumour) is suitable for radical resection at presentation. This involves:

- hepatectomy, including segment 1 (Figure 11.4);
- resection of the portal vein or hepatic artery (if invaded by tumour);
- lymphadenectomy (regional and para-aortic);
- Roux-en-Y hepaticojejunostomy.

There is debate regarding the extent of lymphadenectomy. Proponents of a radical lymphadenectomy, from the coeliac axis to the inferior mesenteric artery, have been successful in

Figure 11.4 ● Liver segments.

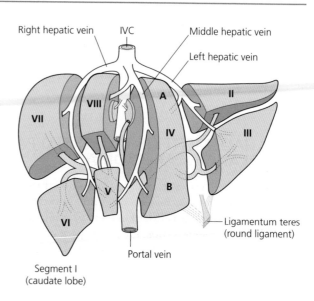

Segment I
(caudate lobe)

achieving negative resection margins in 50 per cent of patients, with 5-year survival of 45 per cent for R0 resection.

Among patients undergoing a laparotomy and who are unresectable, surgical bypass should be considered. This may involve a segment 3 bypass, with the duct being accessed by dividing the liver just to the left of umbilical ligament, but ERCP or PTC-directed biliary stenting may offer similar palliation.

Cholangiocarcinoma of the common hepatic duct or CBD may be treated by bile duct excision and reconstruction by Roux-en-Y hepaticojejunostomy. The role of caudate lobectomy (segment 1 resection) and lymphadenectomy is determined by preoperative and intraoperative findings.

For lower CBD tumours, pancreaticoduodenectomy may be necessary in some patients. If the tumour extends from the lower CBD up to the hilum, then a combined approach of liver resection with bile duct excision, pancreaticoduodenectomy and lymphadenectomy may be considered.

Intrahepatic cholangiocarcinoma requires liver resection, and there is little evidence to support a role for lymphadenectomy in this small group of patients.

Unfortunately, most patients with cholangiocarcinoma are not suitable for curative resection. Biliary decompression is indicated to prevent or treat cholangitis and severe intractable pruritus and to obtain tissue diagnosis. Endoscopic retrograde cholangiopancreatography or PTC and stenting can relieve the obstruction. Metallic stents are associated with a 1-year patency rate of 46 per cent (superior to conventional plastic stents). Endoscopic retrograde cholangiopancreatography and stenting is considered to be less invasive than PTC and, when possible, should be the first choice. The palliative use of radiotherapy and photodynamic therapy remains uncertain.

● SUMMARY

Obstructive jaundice is a common problem that the majority of general surgeons will have to deal with in their careers. The majority of patients with obstructive jaundice will have choledocholithiasis, and the clinician should have a clear algorithm based on local expertise to deal with such patients. Patients with a malignant cause of obstructive jaundice require the facilities that a tertiary referral hepato-pancreato-biliary (HPB) centre has to offer. However, the clinician has an important role in facilitating initial investigations and management of the acutely jaundiced patient.

● QUESTIONS

1 What is the role of ERCP in the management of CBD stone?
2 What are the indications of CBD decompression in patient with pancreatic adenocarcinoma?
3 Describe the palliative management of a patient with advanced Klatskin tumour.

● REFERENCES

Choudari CP, Sherman S, Fogel EL, *et al*. (2000). Success of ERCP at a referral center after a previously unsuccessful attempt. *Gastrointest Endosc* **52**: 478–83.

Christensen M, Matzen P, Schulze S, Rosenberg J (2004). Complications of ERCP: a prospective study. *Gastrointest Endosc* **60**: 721–31.

Csendes A, Burdiles P, Maluenda F, *et al*. (1996). Simultaneous bacteriologic assessment of bile from gallbladder and common bile duct in control subjects and patients with gallstones and common duct stones. *Arch Surg* **131**: 389–94.

Frank BB (1989). Clinical evaluation of jaundice: a guideline of the Patient Care Committee of the American Gastroenterological Association. *J Am Med Assoc* **262**: 3031–4.

Gastrointestinal Tumor Study Group (1987). Further evidence of effective adjuvant combined radiation and chemotherapy following curative resection of pancreatic cancer. *Cancer* **59**: 2006–10.

Lai EC, Mok FP, Tan ES, *et al*. (1992). Endoscopic biliary drainage for severe acute cholangitis. *N Engl J Med* **326**: 1582–6.

Sung JJ, Lyon DJ, Suen R, *et al*. (1995). Intravenous ciprofloxacin as treatment for patients with acute suppurative cholangitis: a randomised, controlled clinical trial. *J Antimicrob Chemother* **35**: 855–64.

Thompson JE, Jr, Pitt HA, Doty JE, Coleman J, Irving C (1990). Broad spectrum penicillin as an adequate therapy for acute cholangitis. *Surg Gynecol Obstet* **171**: 275–82.

Yeh TS, Jan YY, Tseng JH, *et al*. (2000). Malignant perihilar biliary obstruction: magnetic resonance cholangiopancreatographic findings. *Am J Gastroenterol* **95**: 432–40.

Upper gastrointestinal bleeding

Basil J Ammori and Saleh Baghdadi

- Introduction
- Symptoms, causes and diagnosis
- Recommendations for management of patients with non-variceal upper gastrointestinal bleeding (peptic ulcer disease)
- Management of other causes of non-variceal upper gastrointestinal bleeding
- Recommendations for the management of patients with variceal upper gastrointestinal bleeding
- Summary
- Questions
- References

INTRODUCTION

Acute upper gastrointestinal bleeding (UGIB) refers to acute bleeding derived from a source proximal to the ligament of Treitz (duodenojejunal flexure) and has an incidence of 50–150 per 100 000 population each year. Bleeding from the upper gastrointestinal tract is approximately four times more common than bleeding from the lower gastrointestinal tract (Fallah *et al.*, 2000).

SYMPTOMS, CAUSES AND DIAGNOSIS

A cause for UGIB is found in approximately 80 per cent of cases. The underlying causes and their potential frequencies are listed in Table 12.1 (Rockall *et al.*, 1995). The incidence of presenting symptoms in patients with UGIB from the USA is shown in Table 12.2 (Peter and Dougherty, 1999). Most deaths occur in elderly patients who have significant comorbidity.

Our recommendations for the management of patients with UGIB are based on the recommendations issued by the British Society of Gastroenterology Endoscopy Committee (Palmer, 2002), the British Society of Gastroenterology (Jalan and Hayes, 2000), the Canadian Association of Gastroenterology (Barkun *et al.*, 2003) and the French recommendations (Thabut and Bernard-Chabert, 2007).

We review non-variceal haemorrhage (the most common type of UGIB, and most commonly caused by peptic ulcer) and then variceal haemorrhage.

> ■ KEY POINT
> Most deaths occur in elderly patients who have significant comorbidity.

Laboratory tests

- Haemoglobin (Hb) value and blood type and cross-match of 2–6 units of blood should be ordered immediately.
- A marked elevation of blood urea level in the presence of normal creatinine in a patient without renal dysfunction is suggestive of UGIB.
- A coagulopathy and thrombocytopenia may be secondary to massive blood loss or could reflect existing liver disease and possible variceal bleeding. Prolongation of prothrombin time (PT) with an international normalisation ratio (INR) of more than 1.5 may indicate moderate liver impairment.

Table 12.1 Causes of acute upper gastrointestinal bleeding

Diagnosis	Incidence (%)
Peptic ulcer	35–50
Gastric erosions, duodenitis	8–15
Oesophagitis	5–15
Varices	5–10
Mallory–Weiss tear	5
Upper gastrointestinal malignancy	1
Vascular malformations	5
Rare	5

Based on Rockall *et al.* (1995) and Stabile and Stamos (2000).

Table 12.2 Presentations of upper gastrointestinal bleeding

Symptom	Incidence (%)
Haematemesis	40–50
Melaena	70–80
Haematochezia	15–20
Either haematochezia or melaena	90–98
Syncope	14.4
Dyspepsia	18
Epigastric pain	41
Heartburn	21
Diffuse abdominal pain	10
Dysphagia	5
Weight loss	12
Jaundice	5.2

Based on Peter and Dougherty (1999).

A platelet count of less than 50 with active bleeding requires platelet transfusion and fresh frozen plasma in an attempt to replete the lost clotting factors. A fibrinogen level of less than 100 mg/dL indicates advanced liver disease with extremely poor synthetic function.

● Liver function tests as well as PT are needed to calculate the Child–Pugh score (Table 12.3) (Corson and Williamson, 2001).

Endoscopy

Endoscopy should be performed within 24 h to discover whether the bleeding is variceal (from an oesophageal or gastric varix) or not.

Table 12.3 Child–Pugh classification of severity of liver cirrhosis

Parameter	1 point	2 points	3 points
Bilirubin (mg/dL)	< 2	2–3	> 3
Albumin (g/dL)	> 3.5	2.8–3.5	< 2.8
Increase in PT (seconds over control)	1–3	4–6	> 6
Ascites	None	Slight	Moderate
Encephalopathy	None	Grade 1–2	Grade 3–4

Total score: 1–6, grade A; 7–9, grade B; 10–15, grade C.
PT, prothrombin time.
Based on Corson and Williamson (2001).

● RECOMMENDATIONS FOR MANAGEMENT OF PATIENTS WITH NON-VARICEAL UPPER GASTROINTESTINAL BLEEDING (PEPTIC ULCER DISEASE)

A management algorithm for non-variceal UGIB is shown in Figure 12.1 (Dallal and Palmer, 2001; Palmer, 2002).

Risk stratification

The Rockall scoring system for the independent risk factors for mortality from non-variceal UGI is given in Table 12.4 (Rockall *et al.*, 1996). A total score of less than 3 is associated with an excellent prognosis, while a score above 8 is associated with a high risk of death.

Table 12.4 Rockall scoring system for risk of rebleeding and death after admission to hospital for acute upper gastrointestinal bleeding

Variable	Score			
	0	1	2	3
Age (year)	< 60	60–79	≥ 80	
Shock	No shock (systolic BP > 100, pulse <100)	Tachycardia (systolic BP > 100, pulse < 100)	Hypotension (systolic BP < 100, pulse > 100)	
Comorbidity	Nil major		Cardiac failure, ischaemic heart disease, any major comorbidity	Renal failure, liver failure, disseminated malignancy
Diagnosis	Malloy–Weiss tear, no lesion, no SRH	All other diagnoses	Malignancy of upper GI tract	
Major SRH	None, or dark spot		Blood in upper GI tract, adherent clot, visible or spurting vessel	

BP, blood pressure; GI, gastrointestinal; SRH, stigmata of recent haemorrhage.
Each variable is scored and the total score calculated by simple addition.
Based on Rockall *et al.* (1996).

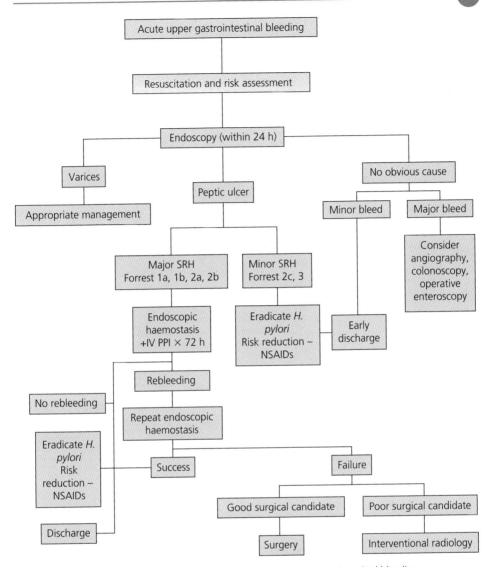

Figure 12.1 ● Algorithm for management of non-variceal upper gastrointestinal bleeding.

NSAID, non-steroidal anti-inflammatory drug; IV, intravenous; PPI, proton-pump inhibitor; SRH, stigmata of recent haemorrhage.

Resuscitation

Resuscitation should precede further diagnostic and therapeutic measures. Resuscitate and admit patients with severe bleeding and those with significant comorbidity or old age (> 60 years) to a high dependency unit (HDU).

Intravenous fluid replacement

A guide to the estimated blood loss and fluid replacement is given in Table 12.5.

Table 12.5 Estimated fluid and blood losses in shock

	Class 1	Class 2	Class 3	Class 4
Blood loss (mL)	≤ 750	750–1500	1500–2000	> 2000
Blood loss (% blood volume)	≤ 15	15–30	30–40	> 40
Pulse rate (beats/min)	< 100	> 100	> 120	> 140
Blood pressure	Normal	Normal	Decreased	Decreased
Pulse pressure	Normal or increased	Decreased	Decreased	Decreased
Respiratory rate	14–20	20–30	30–40	> 35
Urine output (mL/h)	> 30	20–30	10–20	< 10
Mental status	Slightly anxious	Mildly anxious	Anxious and confused	Confused and lethargic
Fluid replacement	Crystalloid	Crystalloid	Crystalloid and blood	Crystalloid and blood

Based on American College of Surgeons Committee on Trauma (1997).

Endoscopy

Endoscopy should be performed within 24 h. The risk of rebleeding and mortality based on endoscopic findings should be assessed, as shown in Table 12.6 (Forrest *et al.*, 1974; Laine and Peterson, 1994).

> ■ KEY POINT
> Endoscopy should be performed within 24 h and used to assess the risk of rebleeding and mortality.

Table 12.6 Forrest classification of stigmata of recent haemorrhage (SRH) from peptic ulcer and risk of rebleeding and mortality

Forrest classification of SRH	Risk of rebleeding (%)	Risk of mortality (%)
Ia Spurting bleeding	55	11
Ib Non-spurting active bleeding		
IIa Visible vessel (no active bleeding)	43	11
IIb Non-bleeding ulcer with overlying clot (no visible vessel)	22	7
IIc Ulcer with haematin-covered base	10	3
III Clean ulcer ground (no clot, no vessel)	5	2

Major SRH, Forrest Ia, Ib, IIa and IIb; minor SRH, Forrest IIc and III.
Based on Forrest *et al.* (1974) and Laine and Peterson (1994).

Endoscopic haemostasis

Endoscopic haemostasis has been shown to significantly reduce rebleeding rates, the need for surgery, and mortality when compared with drug or placebo treatment.

■ KEY POINT

Endoscopic haemostasis has been shown to significantly reduce rebleeding rates, the need for surgery, and mortality when compared with drug or placebo treatment.

The finding of a clot in an ulcer bed warrants targeted irrigation in an attempt to dislodge and treat the underlying lesion. The finding of high-risk endoscopic stigmata (active bleeding or visible vessel in an ulcer bed) is an indication of immediate endoscopic haemostatic therapy (Barkun *et al.*, 2003). Endoscopic therapies may include the following:

- *Injection of 1 : 10 000 adrenaline solution in normal saline in quadrants around the bleeding point, and then into the bleeding vessel, using a total of 4–16 mL*: this approach achieves primary haemostasis in up to 95 per cent of patients, although bleeding will recur in 15–20 per cent of these patients. There is little evidence that addition of other agents such as sclerosants (e.g. sodium tetradecyl sulphate STD, 1% polidocanol, 5% ethanolamine) reduces the rate of rebleeding. However, there is no consensus regarding the recommended dose or frequency of these substances. The injection of agents that directly stimulate clot formation, such as fibrin glue and thrombin, has been shown to be effective, but these agents are not freely available.
- *Thermal haemostasis with either heater probe or multipolar coagulation (bipolar current electrocoagulation, BICAP)*: this is as effective as adrenaline injection. The combination of injection and thermal coagulation is superior to either treatment alone (Barkun *et al.*, 2003). Laser therapy is no longer used because of its high cost and the poor portability of equipment.
- *Mechanical clips (Haemoclips®)*: these can be applied to bleeding points and are particularly useful for actively bleeding large vessels. They may be difficult to apply to awkwardly placed ulcers. Endoscopic clips are usually placed over a bleeding site (e.g. visible vessel) and left in place. Clips are currently available in two- and three-pronged configurations. They can be affixed to bleeding sites and typically slough off days to weeks after placement.

Management following endoscopy

Although routine second-look endoscopy is not recommended (Barkun *et al.*, 2003), repeat endoscopy should be considered if there is clinical evidence of active rebleeding, in order to endoscopically confirm and retreat rebleeding, and if there are concerns regarding optimal initial endoscopic therapy due to technical reasons such as excessive blood (consider re-endoscopy within 12–24 h) (Palmer, 2002).

■ KEY POINT

Although routine second-look endoscopy is not recommended, repeat endoscopy (within 12–24 h) should be considered if there is clinical evidence of active rebleeding and if there are technical concerns with regard to the initial endoscopic therapy.

Pharmacotherapy

An intravenous bolus followed by continuous infusion proton-pump inhibitor (PPI) is effective in decreasing rebleeding and mortality in patients who have undergone successful endoscopic therapy (Barkun *et al.*, 2003).

> ■ KEY POINT
> Intravenous bolus followed by continuous infusion PPI is effective in decreasing rebleeding and mortality in patients following successful endoscopic therapy.

There are no convincing data to support the use of H_2 receptor antagonists (Palmer, 2002). In patients awaiting endoscopy, empirical therapy with a high-dose PPI should be considered (Barkun *et al.*, 2003).

Somatostatin, octreotide and interleukin 2 receptor antagonists are not recommended in the routine management of patients with acute UGIB (Barkun *et al.*, 2003).

Surgery

Patients who continue to actively bleed after endoscopy require urgent surgery. Early surgical consultation in patients at high risk of rebleeding and for those who rebleed after endoscopic therapy is indicated. Timing of an operation should, if possible, avoid the hours between midnight and 7 a.m., as supportive medical services tend to have minimal staffing during this period.

> ■ KEY POINT
> Patients who continue to actively bleed after endoscopy require urgent surgery.

The indications for surgery in patients with bleeding peptic ulcers are:

- severe life-threatening haemorrhage not responsive to resuscitation;
- failure of medical therapy and endoscopic haemostasis with persistent recurrent bleeding;
- coexisting indication for surgery, such as perforation, obstruction or malignancy;
- prolonged bleeding with loss of 50 per cent of blood volume;
- second hospitalisation for peptic ulcer bleeding.

A bleeding duodenal ulcer should be under-run with specific ligation of the gastroduodenal and right gastroepiloic arteries. In the present era of PPI therapy, the addition of a vagotomy is unnecessary. Vagotomy with antrectomy is reserved for patients who rebleed after simple under-running of the duodenal ulcer and for those with other ulcer complications such as gastric outlet obstruction. Highly selective vagotomy with anatomical closure of the duodenostomy or the pyloroduodenostomy in order to preserve the normal pyloric sphincter muscle is an operation reserved for young, stable, low-risk patients with a low risk of recurrent ulcer rate (< 10% at a mean follow-up of 3.5 years), although this procedure is now uncommon.

The surgical management of bleeding gastric ulcer is slightly different and should exclude malignancy as well as control and prevent recurrent bleeding or ulceration. A bleeding gastric ulcer is most commonly managed by a distal gastrectomy that incorporates the ulcer with a gastroduodenostomy (Billroth I) or a gastrojejunostomy (Billroth II) reconstruction. Alternative options include wedge resection of the ulcer with or without truncal vagotomy and drainage procedure. The type of operative approach relies on the location of the ulcer and the patient's fitness and haemodynamic stability. Ulcer biopsy and oversewing, thus leaving the ulcer in situ, carries a high risk of rebleeding (20–40%) (Corson and Williamson, 2001) but may be justified in high-risk patients who cannot withstand resection.

Arterial embolisation

This is an effective option to control massive bleeding from peptic ulcers in patients with failed endoscopic therapy and in poor surgical candidates. Acute transpapillary bleeding is best addressed by radiological means.

Follow-up

- Test for and eradicate *Helicobacter pylori* in order to prevent rebleeding (Barkun *et al.*, 2003).
- Stop non-steroidal anti-inflammatory drugs (NSAIDs) and aspirin. If the patient needs to continue taking NSAIDs after an episode of ulcer bleeding, the least damaging medication (ibuprofen) should be used with a PPI; alternatively, consider cyclo-oxygenase 2 (COX2)-specific anti-inflammatory drugs.
- In patients with gastric ulcer, continue PPI therapy for 6 weeks and then repeat endoscopy to confirm healing and to exclude malignancy (Palmer, 2002).
- In patients with duodenal ulcer, continue PPI therapy for 6 weeks and consider re-endoscopy only in patients who need to continue NSAID therapy (Palmer, 2002).

■ KEY POINT

Test for and eradicate *H. pylori* to prevent rebleeding, and stop NSAIDs and aspirin.

Treatment regimens for *H. pylori* infection include the following (Corson and Williamson, 2001):

- Omeprazole 40 mg/day + clarithromycin 500 mg every 8 h for 2 weeks; then omeprazole 20 mg/day for 2 weeks.
- Ranitidine bismuth citrate 400 mg every 12 h + clarithromycin 500 mg every 8 h for 2 weeks; then ranitidine bismuth citrate 400 mg every 12 h for 2 weeks.
- Bismuth subsalicylate 525 mg every 6 h + metronidazole 250 mg every 6 h + tetracycline 500 mg every 6 h for 2 weeks, + an H_2-receptor antagonist for 4 weeks.
- Lansoprazole 30 mg every 12 h + amoxicillin 1 g every 12 h + clarithromycin 500 mg every 12 h for 2 weeks.

● MANAGEMENT OF OTHER CAUSES OF NON-VARICEAL UPPER GASTROINTESTINAL BLEEDING

Mallory–Weiss tear

Mallory–Weiss tear is a linear mucosal laceration involving the gastric cardia, often extending to no more than 2.5 cm. It is the result of forceful vomiting, retching, coughing or straining. It accounts for 5 per cent of acute UGIB (Stabile and Stamos, 2000).

It is critical to distinguish Mallory–Weiss tear from Boerhaave syndrome, which represents a full-thickness laceration with perforation of the oesophagus. The latter may be suspected on chest X-ray and can be confirmed with either a gastrograffin swallow or computed tomography (CT) scan with oral contrast, and it requires prompt surgical intervention; bleeding from a Mallory–Weiss tear, however, ceases spontaneously in 50–80 per cent of patients by the time endoscopy is performed, and surgery (oversewing through an anterior gastrostomy) is required to achieve haemostasis in only 10 per cent of cases. If bleeding from a Mallory–Weiss tear is visualised at endoscopy, then electrocoagulation, heater-probe application and sclerotherapy are viable options. The overall mortality rate of patients who require emergency surgery is 15–25 per cent, in contrast to less than 3 per cent in those whose bleeding stops by the time of initial endoscopy.

Dieulafoy lesion

This is a vascular malformation of the proximal stomach, usually within 6 cm of the gastro-oesophageal junction and along the lesser curvature; however, it can occur anywhere along the gastrointestinal tract. Dieulafoy lesion accounts for 2–5 per cent of acute UGIB. Endoscopically, the lesion appears as a large submucosal vessel that has become ulcerated; the bleeding can be massive and brisk.

Endoscopic management options include contact thermal ablation with heater probe (with or without prior injection with adrenaline) as first choice, band ligation and sclerotherapy. Rebleeding after endoscopic therapy occurs in 15 per cent of patients and can be managed in most cases by repeated endoscopy with suture ligation or, more preferably, surgical excision of the lesion reserved for endoscopic failures.

Angiodysplasia

Angiodysplasia most commonly involves the stomach and duodenum and accounts for 2–4 per cent of acute UGIB. Histologically, angiodysplasias are dilated, thin-walled vascular channels that appear macroscopically as a cluster of cherry spots. Angiodysplasia can be acquired or congenital, as in hereditary haemorrhagic telangiectasia and Rendu–Osler–Weber syndrome (an autosomal dominant disorder typically identified by the triad of telangiectasia, recurrent epistaxis and a positive family history). Most lesions are smaller than 1 cm in diameter; they are multiple in two-thirds of patients. These lesions may be readily eradicated endoscopically with contact heater probes, argon plasma coagulation, or band ligation with surgery reserved for endoscopic failure. Alternatively, catheter-directed vasopressin may avoid the need for surgery. When the diagnosis is unknown and a vascular lesion is suggested, combined hormonal therapy with oestrogen and progesterone may be beneficial.

Aortoenteric fistula

An aortoenteric fistula results from the erosion of the aortic graft into the bowel lumen, usually at the third or fourth part of the duodenum. Most of the fistulae involve the proximal aortic anastomotic suture line. Patients usually present with self-limiting sentinel bleeding followed by exsanguinating massive gastrointestinal bleed. Diagnosis may be established at an upper gastrointestinal endoscopy to the ligament of Treitz and occasionally by CT scanning, which might show air bubbles in relation to the graft. Angiography requires active bleeding (1 mL/min) in order to be diagnostic. Emergency surgery to remove the aortic graft and debride and close the duodenum and the aorta, followed by bilateral extra-anatomic vascular bypass (e.g. axillo-bifemoral), is required. Alternatively, an endovascular stent to repair the fistula with prolonged antibiotic therapy (for at least 3 months) may be considered as a bridge to more definitive treatment after haemodynamic stabilisation in high-risk surgical patients.

● RECOMMENDATIONS FOR THE MANAGEMENT OF PATIENTS WITH VARICEAL UPPER GASTROINTESTINAL BLEEDING

Variceal haemorrhage is defined as bleeding from an oesophageal or gastric varix at the time of endoscopy or the presence of large oesophageal varices with blood in the stomach and no other identifiable source of bleeding. An episode of bleeding is considered significant when there is a transfusion requirement of 2 units of blood or more within 24 h of time zero, together with a systolic blood pressure of less than 100 mmHg or a postural change of more than 20 mmHg and/or pulse greater than 100 beats/min at time zero. (Time zero is the time of first hospital admission.)

The acute bleeding episode encompasses an interval of 48 h from time zero with absence of evidence of clinically significant bleeding between 24 h and 48 h. Evidence of any bleeding after 48 h is the first rebleeding episode. Variceal rebleeding is defined as the occurrence of new haematemesis or melaena after a period of 24 h or more from the 24-h point of stable vital signs and haematocrit/haemoglobin. All bleeding episodes regardless of severity should be counted in evaluating rebleeding.

The definition of failure to control active bleeding can be divided into two time frames:

- *Failure to control bleeding within 6 h:* this is represented by a transfusion requirement of 4 units of blood or more and inability to achieve an increase in systolic blood pressure by 20 mmHg or to 70 mmHg or more, and/or inability to achieve a pulse rate reduction to less than 100 beats/min or a reduction of 20 beats/min from baseline pulse rate.
- *Failure to control bleeding after 6 h:* this is defined as occurrence of haematemesis from the 6-h point or a reduction in blood pressure of more than 20 mmHg from the 6-h point and/or increase in pulse rate of more than 20 beats/min from the 6-h point on two consecutive readings 1 h apart, transfusion of 2 units of blood or more (over and above the previous transfusions) required to increase the haematocrit to above 27 per cent, or haemoglobin to above 9 g/L.

Development of varices

The rise in portal pressure is associated with the development of collateral circulation that allows the portal blood to be diverted into the systemic circulation. These spontaneous shunts occur:

- at the cardia through the intrinsic and extrinsic gastro-oesophageal veins;
- in the anal canal where the superior haemorrhoidal vein belonging to the portal system anastomoses with the middle and inferior haemorrhoidal veins that belong to the caval system;
- in the falciform ligament of the liver through the para-umbilical veins, which are the remains of the umbilical circulation in the fetus;
- in the abdominal wall and the retroperitoneal tissues, from the liver to the diaphragm, veins in the lienorenal ligament, in the omentum and lumbar veins;
- as blood diversion from the diaphragm, gastric, pancreatic, splenic and adrenal veins, which may drain into the left renal vein.

Current evidence suggests that varices develop and enlarge with time. The two factors that appear to determine the development of varices are continued hepatic injury and the degree of portosystemic shunting.

The factors that predispose to and precipitate variceal haemorrhage are still not clear. Currently the following are the most important factors:

- Portal pressure: usually reflects the intravariceal pressure. A hepatic venous pressure gradient (HPVG) greater than 12 mmHg is necessary for the development of and bleeding from oesophageal varices, but there is no linear relationship between the severity of portal hypertension and the risk of variceal haemorrhage. However, the HVPG tends to be higher in bleeders and in patients with large varices.
- Variceal wall size: this is best assessed endoscopically. The literature varies in its scoring of the relevance of this point, due largely to the lack of clear definition regarding the distinction between large and small varices.
- Variceal wall and tension: endoscopic features such as 'red spots' and 'wale' markings have been described as significant in the prediction of variceal bleeding. These features represent changes in variceal wall structure and tension associated with the development of micro-telangiectasias.
- Severity of liver disease and bleeding indices.

The two most important factors that determine the risk of variceal bleeding are the severity of liver disease and the size of the varices.

In summary, some 30–50 per cent of patients with portal hypertension will bleed from varices, and this is related to the severity of liver disease measured by Child–Pugh class (see Table 12.3) and the size of the varices. The average mortality rate of the first episode of variceal bleeding is around 50 per cent. The average mortality from a subsequent variceal haemorrhage is 5 per cent in Child class A patients, 25 per cent in Child class B patients and 50 per cent in Child class C patients.

Control of active variceal bleeding

The following summarises the management recommendations for control of active variceal bleeding in patients with cirrhosis:

- Treatment should ideally be undertaken by a dedicated appropriately equipped and staffed unit.
- Resuscitate in a setting appropriate to the severity of bleeding. Maintain mean arterial pressure at 80 mmHg and Hb at around 8 g/dL. Use gelatine-based colloids and packed red blood cells for volume replacement. Avoid dextrans (may increase bleeding times), hydroxyethyl starch (can worsen liver function) and Ringer's lactate solution.
- Electively intubate patients with severe uncontrolled variceal bleeding, severe encephalopathy, oxygen saturation below 90 per cent and aspiration pneumonia.
- Place a nasogastric tube for repeated gastric lavage or administer intravenous low-dose erythromycin in order to clear the stomach for endoscopy.
- Start vasoactive therapy as soon as possible. Intravenous octreotide, a synthetic analogue of somatostatin, is often begun as soon as the diagnosis is certain. This newer agent has mostly replaced vasopressin, due to its ease of use. Vasopressin's mechanism of action is thought to be splanchnic arteriolar vasoconstriction, resulting in decreased portal pressure, although it remains controversial whether this effect is maintained in the face of severe haemorrhage. The usual dose for vasopressin is 0.2–0.4 units/min, although high-dose therapy (1.0–1.5 units/min) has been advocated. The potential side effects of vasopressin are primarily cardiovascular and increase with higher doses. Sublingual nitroglycerine administered simultaneously with vasopressin significantly decreases the complication rate of vasopressin. The control of bleeding with this combination therapy is superior to that achieved with vasopressin alone. An alternative to vasopressin for control of variceal haemorrhage is the synthetic analogue terlipressin (1–2 mg, depending on body weight, given by bolus every 4 h for 2–5 days); this is more effective than vasopressin. The most commonly used drug for treating variceal bleeding is somatostatin (an initial bolus of 250 µg followed by intravenous infusion at a rate of 250 µg/h for 2–5 days). This has been shown to be equally efficacious with terlipressin and vasopressin. Although concerns over potential effects on renal function have been raised, octreotide (continuous intravenous infusion of 25 µg/h for 2–5 days) is a widely used alternative to vasopressin and nitroglycerine because of the simplicity of single-agent use.
- Start ciprofloxacin (1 g/day for 7 days) in order to prevent bacterial infections such as spontaneous peritonitis and bacteraemia.
- Upper gastrointestinal endoscopy should be performed by an experienced endoscopist as soon as the patient is haemodynamically stable.
- Variceal band ligation is the method of first choice for endoscopic therapy. Failing that, endoscopic intravariceal or paravariceal injection sclerotherapy should be performed. Its risks include oesophageal perforation, ulceration and stricture. Alternatively, a tissue adhesive (e.g. cyanoacrylate) can be injected into bleeding varices to plug the lumen; this is 90 per cent successful in achieving haemostasis. Its risks include pulmonary embolisation, portal vein embolisation, splenic infarction, and permanent damage to the lens of the endoscope.
- Combined endoscopic and vasoactive therapy is superior to either treatment in the control of bleeding.

In clinical practice, the choice of sclerosant has largely remained a matter of personal preference and has depended on the availability of the particular sclerosants in various countries. In the USA, sodium morrhuate and sodium tetradecyl have been those used most widely. Ethanolamine, which is also available in the USA, has been used exclusively in the UK and South Africa. Polidocanol is the sclerosant of choice in Austria and Germany. Sodium morrhuate, sodium tetradecyl sulphate, ethanolamine or ethanol is usually injected directly into the varix. Depending on the size of the varix, 0.5–2 mL of the selected sclerosant is used in each injection. The total volume used per sclerotherapy session is usually around 10–20 mL. Polidocanol, on the other hand, is injected into the submucosa around the varix. At each injection, 0.5–1.5 mL may be delivered, and 40–60 mL of polidoconal may be used per sclerotherapy session. Isobutyl 2-cyanoacrylate, a liquid tissue adhesive, has been used for intravariceal injections into bleeding oesophageal and gastric varices. This liquid polymer solidifies instantly in blood and obliterates the varix immediately. This adhesive plug sloughs off in a few weeks, leaving a fibrotic scar at the injection site. Cyanoacrylate is diluted with lipiodol (0.5 : 0.8 mL) before injection in order to prevent the adhesive from hardening too fast and to allow fluoroscopic monitoring. The biopsy channel and tip of the endoscope should be treated with silicone oil to prevent sticking of cyanoacrylate to the instrument. A single 0.5-mL dose of this solution may be injected intravascularly into each oesophageal variceal channel through a regular sclerotherapy needle. Two to three injections of 0.5 mL each are often required for large varices in the gastric fundus. After each injection of 0.5 mL of the cyanoacrylate solution, the sclerotherapy needle must be rinsed thoroughly with distilled water.

There are differences in opinion regarding the correct injection site. Intravariceal injection was the first method described and is still used by most endoscopists around the world, especially in the USA and the UK. Injection is performed initially at the bleeding site. All the variceal channels are then injected at the bottom of the varix, which is usually located at or just below the gastro-oesophageal junction. Finally, the variceal channels are injected 3–5 cm proximally. Cyanoacrylate must be injected directly into the varix. Inadvertent injection of this chemical into surrounding tissue causes severe ulceration.

Some endoscopists inject the sclerosant alongside the varix or paravariceally. The aim of paravariceal injection is to create a layer of fibrosis covering the variceal channels. Injections are performed starting at the cardia and repeated 30–50 times, producing a helical arrangement of wheals as the endoscope is withdrawn. The injections are limited to the distal oesophagus unless there is a more proximal bleeding site. This technique is currently the method of choice in Germany, Austria and some other European countries.

Sclerotherapy as a long-term treatment requires repeated injection sessions in order to achieve obliteration of varices. Despite the popularity of the procedure since the 1970s, no uniform follow-up sclerotherapy schedule has emerged. After the initial treatment, subsequent sclerotherapy sessions have been scheduled at various intervals, ranging from a few days to a few weeks.

In summary, although the concept of endoscopic sclerotherapy for varices appears to be straightforward, the clinical practice of the technique has not been standardised. The overall importance of the multiple technical variables outlined above is not well understood. Many investigators believe that these factors are of secondary importance when compared with the patient's overall clinical status at the time of sclerotherapy. The sclerotherapy patient should usually anticipate a long-term treatment programme. In the USA, the patient will probably undergo two to three sclerotherapy sessions during the index hospitalisation for an acute episode of variceal haemorrhage. Two to three subsequent sessions will be performed in the following 4–8 weeks before the variceal channels are obliterated. The patient will return for follow-up endoscopies every 3–6 months, presumably for the rest of their life, because oesophageal varices recur in up to 60 per cent of patients.

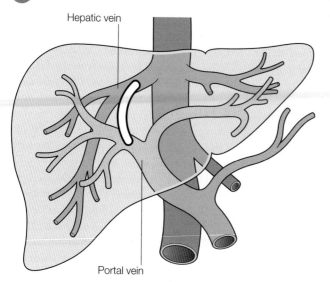

Hepatic vein

Portal vein

Figure 12.2 ● Transjugular intrahepatic portosystemic shunt (TIPS) is an expandable stent placed angiographically between a branch of the hepatic vein and a branch of the portal vein to create a non-surgical shunt.

If endoscopic therapy is unavailable, vasoconstrictors such as octreotide (unlicensed) or terlipressin are administered, or a Sengstaken–Blackmore or Minnesota tube (with both gastric and oesophageal balloons) or a Linton–Nachlas tube (with gastric balloon only) with adequate provision for airways protection can be placed until definitive therapy is arranged. The tube is inserted into the stomach and the gastric balloon partially inflated with 40–50 mL of air. The balloon position within the stomach and below the diaphragm is confirmed with abdominal radiography before its further inflation with 300 mL of air. Upward traction is then applied to the tube. If bleeding continues, the oesophageal balloon is inflated to a pressure of 35–40 mmHg. The oesophageal balloon should be deflated every 4 h for 15 min in order to avoid oesophageal necrosis, and the entire tube should not be left in place for more than 24–48 h. Unlike the Sengstaken tube, which has three lumens, the Minnesota tube has a fourth lumen that enables oesophageal drainage above the inflated oesophageal balloon. These tubes are successful in 85 per cent of cases, but recurrent bleeding after balloon deflation is common. Tube-related complications, such as airway obstruction, aspiration and oesophageal necrosis with rupture, occur in 20 per cent of patients.

If endoscopic control of bleeding cannot be achieved, then a Sengstaken or Minnesota tube can be inserted until further endoscopic treatment, transjugular intrahepatic portosystemic shunt (TIPS) or surgical treatment is possible. The TIPS procedure involves the transjugular insertion of a self-expanding nitinol stent in the liver to connect the portal and hepatic veins, thus creating a portosystemic shunt (Figure 12.2). Specialist help should be sought at this time, and transfer to a specialist centre should be considered, where the choice of definitive intervention is determined by the preference of that centre.

Transjugular intrahepatic portosystemic shunt with or without transvenous variceal embolisation is the standard therapy for patients with bleeding oesophagogastric varices that are unresponsive to, or who rebleed severely soon after, endoscopic and pharmacological first-line therapy. Patients with marginal liver function (Child class B or C cirrhosis) may also receive TIPS as a bridge to liver transplantation. Transjugular intrahepatic portosystemic shunt controls variceal bleeding in more than 90 per cent of patients but risks hepatic encephalopathy in 25–35 per cent of patients and a mortality of 15 per cent (due mainly to multisystem organ failure in Child class C patients).

Liver transplantation should be considered in patients with Child class C cirrhosis, although this is often an unavailable option due to organ shortages. Transjugular intrahepatic porto-systemic shunt can be used as a bridge to transplantation. Portal decompression (e.g. TIPS) is preferable to transplantation in patients with Child class A or B cirrhosis.

Surgical decompression of the portal system is reserved for patients with failed initial non-surgical treatment who still have preserved liver function and in patients who are bleeding from colonic and stomal varices. Surgical shunts carry a success rate greater than 90 per cent and a rebleeding rate of less than 10 per cent, but they risk encephalopathy in 25 per cent of patients. In the presence of actively bleeding varices, non-selective shunts such as portocaval or mesocaval shunt or interposition graft are favoured over selective distal splenorenal (Warren) shunt (DSRS). Gastro-oesophageal decongestion and splenectomy (GEDS; Hassab operation), when done properly, is as effective in controlling bleeding as DSRS with higher survival and minimal or no encephalopathy. Combined with sclerotherapy, GEDS could be an ideal therapy for bleeding varices. Oesophagogastric devascularisation with oesophageal tran-section and re-anastomosis with (the 'modified Sugiura procedure') or without splenectomy

---

Box 12.1 Prophylaxis of variceal bleeding in cirrhosis

Primary prophylaxis
- Pharmacological therapy with propranolol is the best available modality to prevent variceal bleeding.
- In case of contraindication or intolerance to propranolol, variceal band ligation is the treatment of choice.
- Where neither propranolol nor variceal band ligation can be used, isosorbide mononitrate is the treatment of first choice.
- All patients with cirrhosis should undergo regular endoscopy at the time of diagnosis (yearly if varices are detected, or every 3 years if no varices are found).

> **KEY POINT**
> All patients with cirrhosis should undergo regular endoscopy at the time of diagnosis.

Secondary prophylaxis
- Following control of active variceal bleeding, the varices should be eradicated using endoscopic methods. The method of first choice is variceal band ligation. If banding is not available, sclerotherapy should be used.
- It is recommended that endoscopic variceal therapy is delivered at weekly intervals until variceal eradication, and that endoscopy is repeated at 3 months and every 6 months thereafter.
- Either combination treatment of sclerotherapy and non-selective beta-blocker or either of these alone may be used. If the latter strategy is used, then it is recommended that the hepatic venous pressure gradient is measured in order to confirm that this has been successfully reduced to less than 12 mmHg.
- Transjugular intrahepatic portosystemic shunt (TIPS) is more effective than endoscopic treatment in reducing variceal rebleeding but does not improve survival and is associated with more encephalopathy. It is a treatment option that may be used in certain centres with particular expertise.

may have a role in patients with Child class A or B cirrhosis with well-preserved liver function and contraindications for Warren shunt, TIPS and liver transplantation.

In order to prevent encephalopathy, the use of intravenous flumazenil, a benzodiazepine receptor antagonist, appears beneficial; the use of lactulose remains controversial.

Primary and secondary prophylaxis against variceal bleeding

A summary of the management recommendations for primary and secondary prophylaxis against bleeding from varices is shown in Box 12.1.

● SUMMARY

The management of UGIB has been a challenge to the gastroenterologist and surgeon. Although there is a wide range of treatment options available, this chapter describes only the best current and evidence-based options.

All patients with UGIB should first be resuscitated and stabilised. Early endoscopy (within 24 h) should be performed in order to stratify the patient's risk and achieve haemostasis when required. A proton pump inhibitor should be prescribed for patients with peptic ulcer disease, and *H. pylori* should be eradicated when present. When rebleeding occurs after the initial endoscopic management of a peptic ulcer, a second-look endoscopy should be performed, with early liaison with the surgical team for consideration for surgery should the second procedure fail. The choice between surgery and radiological intervention relies on the patient's fitness for surgery and the diagnosis.

The management of variceal UGIB prompts vasoactive treatment with octreotide as soon as possible. The first-choice endoscopic management is variceal band ligation. If this fails, endoscopic injection sclerotherapy should be tried. Failing that, a Sengstaken or Minnesota tube should be inserted until further endoscopy, TIPS or surgery is performed.

● QUESTIONS

1 What is the investigation of choice in a stable patient with melaena?
2 What best characterises a Dieulafoy's lesion?
3 What is haemobilia? Describe its clinical presentation and endoscopic findings.
4 Describe the clinical presentation and chest X-ray findings in Boerhaave syndrome.
5 How would you achieve control of an active variceal bleeding in a cirrhotic patient?
6 What is the best treatment of choice in a 40-year-old man with large, actively bleeding oesophageal varices on upper gastrointestinal endoscopy?
7 What are the indications for TIPS procedure?
8 What is the Child classification of a patient with slight ascites, no encephalopathy, a serum bilirubin of 8 mg/dL, albumin 2, and increased prothrombin time (5 s over control)?

● REFERENCES

American College of Surgeons Committee on Trauma (1997). *Advanced Trauma Life Support Course Manual*. Chicago, IL: American College of Surgeons.

Barkun A, Bardou M, Marshall JK (2003). Nonvariceal Upper GI Bleeding Consensus Conference Group. Consensus recommendations for managing patients with nonvariceal upper gastrointestinal bleeding. *Ann Intern Med* **139**: 843–57.

Corson JD, Williamson RCN (eds) (2001). *Surgery*. London: Mosby-Year Book.

Dallal HJ, Palmer KR (2001). ABC of the upper gastrointestinal tract: upper gastrointestinal haemorrhage. *Br Med J* **323**: 1115–17.

Fallah MA, Prakash C, Edmundowicz S (2000). Acute gastrointestinal bleeding. *Med Clin North Am* **84**: 1183–208.

Forrest JA, Finlayson ND, Shearman DJ (1974). Endoscopy in gastrointestinal bleeding. *Lancet* **2**: 394–7.

Jalan R, Hayes PC (2000). UK guidelines on the management of variceal haemorrhage in cirrhotic patients. *Gut* **46**: iii1–15.

Laine L, Peterson WL (1994). Bleeding peptic ulcer. *N Engl J Med* **331**: 717–27.

Palmer KR (2002). Non-vaiceal upper gastrointestinal haemorrhage: guidelines. *Gut* **51**: iv1–6.

Peter DJ, Dougherty JM (1999). Evaluation of the patient with gastrointestinal bleeding: an evidence based approach. *Emerg Med Clin North Am* **17**: 239–61.

Rockall TA, Logan RF, Devlin HB, Northfield TC (1995). Incidence of and mortality from acute upper gastrointestinal haemorrhage in the United Kingdom. Steering Committee and members of the National Audit of Acute Upper Gastrointestinal Haemorrhage. *Br Med J* **311**: 222–6.

Rockall TA, Logan RF, Devlin HB, Northfield TC (1996). Risk assessment after acute upper gastrointestinal haemorrhage. *Gut* **38**: 316–21.

Stabile BE, Stamos MJ (2000). Surgical management of gastrointestinal bleeding. *Gastroenterol Clin North Am* **29**: 189–222.

Thabut D, Bernard-Chabert B (2007). Management of acute bleeding from portal hypertension. *Best Pract Res Clin Gastroenterol* **21**: 19–29.

Lower gastrointestinal bleeding

Nigel A Scott

- Introduction
- Rectal bleeding in the outpatient department
- Rectal bleeding in the emergency room
- Summary
- Questions
- References

● INTRODUCTION

Passing blood from the anus is an alarming but not uncommon symptom. Of 4006 respondents to a postal survey, 18 per cent reported rectal bleeding in the previous year (Thompson *et al.*, 2000). Young women (age 16–40 years) were significantly more likely to report rectal bleeding than young men (26% v. 16%). For 25 per cent, this was their first episode of rectal bleeding, but 63 per cent had experienced rectal bleeding in the previous year. Extrapolation of these findings to the total population of Portsmouth and south-east Hampshire (n = 540 290) indicates that 145 in every 1000 people experience rectal bleeding each year; in a notional district general hospital catchment of 250 000 people, that is nearly 40 000 individuals per year.

> ■ KEY POINT
> Passing blood from the anus is alarming but not uncommon.

● RECTAL BLEEDING IN THE OUTPATIENT DEPARTMENT

Assessment

For the patient referred by their general practitioner (GP) as an outpatient with rectal bleeding, there are three possible concerns, and therefore three possible medical responses to the consultation for rectal bleeding (Table 13.1).

History

Included in the outpatient history are details of the colour of the blood, whether it is mixed in with the stool, change in bowel habit and the presence or absence of anal symptoms.

Painless bright-red bleeding is most commonly due to haemorrhoids, while severe pain and red bleeding on defecation indicate an anal fissure. Loose frequent stools with blood and mucus may be due to an acute proctitis.

Table 13.1 Expectations and rectal bleeding

Patient concern	Medical response
Is it bowel cancer?	Definitive yes or no
Can the bleeding be fixed?	Possibly
Is rectal bleeding something I may see on and off, indefinitely?	Possibly/probably

---

Box 13.1 Higher-risk symptom combinations

- Rectal bleeding and a change in bowel habit have a three to five times greater risk of colorectal cancer compared with patients presenting with either symptom alone.
- Rectal bleeding and no anal symptoms have a three to four times greater risk than anal symptoms alone.
- Dark-red bleeding has only a slightly higher predictive value (9–13%) when compared with bright red rectal bleeding.

Box 13.2 Outpatient anorectal examination

Setting
- *Always* obtain consent
- Privacy – keep patient covered
- Use a chaperone
- Left lateral position.

Rectal examination
1 Separate buttocks – inspect perineum and perianal skin.
2 Separate anal margin to visualise fissure if relevant.
3 Insert lubricated finger – systematic 360 degree palpation; note prostate and sacral hollow.
4 Withdraw finger and observe for blood and mucus.

Rigid sigmoidoscopy
1 Insert with obturator tip directed towards umbilicus.
2 Withdraw obturator – attach lens and insufflator.
3 Warn patient that rectum will feel full as air insufflated.
4 Observe mucosa – biopsy abnormality (having checked patient not anticoagulated).
5 Document extent of examination and any pathology in centimetres from anal verge.
6 Wipe perineum clean at end of examination.

Communication
Allow patient time to get dressed and comfortable before discussing findings.

It is the possible diagnosis of colorectal cancer, however, that dominates the initial consultation for most patients. In practice all patients referred for hospital evaluation of rectal bleeding require an endoscopic examination of the rectum, but certain symptom combinations make a diagnosis of colorectal cancer more likely (Box 13.1) (Thompson, 2002).

Examination
Examination includes general clinical inspection for signs of anaemia, abdominal palpation for masses and a digital rectal examination. In many clinics this is followed by rigid sigmoidoscopy of the unprepared rectum (Box 13.2).

In the large majority of patients, at the end of this sequence a positive diagnosis of haemorrhoids, anal fissure, rectal neoplasm or proctitis can be made. Patients with anal fissure may require a short period of topical glyceryl trinitrate (GTN) therapy before tolerating sigmoidoscopy. A few patients with rectal bleeding and a painful anus may require examination under anaesthetic in order to complete their assessment.

Table 13.2 Flexible sigmoidoscopy and common diagnoses by age

Diagnosis	Patients aged ≥ 45 years (n = 1033)	Patients aged < 45 years (n = 242)
Nothing abnormal detected	214 (20.7)	108 (44.6)
Haemorrhoids	301 (29.1)	89 (36.8)
Diverticular disease	218 (21.1)	9 (3.7)
Colitis	49 (4.7)	6 (2.5)
Polyps	171 (16.6)	19 (7.9)
Carcinoma (confirmed on histology)	36 (3.5)	0
Other (melanosis coli, anal polyp, radiation proctitis, submucous lipoma, solitary rectal ulcer, anal fissure)	44 (4.3)	10 (4.1)

Based on Mathew *et al.* (2004).

Flexible sigmoidoscopy for everybody?

In many UK colorectal departments, all patients with rectal bleeding are evaluated by flexible sigmoidoscopy, after suitable bowel preparation. However, although this policy may be justified in the older patient (Table 13.2), the diagnostic yield in younger patients has led some authors to question this policy on the basis of cost (Mathew *et al.*, 2004) – approximately £330 per examination – versus the low yield of colorectal neoplasia in patients under the age of 45 years.

On the other hand, at least one health economics analysis of the endoscopic evaluation of the colon in young patients (age 25–45 years) with symptomatic rectal bleeding, found an increased life expectancy in these patients – at a cost comparable with colon cancer screening (Lewis *et al.*, 2002). Furthermore, the majority of patients who attend with the symptom of rectal bleeding seek and expect the reassurance of a normal lower gastrointestinal endoscopy.

> ■ KEY POINT
> The majority of patients who attend with rectal bleeding seek the reassurance of a normal lower gastrointestinal endoscopy.

Haemorrhoids

Haemorrhoids are a specialised ring of vascular 'cushions' containing a venous plexus with arteriovenous communications. A key point to emphasise to all patients before any haemorrhoid therapy is that this ring of vascular tissue is not a disease but part of the normal anal canal. It is only when these normal vascular cushions produce symptoms – bleeding or prolapse – that they earn the sobriquet 'haemorrhoid' or 'pile'.

Haemorrhoids are classified as follows:

First *degree:* bleeding only
Second *degree:* prolapse, reduce spontaneously
Third *degree:* prolapse, need to be pushed back
Fourth *degree:* permanently prolapsed.

Outpatient therapy

First-degree piles are defined by bleeding alone and are usually managed on an outpatient basis as follows:

- Fibre supplementation can reduce episodes of haemorrhoidal bleeding (Nisar and Scholefield, 2003).
- Sclerotherapy with 5% phenol in oil carries the principal hazard of accidental prostatic injection. Among 189 patients managed by single-session large-dose oily phenol injection (3 × 5 mL), and followed for 4 years, only 53 (28%) considered themselves cured (Santos *et al.*, 1993). Infrared coagulation has been described as achieving better symptom relief than injection sclerotherapy at 3 months, but with no difference between the two techniques at 1 year's and 4 years' follow-up (Walker *et al.*, 1990).
- Rubber-band ligation (RBL) is the dominant outpatient intervention for bleeding haemorrhoids. Meta-analyses of randomised controlled trials have demonstrated superior outcomes for RBL compared with both injection sclerotherapy and infrared coagulation (MacRae and McLeod, 1995). Potential banding problems include discomfort, vasovagal episodes and urinary symptoms, all of which are worsened by multiple banding (Nisar and Scholefield, 2003).

It is unlikely that haemorrhoidal bleeding can be cured by these techniques in all patients. 'Cure' depends on the definition of success, but when defined as permanent relief of symptoms or a marked improvement in symptomatology with rare manifestation of bleeding (< 1/month), the proportion of patients free from haemorrhoid symptoms after RBL decreases as a function of time (Figure 13.1). Thus, living with rectal bleeding is an everyday reality for many people, with or without haemorrhoid therapy.

> ■ KEY POINT
> It is unlikely that haemorrhoidal bleeding can be cured in all patients.

Surgical therapy

Surgical therapy for haemorrhoids is directed largely at the symptom of prolapse – that is, second-, third- and fourth-degree piles. Surgical techniques for haemorrhoids include the following:

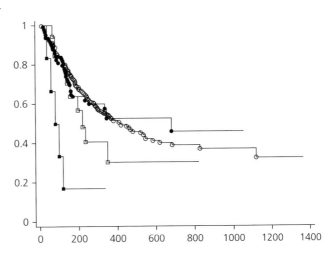

Figure 13.1 ● Success of rubber band ligation (RBL) diminishes with time. Kaplan–Meier curves of patients who are symptom-free after RBL of haemorrhoids. The *x*-axis represents time (days) and the *y*-axis represents the percentage of patients who are symptom-free.

Reproduced, with kind permission of Springer Science and Business Media, from Iyer VS, Shrier I, Gordon PH (2004). Long-Term Outcome of Rubber Band Ligation for Symptomatic Primary and Recurrent Internal Hemorrhoids. *DCR* **47**(8):1364–1370.

○, first RBL; ●, second RBL; □, third RBL; ■, fourth RBL.

- Open (Milligan–Morgan) haemorrhoidectomy
- Closed haemorrhoidectomy
- Stapled haemorrhoidopexy (procedure for prolapse and haemorrhoids, PPH)
- Ligasure haemorrhoidectomy
- Doppler-guided haemorrhoidal artery ligation (DG-HAL).

Excision of haemorrhoids (open technique – UK; closed technique – USA) is designed to remove swollen haemorrhoidal tissue from within the canal and out on to the perianal skin, while preserving sufficient mucosa and anoderm in order to maintain anal canal function.

Ligasure haemorrhoidectomy is an excisional technique that is thought to be associated with less postoperative pain and reduced operative time when compared with conventional techniques.

Stapled haemorrhoidopexy aims to return normal but prolapsed haemorrhoidal tissue to the anal canal by correction of the weakened suspensory ligament. This procedure should be less painful than excisional techniques, as it does not involve the skin of the anal canal.

Doppler-guided haemorrhoidal artery ligation also avoids haemorrhoid excision. A modified proctoscope housing a miniature Doppler transducer locates terminal branches of the superior rectal artery supplying the haemorrhoids. A small window in the device allows a suture to be placed around the artery, thus cutting off the blood supply to the haemorrhoid.

Other causes of outpatient rectal bleeding

Anal fissure

Anal fissure is distinguished clinically from haemorrhoids by the dominant symptom of severe anal pain on defecation. It is diagnosed on inspection of the gently separated anal margin. Rectal examination and sigmoidoscopy may be impossible. Management is initially by topical GTN (Box 13.3) or calcium channel blockers for 4–6 weeks, followed by sigmoidoscopy. If symptoms do not settle, examination and sigmoidoscopy under anaesthetic followed by operative management (injection of botulinum toxin, internal sphincterotomy or advancement flap) may be necessary.

A total of 48 different comparisons of the ability of medical therapies to heal anal fissure have been reported, in 53 randomised controlled trials. Glyceryl trinitrate is marginally better than placebo in healing anal fissure (48.6% v. 37%), but late recurrence of fissure after GTN therapy is common, in the range of 50% of those initially cured by GTN. Botulinum toxin and calcium channel blockers are equivalent in efficacy to GTN, and have fewer adverse events. No medical therapy matches the efficacy of surgical sphincterotomy, with a cure rate in the region of 95 per cent (Nelson, 2006).

Ulcerative proctitis

Ulcerative proctitis is readily diagnosed at initial rigid sigmoidoscopy. The extent and nature are confirmed by subsequent colonoscopy and systematic colonic biopsy. Topical management is with mesalazine or steroids by enema or suppository preparations.

Box 13.3 Glyceryl trinitrate ointment: patient instructions

- Use 0.2% GTN ointment supplied by hospital pharmacy.
- Place a small amount of the ointment on index finger.
- Apply around anus. Do not rub it in.
- Apply three times during the day, and once last thing at night.
- About 30% of patients develop a headache with use.
- Discard ointment after 6 weeks.

● RECTAL BLEEDING IN THE EMERGENCY ROOM

Who requires admission?

The emergent presentation of rectal bleeding has several well-recognised causes, including diverticular disease, colonic angiodysplasia and iatrogenic causes such as recent RBL of haemorrhoids and colonoscopic polypectomy (Table 13.3). The clinical spectrum can vary from a frightened but well patient with minimal volume loss, to a patient in haemorrhagic shock. The first practical decision is which patients with rectal bleeding require admission.

Factors that should be assessed in a patient presenting with emergency room rectal bleeding include the following:

- Patient's, relative's or nursing attendant's account of the bleeding
- Record of comorbidity and social isolation
- Drug history, e.g. aspirin, clopidogrel, warfarin
- Absence or presence of anaemia, rectal examination and bedsheet/bedpan findings
- Pulse rate and blood pressure monitoring
- Haemoglobin and haematocrit estimation
- Urine output if catheterised.

Haemodynamic compromise is an absolute indication for admission. Advanced age, large witnessed blood loss, comorbidity, social isolation, anticoagulant therapy and anaemia all argue in favour of admission for assessment.

Management

Of those patients admitted for observation, two distinct clinical groups can be distinguished:

- *No significant blood loss after admission:* this is the large majority of patients, who spend 48–72 h in hospital, with no further bleeding. Flexible sigmoidoscopy after enema preparation in these patients usually demonstrates some old blood limited to the left colon and excludes any neoplastic lesion. If the patient is on anticoagulants, then these medications should be reviewed against the severity of the initial indication. After discharge, complete colonic examination may be considered as determined by the patient's general fitness and any residual colonic symptoms.
- *Continuing significant rectal blood loss:* this is the minority of patients, but they constitute a difficult problem. As well as resuscitation, blood transfusion and correction of any clotting abnormality, attempts need to be made to localise the bleeding point and arrest continuing haemorrhage. The principal diagnostic and therapeutic modalities for these patients include colonoscopy, selective mesenteric angiography, technetium-labelled red blood cell scan and helical computed tomography (CT) scanning.

Colonoscopy

This must be combined with gastroscopy and can be performed in the unprepared colon, after enema preparation or after a colonic purge with oral polyethylene glycol (PEG) solution (Hoedema and Luchtefield, 2005). The overall diagnostic yield of colonoscopy in acute lower gastrointestinal bleeding is 69–80 per cent (Zuccaro, 1998).

Clinical series suggest that colonoscopy has a therapeutic role in diverticular haemorrhage (Jensen *et al.*, 2000). Of 17 patients with definite signs of diverticular haemorrhage (active bleeding in six, non-bleeding visible vessels in four, adherent clots in seven) and no therapeutic intervention, nine patients rebled and six patients required colectomy. By contrast, of a subsequent ten patients with definite signs of diverticular haemorrhage (active bleeding in five, non-bleeding visible vessels in two, adherent clots in three) and treated endoscopically

Table 13.3 Common causes of acute lower gastrointestinal bleeding

Lesion	Frequency	Comments
Diverticular disease	17–40%	Stops spontaneously in 80% of patients
		Surgery unlikely if < 4 units red cell transfusion given in 24 h, but required in 60% of patients receiving > 4 units in 24 h
Colonic angiodysplasia	2–30%	Frequency varies widely in clinical series
		Acute bleeding appears to be due more frequently to lesion in proximal colon
Colitis (ischaemic, infectious, inflammatory bowel disease, radiation enteritis)	9–21%	Ischaemic colitis often presents with abdominal pain and self-limited rectal bleeding; colitis is segmental, most often affecting splenic flexure
		Bloody diarrhoea is most frequent symptom of infectious colitis and inflammatory bowel disease of the colon
Colonic neoplasia, post-polypectomy bleeding	11–14%	Post-polypectomy bleeding is frequently self-limiting and may occur up to 14 days after polypectomy
Anorectal causes (e.g. haemorrhoids, secondary haemorrhage after RBL, rectal varices)	4–10%	Anoscopy/proctoscopy should be included in initial evaluation
Upper gastrointestinal sites (including duodenal/gastric ulcer, varices)	0–11%	Gastroscopy mandatory in severe lower gastrointestinal bleeding
Small bowel sites (including Crohn's ileitis, vascular ectasia, Meckel's diverticulum, tumours)	2–9%	Diagnosed by radiological studies or enteroscopy after acute bleeding episode has resolved

RBL, rubber-band ligation.
Based on Zuccaro (1998).

(injection of adrenaline or bipolar coagulation), none had recurrent bleeding and none required surgery.

Colonic angiodysplasia is usually found in the right colon (Ghosh *et al.*, 2002). Bipolar probe coagulation, argon plasma coagulation or laser therapy may be used to ablate angiodysplastic lesions. Possible complications of therapy include perforation, delayed haemorrhage and post-coagulation syndrome (self-limited abdominal pain and peritonism caused by serosal burns).

Selective mesenteric angiography

Angiography localises the site of bleeding in 40–84 per cent of patients presenting with lower gastrointestinal bleeding. Provocative measures, such as vasodilators, heparin and thrombolytic agents, may further increase the yield (Hoedema and Luchtefield, 2005). Diverticular haemorrhage is most likely to produce extravasation of contrast; this is less likely with bleeding angiodysplasia. Angiographic haemostasis may be possible using vasopressin or superselective embolisation (Zuccaro, 1998).

Technetium-labelled red blood cell scanning

Although this technique is well described (Jensen *et al.*, 2000) the author has never seen this technique be of practical value in acute lower gastrointestinal haemorrhage. Widely divergent results have been reported, and many surgeons are reluctant to proceed to colectomy on the basis of one such study alone. In UK practice, moreover, the availability of this technique does not lend itself to managing a patient with recurrent haemorrhagic shock.

Helical computed tomography scanning

The rapidity of helical CT scanning (Sabharwal *et al.*, 2006) permits the maintenance of intravascular concentration of contrast throughout a scan and provides accurate visualisation of vessels. In a pilot comparison of helical CT (2 h after admission), conventional angiography (3 h after admission) and colonoscopy (4 h after admission), five of seven patients with lower gastrointestinal bleeding had positive CT scans. By contrast, conventional angiography was positive in only two of seven patients. This experience suggests that, in acute lower gastrointestinal haemorrhage, helical CT may have a role as a screening tool, allowing patient selection for directed therapeutic angiography.

Surgical resection

Despite the claimed efficacy of colonoscopy and angiography in the management of patients with lower gastrointestinal haemorrhage, it is estimated that an emergency operation is ultimately required in 10–25 per cent of patients (Hoedema and Luchtefield, 2005). The likelihood of surgical intervention is related directly to transfusion requirement (Table 13.4) (McGuire, 1994).

Thus, the surgeon has on the operating table the patient who has failed endoscopic and angiographic localisation, has had recurrent or persistent haemorrhagic shock, and has undergone large-volume blood replacement. Faced with this challenge, a systematic approach is required:

1   After anaesthetic induction and stabilisation, repeat gastroscopy.
2   Put the patient in the Lloyd–Davies position.
3   Midline incision: inspect the small and large bowel for any obvious lesions. Note that, in colonic bleeding, some blood in the very distal ileum is not unusual.
4   On-table colonoscopy (Scott *et al.*, 1986):
   • Mobilise the whole of the colon, including the splenic and hepatic flexures.
   • Place a large catheter via the appendix stump into the caecum, and a large proctoscope into the anus, and lavage the colon with warm saline until clear.
   • Remove the proctoscope and perform a colonoscopy with additional lavage as necessary to visualise all of the colonic mucosa.

Table 13.4 Transfusion requirements and colectomy for lower gastrointestinal haemorrhage

Maximum transfusion on any given day	Number of patient episodes of bleeding	Number that stopped spontaneously	Number requiring colonic resection
< 4 units	66	65	1 (1.5%)
≥ 4 units	42	17	25 (60%)
Total	108	82	26

Based on McGuire (1994).

5   *If bleeding lesion is identified,* directed colonic resection with anastomosis or exteriorisation.
6   *If no lesion is visible,* consider the following:
   - Small bowel enteroscopy via terminal ileal enterotomy
   - Finally non-directed colonic resection:
     - Blind right hemicolectomy with end ileostomy and mucous fistula
     - Blind subtotal colectomy with end ileostomy and mucous fistula
     - If patient survives without further haemorrhage, re-anastomosis after 6 months.

● SUMMARY

Rectal bleeding is common. Fortunately, it is rarely the portent of serious or threatening disease. Excluding colorectal cancer as the cause of this bleeding remains the primary task facing the surgeon. Thereafter, in the outpatient setting, reducing haemorrhoidal bleeding with dietary advice and RBL is needed. Promising a cure for the patient's haemorrhoidal bleeding is misleading and can be the source of considerable patient unhappiness.

Hospital admission for significant rectal bleeding is not uncommon. The majority of rectal bleeds stop, but the patient may then require advice on the future use of antiplatelet or anticoagulant therapy. A tiny minority of patients with frightening and persistent colonic haemorrhage require colonic surgery after failed localisation by colonoscopy and mesenteric angiography.

● QUESTIONS

The following are single-best-answer questions on rectal bleeding. Asterisks (*) indicate the correct answers.

1   What symptom combinations with rectal bleeding indicate a higher risk of colorectal cancer?
2   How are haemorrhoids classified and what treatment modalities exist?
3   What is the most effective therapy for anal fissure?
4   Which patients with rectal bleeding should be admitted from the Emergency Room?
5   List three common causes of colonic bleeding.
6   What would you do if at laparotomy the precise site of colonic bleeding could not be identified?

● REFERENCES

Ghosh S, Watts D, Kinnear M (2002). Management of gastrointestinal haemorrhage. *Postgrad Med J* **78**: 4–14.

Hoedema RF, Luchtefield MA (2005). The management of lower gastrointestinal haemorrhage. *Dis Colon Rectum* **48**: 2010–24.

Jensen DM, Machicado GA, Jutabha R, *et al.* (2000). Urgent colonoscopy for the diagnosis and treatment of severe diverticular hemorrhage. *N Engl J Med* 342: 78–82.

Lewis JD, Brown A, Localio AR, Schwartz JS (2002). Initial evaluation of rectal bleeding in young persons: a cost effectiveness analysis. *Ann Intern Med* **136**: 99–110.

MacRae HM, McLeod RS (1995). Comparison of hemorrhoidal treatment modalities. *Dis Colon Rectum* **38**: 687–94.

Mathew J, Shankar P, Aldean IM (2004). Audit on flexible sigmoidoscopy for rectal bleeding in a district general hospital: are we over-loading the resources? *Postgrad Med J* **80**: 38–40.

McGuire HH (1994). Bleeding colonic diverticula: a reappraisal of natural history and management. *Ann Surg* **220**: 653–6.

Milewski PJ, Schofield PF (1989). Massive colonic haemorrhage: the case for right hemicolectomy. *Ann R Coll Surg Engl* **71**: 253–9.

Nelson R (2006). Non surgical therapy for anal fissure. *Cochrane Database Syst Rev* (4): CD003431.

Nisar PJ, Scholefield JH (2003). Managing haemorrhoids. *Br Med J* **327**: 847–51.

Sabharwal R, Vladica P, Chou R, Phiilip W (2006). Helical CT in the diagnosis of acute lower gastrointesti-nal haemorrhage. *Eur J Radiol* **58**: 273–9.

Santos G, Novell JR, Khoury G, Winslet MC, Lewis AAM (1993). Long-term results of large-dose, single-session phenol injection sclerotherapy for hemorrhoids. *Dis Colon Rectum* **36**: 958–61.

Scott HJ, Lane IF, Glynn MJ, *et al.* (1986). Colonic haemorrhage: a technique for rapid intra-operative bowel preparation and colonoscopy. *Br J Surg* **73**: 390–91.

Thompson MR (2002). ACPGBI Referral guidelines for colorectal cancer. *Colorectal Dis* **4**: 287–97.

Thompson JA, Pond CL, Ellis BG, Beach A, Thompson MR (2000). Rectal bleeding in general and hospital practice: 'the tip of the iceberg'. *Colorectal Dis* **2**: 288–93.

Walker AJ, Leicester RJ, Nicholls RJ, Mann CV (1990). A prospective study of infrared coagulation, injection and rubber band ligation in the treatment of haemorrhoids. *Int J Colorect Dis* **5**: 113–16.

Zuccaro G (1998). Management of the adult patient with acute lower gastrointestinal bleeding. *Am J Gas-troenterol* 93: 1202–8.

14 Management of severely injured patients

Andrew Lockey and Amjid Mohammed

- Introduction
- Airway with cervical spine control
- Breathing with assisted ventilation
- Circulation
- Dysfunction
- Secondary examination: exposure
- Ongoing care
- Pitfalls in the management of severely injured patients
- Summary
- Questions
- References

● INTRODUCTION

Trauma has been shown to be the fourth most common cause of mortality worldwide. The World Health Organization (WHO) reported 5.18 million deaths worldwide in 2002 as a result of trauma (80 000 in Europe).

The management of the seriously injured patient should follow a structured approach. This approach follows the 'ABCDE' principle and is advocated in courses such as Advanced Trauma Life Support (ATLS®; American College of Surgeons, 2004) and European Trauma Course (ETC®; European Resuscitation Council, 2006). These courses are run internationally and promote a standardised approach to the trauma patient. ABCDE stands for:

- Airway with cervical spine control
- Breathing with assisted ventilation
- Circulation
- Dysfunction
- Exposure.

> ■ KEY POINT
> The management of the seriously injured patient should follow the ABCDE approach.

It is essential that there is seamless communication between the pre-hospital services and the emergency department with regard to victims of trauma. This enables the emergency department to appropriately prepare and mobilise the trauma team. Trauma team call-out criteria include the following:

- Significant poly-trauma
- Spinal injury
- Decreased level of consciousness
- High-energy transfer mechanism of injury:
  - Ejection
  - Fall from >6 m
  - Entrapment

- Any penetrating trunk injury
- Death in same passenger compartment
- Rollover
- Pedestrian thrown or run over
- Pedestrian hit by car travelling at > 20 mph
- High-speed collision (> 40 mph), major vehicle deformity or intrusion
- Motorcycle travelling at > 20 mph.

The trauma team may comprise the following personnel:

- *Team leader:* typically a senior clinician (ideally a consultant and usually an emergency physician) who has the ability to direct the resuscitation without any prejudice regarding ongoing care.
- *Airway/breathing doctor:* usually an experienced anaesthetist or emergency physician.
- *Circulation doctor(s):* usually members of the emergency department team.
- *Surgical doctor:* assesses the patient from a surgical perspective and assists with any immediate surgical interventions; should also help to plan the immediate resuscitation and ongoing care of the patient in conjunction with colleagues.
- *Orthopaedic doctor:* specialist surgical doctor.
- *Nursing staff.*

All trauma patients should be managed as follows:

1 *Primary survey and resuscitation:* a rapid ABCDE assessment is made and immediate resuscitation is instigated. If a team approach is used, then simultaneous assessment and treatment strategies can be used. If there is a lone rescuer, then it is important that 'A' problems are rectified before progressing to 'B' problems (and likewise 'C', 'D' and 'E'). If the patient needs immediate surgical intervention, then it may not be applicable to progress immediately to the next stage of management.
2 *Secondary survey:* it is essential that all trauma patients receive a 'top-to-toe' and 'front-to-back' examination in order to exclude any associated injuries. It is imperative that patients who have received immediate surgical intervention for their injuries receive a full secondary survey as soon as is practically possible.
3 *Definitive care:* if the patient requires admission, they should be admitted to the most appropriate clinical area where appropriate monitoring and treatment can be administered. This can range from a specialty ward to the intensive care unit (ICU).

■ KEY POINT
Primary assessment and resuscitation should always be performed first.

Radiography

The primary survey should include plain radiography of the chest and pelvis. Radiography of the cervical spine is also important, but time should not be wasted getting views if there are more urgent problems. It is safer in this instance to retain spinal immobilisation until further imaging can be obtained.

Focused assessment with sonography for trauma (FAST) scanning can be used in the emergency department as a 'rule-in' investigation for free abdominal fluid (81–88.2% sensitivity, 90–99.7% specificity).

Further imaging may be required, in particular computed tomography (CT) or magnetic resonance imaging (MRI). These imaging modalities require the patient to have some degree of haemodynamic stability.

● AIRWAY WITH CERVICAL SPINE CONTROL

The maintenance of a patent airway is the first priority in the management of any critically unwell patient. In the absence of a patent airway, breathing will become impaired, resulting in reduced levels of oxygenated blood. This in turn will exacerbate shock and lead to a deterioration in the patient's condition. Early management of the at-risk or compromised airway will therefore help to prevent an already unwell patient from deteriorating further. Symptoms and signs of airway obstruction include the following:

- *Difficulty breathing:* the respiratory rate will initially be increased as the body attempts to maintain adequate levels of oxygenation.
- *Altered patterns of respiration:* can range from the use of accessory muscles and 'seesaw respiration' in the partially occluded airway to no chest movement at all in the completely occluded airway.
- *Distress:* conscious and semiconscious patients will be extremely distressed. Associated hypoxaemia may also contribute to aggressive behaviour, leading ultimately to unconsciousness.
- *Choking:* this is a natural response and will hopefully lead to the expulsion of the foreign body.
- *Additional noises:*
  - Stridor – upper airways, inspiratory phase of respiration
  - Wheeze – lower airways, expiratory phase of respiration
  - Snoring – partial occlusion of the airway by the tongue or palate
  - Gurgling – fluid in the oropharynx.

Airway obstruction may be partial or complete and may occur at any level from the upper to the lower airways. Trauma patients are particularly susceptible to airway problems; the following may be a cause of airway compromise:

- Foreign body, e.g. blood, vomit, tooth
- Damage to the facial skeleton
- Soft tissue swelling
- Laryngospasm
- Central nervous system depression.

The immediate management should be to safely open the airway if there is any compromise. Some degree of partial obstruction may need to be tolerated if further manoeuvres endanger the patient.

Neck immobilisation

It is important that the neck is immobilised where there is any suspicion of neck injury. This is particularly pertinent in the pre-hospital setting. Neck immobilisation involves *all* of the following:

- *Hard collar:* this should be appropriately sized. A large collar may lead to excessive neck movement, while a small collar may lead to increased intracranial pressure.
- *Head immobilisation:* achieved by placing blocks either side of the head and using straps to secure the head.
- *Body immobilisation:* without this, the patient will still be able to pivot on the neck.

If the patient is combative, then immobilisation by hard collar alone is acceptable in order to prevent strain against the strapping leading to more neck trauma.

Airway management and interventions

All patients should have high-flow oxygen administered using a mask with a reservoir bag. There are a range of techniques used to open the airway, and it is important that simple airway techniques are attempted first.

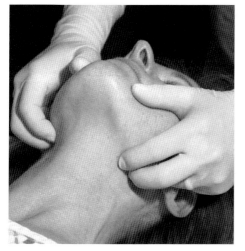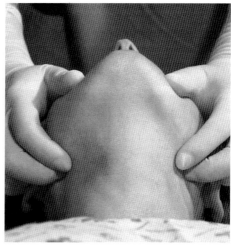

Figure 14.1 ● Airway-positioning manoeuvres (head-tilt, chin-lift and jaw-thrust).

Airway positioning

Where there is no evidence of a neck injury, the manoeuvre of choice is head-tilt and chin-lift (Figure 14.1). This realigns the soft tissues to provide an open airway. Where a neck injury is suspected, a head-tilt should not usually be performed. The only exception to this rule is where the patient has an obstructed airway and all other interventions have been unsuccessful. In this situation, the odds of the patient dying from an obstructed airway far outweigh the risks associated with a gentle, slow head-tilt until airway patency is achieved.

The jaw-thrust is an alternative airway manoeuvre that does not involve any movement of the neck. It is highly effective and involves lifting the soft tissues of the anterior pharyngeal wall upwards to provide an airway. The disadvantage is that it is effective only while the rescuer is performing the manoeuvre. If the rescuer moves on to perform another task, the airway will obstruct again.

Clearance of foreign bodies

Foreign bodies can be removed under direct vision. Rigid suction is used to remove fluid in the oropharynx (e.g. blood, vomit) but should be used only as far as can be visualised in order to avoid further trauma to the airway. Solid and some semisolid foreign bodies can be removed with forceps.

Airway adjuncts

Oropharyngeal

The oropharyngeal airway is used in unconscious patients as an airway adjunct. Its use is not advised in conscious or semiconscious patients as it may stimulate the gag reflex and precipitate vomiting. Caution should be used in the patient with maxillofacial trauma as insertion may precipitate bleeding, leading to further airway compromise.

The airway is inserted in adults upside-down and rotated through 180 degrees (Figure 14.2). In children, it is inserted the correct way round with the assistance of a spatula.

Nasopharyngeal

The nasopharyngeal airway (Figure 14.3) is used in conscious or semiconscious patients, but it can also be used in unconscious patients. Caution should be used in patients with basal skull

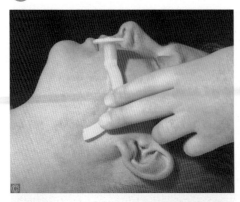

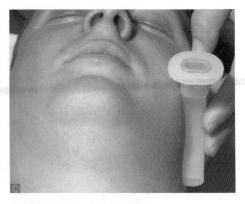

Figure 14.2 ● Sizing and insertion of oropharyngeal airway.

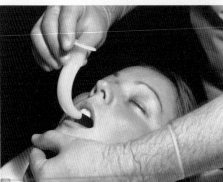

Figure 14.3 ● Insertion of nasopharyngeal airway.

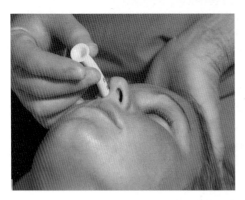

fracture, as aggressive insertion may lead to perforation of the cribriform plate. The airway should be lubricated before insertion in order to avoid epistaxis.

Advanced airway options

If simple airway manoeuvres and/or adjuncts are not successful, then the patient will need an advanced airway manoeuvre. In general, a clinician with advanced airway training performs this. There are two main options:

● *Laryngeal mask airway (LMA)*: this device sits in the back of the oropharynx and overlies the larynx. The tip provides some occlusion to the oesophagus. The level of skill needed to insert an LMA is less than that needed to perform tracheal intubation.

- *Tracheal intubation*: this technique provides full airway protection due to the presence of a cuffed tube in the trachea. The patient is more likely to need a rapid sequence intubation.

Surgical airway options

If none of the above procedures is successful, then a surgical airway can be life-saving. There are two main options:

- *Needle cricothyroidotomy*: a needle is inserted through the cricothyroid membrane and oxygen is insufflated under pressure into the lungs. This immediately life-saving technique provides oxygenation but not ventilation. It is only temporarily beneficial (< 30 min) and the patient will subsequently need to undergo a formal surgical airway.
- *Surgical cricothyroidotomy*: a cuffed tube (either commercially available equipment or a tracheal tube) is placed through an incision in the cricothyroid membrane under local anaesthetic. This enables formal ventilation and access for tracheal suctioning.

Tracheostomy requires skill and is time-consuming. It is therefore not the technique of choice in an emergency.

● BREATHING WITH ASSISTED VENTILATION

The maintenance of breathing is the second priority in the management of any critically unwell patient. Early management of inadequate breathing will prevent an already unwell patient from deteriorating any further.

Symptoms and signs of impaired breathing include the following:

- Tachypnoea
- Shortness of breath, anxiety and irritability
- Decrease in level of consciousness
- Absent or decreased air entry on auscultation
- Altered percussion note – dull with fluid, resonant with air
- Deviated trachea – indicative of mediastinal shift (e.g. tension pneumothorax)
- Cyanosis (late sign).

Breathing problems in the trauma patient may be due to the following causes:

- *Airway compromise*: this should be addressed as a priority.
- *Decreased respiratory drive*: e.g. central nervous system depression.
- *Decreased respiratory effort*: e.g. chest wall damage, burns, spinal injury.
- *Lung disorder*: e.g. haemothorax, pneumothorax.

The immediate management of the patient should be to ensure that the airway is open. High-flow oxygen should be administered and ventilatory support given if necessary. In the first instance, this can be accomplished by use of a self-inflating bag–valve–mask device. Early consideration should be given to tracheal intubation. Any underlying cause of breathing problems should be treated where possible.

Breathing management and interventions

Needle thoracostomy

This procedure is indicated in patients with tension pneumothorax. A needle or wide-bore cannula is inserted on the affected side in the second intercostal space in the mid-clavicular line. A hiss of escaping air confirms the presence of a tension pneumothorax. This procedure treats the tension aspect but does not treat the underlying pneumothorax. The patient will subsequently need a tube thoracostomy.

Tube thoracostomy

This procedure enables drainage of air and fluid from the pleural cavity. In the trauma patient, it is advisable to use a larger tube, as smaller-gauge tubes inserted using the Seldinger technique are unable to drain blood.

The tube is inserted using an aseptic technique. In conscious or semiconscious patients, local anaesthesia (1% lidocaine) should be used. The most sensate areas are the skin and the pleura. The location of insertion is usually the fifth intercostal space in the mid-axillary line. An incision should be made through the skin and then blunt dissection used through the soft tissues across the top of the rib in order to avoid the neurovascular structures. The intercostal nerves and vessels (neurovascular bundle), as in the abdominal wall, run between the middle and innermost layers of muscles of the chest wall. They are arranged in the following order, below the rib, from above downwards: intercostal vein, intercostal artery and intercostal nerve (VAN). Once the pleura has been punctured, a finger should be inserted if possible to clear any adhesions and check for other organs that may have herniated from the abdomen following a ruptured diaphragm. The chest tube is then inserted and connected to an underwater seal or valve to ensure that the movement of air/fluid is only one-way. A chest X-ray should be performed to check the position and efficacy of the tube.

Chest escharotomy

The restrictive effects of full-thickness burns to the chest wall can cause respiratory embarrassment. The burns do not have to be completely circumferential for this complication to ensue.

The indication for escharotomy (after consultation with the local burns unit) is the presence of all of the following:

- Large area of full-thickness burn to the chest wall crossing the mid-line
- Reduced level of respiratory excursion
- Deterioration of arterial blood gases.

This type of procedure should not be undertaken lightly, as complications can cause the patient to deteriorate further.

Escharotomies are usually done in the supine position and are done only through full-thickness burns that are insensate. The field should be cleaned with iodine. It is important to ensure that the patient has been cross-matched previously, as the amount of blood loss can be extensive and a blood transfusion may be required to prevent exacerbation of underlying shock. A standard chequerboard (grid) incision is no longer justifiable as the amount of blood loss can be extensive. As Figure 14.4 indicates, escharotomy scars should be well placed, starting laterally just anterior to the mid-axillary line in a coronal manner (Hettiaratchy and Papini, 2004). The depth of the scar should be to the point at which constriction is relieved and subcutaneous tissues bulge into the wound. This will be accompanied by bleeding. Only the burn tissue – not any underlying fascia – is divided, differentiating this procedure from a fasciotomy. The aim of a thoracic escharotomy is to remove skin tension in order to enable chest excursion to occur.

● CIRCULATION

Hypovolaemia is the most common cause of shock in the traumatised patient. Although the amount of blood loss is one of the components of classification of shock (Table 14.1), the degree to which a person can cope with volume loss depends on their physiological reserve.

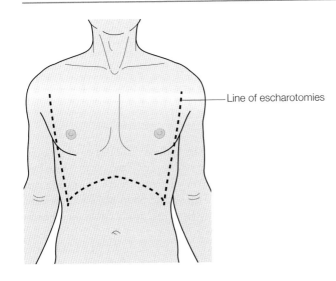

—Line of escharotomies

Figure 14.4 ● Site for escharotomy scar.

From Hettiaratchy S, Papini R (2004). Initial management of a major burn: II – assessment and resuscitation. *Br Med J* 329: 101–3. Adapted by permission from BMJ Publishing Group Limited.

Table 14.1 Classes of shock

Class	I	II	III	IV
Blood loss (mL)	< 750	750–1500	1500–2000	> 2000
Blood loss (%)	< 15	15–30	30–40	> 40
Pulse rate (beats/min)	< 100	> 100	> 120	> 140 or decreasing
Blood pressure	Normal	Normal	Decreased	Decreased
Pulse pressure	Normal	Decreased	Decreased	Decreased
Respiratory rate (breaths/min)	14–20	20–30	30–40	> 35 or decreasing
Urine output (mL/h)	> 30	20–30	5–15	Negligible
Mental status	Slightly anxious	Increasing anxiety	Anxious and confused	Confusion and lethargy
Pelvis	> 2 L			

Patients at the extremes of age behave differently. Children have a significantly better physiological reserve and so the decompensation point can appear suddenly and without warning. Conversely, elderly people may have very little reserve and may be on medication that prevents a compensatory response. The decompensation point may occur sooner, resulting in earlier symptoms of shock.

The ultimate aim of treatment of haemorrhage is to restore normovolaemia. This has two elements:

● Prevention of further loss
● Fluid resuscitation.

Prevention of further loss

The common compartments into which a large-volume haemorrhage can occur are as follows:

- External haemorrhage
- Thoracic cavity
- Peritoneal cavity
- Retroperitoneal
- Pelvic fracture
- Multiple long-limb fracture sites.

External haemorrhage

If the haemorrhage is obvious, external pressure needs to be applied. The degree of pressure depends upon whether the bleeding is venous or arterial.

If ongoing external blood loss continues despite the above attempts, then a tourniquet can be used temporarily to attempt to arrest limb bleeding. This should be in place for less than 60 min in order to prevent complications, e.g. rhabdomyonecrosis, crush syndrome or limb gangrene in extreme cases.

Thoracic cavity

Major vessel injury including aortic disruption usually results in rapid fatal haemorrhage. The absence of solid structures within the chest cavity prevents early tamponade, and ensuing haemorrhage can be unrestrained. Any visible foreign body causing a penetrating chest injury should be left in situ until the patient reaches theatre, as it may be tamponading a major vessel.

Volume replacement should be instituted before chest drainage is undertaken, as decompensation may occur quickly due to the release of the tamponade effect. The degree of volume loss from a chest tube dictates further management. Blood loss of more than 200 mL/h from the time of insertion or an initial loss of more than 1500 mL of blood should alert the clinician to the requirement for a thoracotomy.

Cardiac tamponade causes shock due to mechanical obstruction. Penetrating precordial wounds are the usual cause of tamponade, but it can also occur in blunt trauma. Blood accumulates in the pericardial space, causing restriction of diastolic filling. This leads to a reduction in the end diastolic volume, which leads to a reduction of stroke volume. Beck's triad (low blood pressure, muffled heart sounds, raised jugular venous pressure) may help in the diagnosis, although these signs may not always be present, due to ongoing volume loss. Treatment of cardiac tamponade requires relief of the obstruction to enable cardiac filling to occur. This can be done using either a percutaneous (needle aspiration with insertion point to the left of the xiphichondral junction, 45° to the skin, aiming towards the tip of the left scapula) or open thoracotomy approach (see below).

Peritoneal cavity

Fluid loss into the peritoneal cavity in an obtunded patient may be difficult to determine and may be missed. FAST ultrasound scanning in the resuscitation room may help in the diagnosis.

If the patient is stable and resuscitative measures are in situ, then CT scanning may be of use. In a critically injured patient, CT scanning is not without its pitfalls and marked deterioration can occur during the process of undertaking a scan. A clinical decision should therefore be taken with regard to an urgent laparotomy.

In the absence of readily available CT scanning, a diagnostic peritoneal lavage (DPL) may be indicated (see below).

Retroperitoneal haemorrhage

The retroperitoneal space is a large potential space that can accommodate volume loss from major vessels or viscera or from significant musculoskeletal injury such as pelvic fractures. This area is usually well contained and therefore self-tamponades. If time allows, CT scanning will enable the diagnosis to be made and an appropriate surgical strategy to be instituted.

Pelvic fractures

Pelvic fractures can bleed torrentially due to a combination of venous and arterial bleeding. Any injury that increases the volume of the pelvis is at risk of significant blood loss. The degree of bleeding depends on the structures injured and the space into which bleeding occurs but can easily result in more than 30 per cent blood volume loss. Fatal exsanguination can occur with an isolated open-book pelvic fracture.

Plain X-rays of the pelvis are used as part of the initial trauma series to identify the type of injury. It is also recommended by some authorities that a single pelvic spring be performed to determine the stability of the pelvis. In non-expert hands, this is unnecessary and possibly a dangerous intervention, due to disruption of clots.

The options for managing pelvic fractures include the following:

- External fixation – requires skill and expertise and, although useful in bringing together the bony edges, does not guarantee pelvic stability or arrest of bleeding
- Pelvic sling – by using canvas sheets and towel clips, this can bring the pelvic edges together
- Open surgery
- Interventional radiology.

Long-limb fractures

The average amount of blood loss per fracture site is shown in Table 14.2.

The degree of haemorrhage is usually contained by the surrounding structures, as long as their integrity is not breached. In a closed limb fracture, the degree of bleeding can be reduced by splintage and alignment, as this brings the fracture ends in close proximity to decrease the potential space of bleeding. There is also a significant risk of compartment syndrome due to the build-up of pressure in a contained space.

Fluid resuscitation

The aim is first to restore normal perfusion to vital organs in the first instance and then to ultimately restore normal volume in the vascular compartment.

Guidelines from the National Institute for Health and Clinical Excellence (NICE, 2004) suggest that, in the setting of trauma, pre-hospital fluid should be administered to adults and older children if there is no palpable radial pulse (or for penetrating torso injuries, if a central pulse cannot be felt). Crystalloid should be given in boluses of no more than 250 mL at a time. This avoids the pitfall of excessive fluid resuscitation raising central pressures and causing further bleeding due to disruption of clots and/or dilution of clotting factors.

The type of fluid used for resuscitation is controversial. The risks of colloid administration (e.g. allergic reactions, clotting abnormality) can be alleviated by the use of crystalloids. In a

Table 14.2 Average blood loss per fracture site

Fracture site	Average blood loss
Humerus	750 mL
Femoral fracture	
Closed	1.5 L
Open	> 2 L

Cochrane review, Alderson *et al.* (2004) found there to be no difference in mortality between critically ill/injured patients given colloids and those given crystalloids. They suggest that colloids are not associated with an improvement in survival and, as they are more expensive, they should not be used in this setting.

Two large-bore intravenous cannulae should be inserted and blood taken for full blood count, cross-match, urea, creatinine and lactate. Other tests indicated may include amylase and arterial blood gases. Consideration should be given as to whether to perform a beta human chorionic gonadotrophin (β-HCG) test in women of childbearing age.

An initial bolus of 2 L of crystalloid is administered to any major traumatised patient. Ongoing resuscitation then depends upon the response to this initial fluid bolus:

- *Immediate response and normalisation:* resuscitation has been adequate.
- *Initial response but further deterioration:* suggests there is ongoing loss that has been partially treated by fluid resuscitation. The source of the haemorrhage should be sought and controlled, along with ongoing crystalloid and blood transfusion.
- *Non-response:* may be due to one of two causes:
  - Shock is not due to haemorrhagic volume loss
  - There is catastrophic bleeding occurring that is not amenable to fluid resuscitation. In this circumstance, the need to identify the bleeding site is urgent if fatality is to be avoided. Blood will be required, but most importantly the patient requires surgical intervention.

Patients with major burns require fluid for replacement of losses. It is rare for burns alone to cause hypovolaemic shock within the first few hours, and other causes (e.g. coincidental injuries) should be sought and treated accordingly.

The Parkland formula provides a guide to fluid resuscitation in the first 24 h based upon the percentage of body surface area (%BSA) affected by second- or third-degree burns:

$$\text{Amount of intravenous fluid in first 24 h} = \text{weight in kg} \times 4 \text{ mL} \times \text{\%BSA burned}$$

The %BSA can be estimated in one of two ways. Small burns can be estimated by considering the area of the closed palm of the patient's hand to represent 1 per cent. Alternatively, the 'rule of nines' can be used for adults with extensive burns.

The fluid administered is crystalloid. One-half of the amount is administered in the first 8 h following the burn and the remainder over the subsequent 16 h. Young children should receive maintenance fluid as well.

Circulation interventions

Resuscitative thoracotomy

Indications when there is not a cardiothoracic surgery unit on site are as follows:

- *Penetrating chest trauma in extremis or pulseless electrical activity (PEA) cardiac arrest in the emergency department:* the thoracotomy can be used to treat a cardiac tamponade, repair a myocardial injury and repair a great vessel injury.
- *Penetrating infradiaphragmatic trauma in extremis or in PEA on arrival at the emergency department:* this enables the surgeon to cross-clamp the descending aorta at the supradiaphragmatic level in order to redirect blood flow.

Once a thoracotomy is indicated, it should be done expeditiously. There are two approaches:

- Left anterolateral approach through the fifth intercostal space
- Clam procedure – an extension of a one-sided thoracotomy across the mid-line and into the same intercostal space on the opposite side.

If the heart has been injured, then a pericardial tamponade may be obvious, which will need to be evacuated. A hole should be made in the pericardium to evacuate the clot. Avoid the left phrenic nerve, which lies along the lateral border of the heart.

Myocardial injuries should be stitched by non-absorbable sutures. This can be done on a beating heart. A Foley catheter can often be used to stem blood flow initially. Great vessel injuries can be temporarily repaired similar to a cardiac injury.

Cross-clamping the descending aorta requires the left lung to be lifted anteriorly and collapsed down. The mediastinal pleura should be dissected from the surface of the aorta, and a window needs to be made with blunt dissection behind the aorta where it rests on the vertebral column. A soft aortic clamp can then be introduced just above the level of the diaphragm. (This procedure is performed in the resuscitation room before transfer to theatre.) The wound can then be closed temporarily and a chest drain left in situ before the patient is transferred to theatre or a specialist centre for ongoing care. The clamp should not be in situ for more than 30 min.

Focused assessment with sonography for trauma

FAST was introduced in the early 1990s. It can be performed in the emergency department. The aim is to look for free fluid. Four views are utilised:

- Perihepatic space
- Perisplenic space
- Pelvis
- Pericardium.

FAST has a sensitivity of 81–88 per cent and a specificity of 90–99.7 per cent. It is therefore a 'rule-in' tool; the absence of a positive scan does not mean that there is no free fluid in the abdomen or pericardial space.

The advantages of FAST are that it is non-invasive, can be performed at the bedside in the resuscitation room, is relatively cheap, does not involve irradiation, and can be carried out by surgeons and emergency physicians. The disadvantages are that there may be technical limitations and it is operator-dependent.

Venous cut-down

This procedure is of value if percutaneous attempts at cannulation have failed. This technique is not used as much since the advent of ultrasound guided cannulation. The most common site for a cut-down is the great saphenous vein just above the medial malleolus.

Diagnostic peritoneal lavage

This procedure involves inserting a peritoneal dialysis catheter into the peritoneal cavity once the stomach and bladder have been decompressed with a catheter and gastric tube respectively. Then 10 mL/kg of warmed normal saline is instilled and then drained. The test is positive if laboratory analysis indicates more than 100 000 red blood cells per cubic millimetre, or more than 500 white blood cells per cubic millimetre. Retroperitoneal injuries cannot be excluded by a negative test. Complications of this procedure include haemorrhage, peritonitis, damage to intra-abdominal structures, and wound infection. The common availability of fast CT scanning has largely superseded DPL.

● DYSFUNCTION

The assessment of the conscious state of a critically injured patient is an important part of the initial management of the patient. It not only gives a clue to the immediate conscious level of the patient but also is a dynamic measure that, when recorded recurrently, gives vital clues to the state of the patient.

Dysfunction can be measured using the following:

- AVPU score (see below)
- Glasgow coma score (GCS)
- Examination of pupils.

Both GCS and pupillary reactivity need to be reassessed frequently in critically injured patients.

AVPU score

A patient's AVPU score is assessed as follows:

A – alert
V – responds to voice
P – responds to pain
U – unresponsive.

The system is simple, repeatable and easy to use. It has little intra- and intra-rater variability and forms the basis of the conscious level score in the Medical Early Warning Score (MEWS) tool. It does not provide the same amount of information as the GCS, but it is a useful tool for the initial assessment of the patient. It is accepted that patients who score P or U have a GCS of 8 or less.

Glasgow coma score

The GCS (Table 14.3) requires expertise and skill to use, and it suffers from some intra- and inter-rater variability. However, it is singularly the most important measure of consciousness that is universally accepted. GCS 15 is normal and GCS 3 is the minimum that can be achieved. A GCS of 8 or less is coma and requires immediate assessment of the airway.

Table 14.3 Glasgow coma score (GCS)

Eyes open	Spontaneously	4
	To speech	3
	To pain	2
	None	1
Verbal response	Normal conversation	5
	Confused conversation	4
	Inappropriate words	3
	Inappropriate sounds	2
	None	1
Best motor response	Obey commands	6
	Localise to pain	5
	Withdraws	4
	Flex to pain	3
	Extension to pain	2
	None	1
GCS	Total	15

Examination of pupils

The pupillary response is an important part of the disability assessment of a patient. Pupils should be assessed for the following:

- *Size:*
  - Small – consider opioids, brainstem injury
  - Large – consider hypoxia, hypothermia, drugs (adrenaline, atropine, barbiturates), postictal state.
- *Equality:* unilateral dilated pupil – ipsilateral lesion, third nerve lesion.
- *Reactivity.*

● SECONDARY EXAMINATION: EXPOSURE

Once the initial assessment has been undertaken and the patient is stable, a thorough evaluation of the entirety of the patient should be undertaken as soon as possible. This may be delayed if the patient has to have a critical intervention to maintain the airway, breathing or circulation.

> ■ KEY POINT
> A full secondary survey should be performed as soon as possible after the initial assessment and stabilisation of the patient.

This detailed evaluation requires the patient to be exposed and examined from head to toe and from front to back while maintaining normothermia. All clothing, particularly if wet, needs to be removed, and debris around the patient such as broken glass or soil needs to be cleared. If the patient has arrived on a long board, it is important to log-roll the patient off the board as soon as practically possible in order to prevent pressure sores. At the same time, an examination of the spine and a rectal examination can be performed. All clothing removed should be kept to one side, as they may be required for forensic examination by the police.

● ONGOING CARE

Patient transfer

Once the patient has left the emergency department they will be transported to theatre, a critical care facility such as ICU or high dependency unit (HDU) or a ward. The patient may also be transferred out of the receiving hospital to a tertiary centre for ongoing management.

Ideally, the patient should be haemodynamically stable before transfer. Patients who are being transferred to theatre for an emergency surgical procedure may not be stable. In all other cases, it is essential that adequate preparation is made before transfer. The patient should be monitored fully, and appropriate resuscitation equipment should be available throughout the transfer. The transfer team should be fully trained and capable of performing further resuscitation if necessary.

All notes and X-rays should accompany the patient, and the receiving ward should have prior warning so that they are expecting the patient. On arrival, the patient should be reassessed. If the patient needs to go to theatre before a thorough secondary survey, this survey should be performed as soon as is practically possible.

Monitoring

The trauma patient needs the following minimum monitoring performed on a continuous or recurrent basis:

- Electrocardiogram (ECG)
- Pulse oximetry
- Blood pressure
- Urine output
- GCS.

Other monitoring depends on the severity of the conditions, e.g. invasive blood pressure, central venous pressure, pulmonary artery catheter and intracranial pressure.

PITFALLS IN THE MANAGEMENT OF SEVERELY INJURED PATIENTS

- Senior input is essential. A single poly-traumatised patient can often tax the resources of a hospital. This is due to the complexity of the injuries and the fact that certain specialist care may not be available immediately on site. Senior input ensures that timely and correct decisions are made.
- Documentation and communication need to be meticulous. The circumstances surrounding the injuries may be subject to police investigation.
- Every patient should receive a thorough secondary survey. Patients who are transferred to theatre before this survey can be completed should receive a secondary survey at the earliest opportunity. Repeat examinations, ideally by the same clinician, do the patient no harm and may highlight a slowly evolving pathology.
- The additional effects of alcohol and drugs on patients who are traumatised can make the assessment even more difficult. It should never be assumed that a head-injured patient is drunk; rather, assume that the intoxicated patient has a head injury and needs further investigation.
- Patient monitoring should be performed in a clinical area that has the necessary expertise. Changes in physiological parameters should be acted upon swiftly.

SUMMARY

- We recommend the ABCDE approach to assessment and management of the severely injured patient: airway with cervical spine control, breathing with assisted ventilation, circulation, dysfunction and exposure.
- Primary assessment and resuscitation should be performed first.
- A full secondary survey should be performed as soon as is practically possible.

QUESTIONS

1 What is the order of priority of management in the standardised approach to a trauma victim?
2 What radiological modalities assist the clinical assessment?
3 Describe the interventions available for the management of airway compromise.
4 Name the compartments that large-volume haemorrhage can occur into.
5 What fluids are recommended for the management of hypovolaemic shock?
6 What fluid regime should be used in the first 24 h for a 70-kg male with 50 per cent body surface area burns?

REFERENCES

Alderson P, Bunn F, Lefebvre C, et al. (2004). Human albumin solution for resuscitation and volume expansion in critically ill patients. *Cochrane Database Syst Rev* (4): CD001208.

American College of Surgeons (2004). *Advanced Trauma Life Support for Doctors*, 7th edn. Chicago, IL: American College of Surgeons.

European Resuscitation Council (2006). *Advanced Life Support (ALS): The European Trauma Course Manual*. Antwerp: European Resuscitation Council.

Hettiaratchy S, Papini R (2004). Initial management of a major burn: II – assessment and resuscitation. *Br Med J* **329**: 101–3.

National Institute for Health and Clinical Excellence (NICE) (2004). *Trauma: Fluid Replacement Therapy*. Technology appraisal TA74. London: National Institute for Health and Clinical Excellence. www.nice.org.uk/guidance/index.jsp?action=byID&o=11526.

15 — Management of abdominal trauma

JEF Fitzgerald and Mike Larvin

● INTRODUCTION

Abdominal trauma is a frequent occurrence and must always be considered in the assessment of a severely injured patient. Approximately 15 per cent of all trauma patients suffer abdominal injuries, and of these over 25 per cent require exploratory surgery. It has been shown that the majority of preventable deaths from trauma result from unrecognised intra-abdominal haemorrhage. The timely recognition and appropriate surgical management of abdominal trauma is an essential lifesaving skill that can dramatically impact on outcomes. However, outside of major trauma centres, the relevant expertise may be lacking, making abdominal trauma one of the most challenging conditions a surgeon can face.

> ■ KEY POINT
> About 15 per cent of all trauma patients have abdominal injuries; of these, over 25 per cent require exploratory surgery.

● MECHANISMS OF ABDOMINAL TRAUMA

Consideration of the underlying mechanism is important in establishing potential patterns of injury, together with decisions regarding subsequent management.

Blunt injury

Visceral injury resulting from a non-penetrating mechanism is the most common cause of abdominal trauma in the UK. Blunt injury frequently arises from falls, assaults and road traffic incidents, with the patient as either a pedestrian or an occupant of a vehicle. In the latter case the vehicle occupant suffers a sudden deceleration injury, which creates significant shear forces within the abdomen. This may give rise to a spectrum of potential complications from torn mesentery to complete avulsion of organs on their attachments, or tearing of the organs themselves. This may result in immediate and catastrophic haemorrhage. Injury may also occur from the direct application of pressure on to the abdominal compartment. Such crush patterns are also commonly seen in combination with deceleration-type injuries in motor vehicle incidents where vehicle occupants have been restrained by a lap-belt. This direct trauma may be sufficient to cause rupture of the underlying organs. It is important to note that there may be an initial absence of overt clinical signs to indicate that blunt abdominal injury has occurred, making recognition and assessment considerably more challenging than that for penetrating trauma.

Penetrating injury

Penetrating injury is more common in North America than the UK. In North America, it accounts for 35 per cent of all cases admitted to urban trauma centres. Penetrating injury typically arises from stabbings, ballistic injuries (shooting) and industrial accidents. The standard management of penetrating abdominal injury was, for many years, based on mandatory laparotomy, greater consideration of the mechanisms underlying the injury have led to a more selective strategy. Stab wounds arise from a low-energy penetration, with a limited and more predictable pattern of injury localised to the immediately surrounding structures. Ballistic injury involves high-velocity, high-energy projectiles, with unpredictable and diffuse patterns of underlying damage. In addition to the direct laceration caused by the penetrating projectile, the massive dissipation of energy associated with this causes widespread compression shockwaves through the surrounding tissues. Cavitation injuries may therefore arise as part of this process, causing damage at considerable distance from the impact site. The degree and pattern of injury arising from shooting incidents are related to the type of firearm involved. High-velocity rifled firearms have the greatest capacity for cavitation-related tissue damage, while smoothbore shotgun injury is more likely to result in direct localised tissue laceration.

● RECOGNITION AND ASSESSMENT OF ABDOMINAL TRAUMA

Initial management of the severely injured patient is described in Chapter 14. With the exception of stopping immediately life-threatening external haemorrhage, initial resuscitation should follow the accepted primary survey convention of airway–breathing–circulation. The abdomen may need to be considered when circulatory problems are addressed, if it is thought that bleeding here may be the source of hypovolaemic shock. In other situations, appropriate abdominal assessment must take place as part of a secondary survey.

The history surrounding the injury is essential. Information should be sought from witnesses and paramedics at the scene and should include details such as the mechanism of injury, height of fall, estimated speed of vehicle, type of weapon, distance from firearm, and estimated blood loss at scene, as appropriate to the cause. Objective clinical assessment of the abdomen on the basis of history and examination is essential but unreliable, even in the awake patient. This may be due to the presence of distracting injuries, impaired level of consciousness or altered sensation. In the absence of indicators for immediate surgical intervention, serial examination of the abdomen at regular intervals by the same clinician may provide useful information.

Initial examination should focus as closely on indicators of haemodynamic stability as much as on abdominal findings on examination. It must be remembered that the abdominal cavity runs from the groin crease to the nipple anteriorly, and any penetrating injury in this region should be considered to have entered the abdomen. However, a patient also has flanks and a back, and injuries in these areas may be missed without adequate inspection where appropriate. In the early mild to moderate blunt injury, there may be no positive findings on initial abdominal examination. Further objective assessment must therefore be guided by the haemodynamic parameters of the patient; if these are of concern, then a decision must be made as to whether the abdomen is the likely cause.

In a shocked patient who is unresponsive to adequate resuscitation, and where other causes of bleeding are not suspected (e.g. thoracic, long bone, external haemorrhage), further investi-

---

> ## Box 15.1 Indicators of significant intra-abdominal injury
>
> - Mechanism of injury
> - Positive examination findings
> - Associated chest or pelvic trauma
> - Unexplained hypovolaemic shock
> - Unexplained haemodynamic instability.

gation is inappropriate and the bleeding must be controlled with immediate surgical intervention.

In blunt abdominal trauma, given potentially equivocal findings on examination, a significant contributor to the subsequent morbidity and mortality is a delay in establishing the abdomen as the cause. If indicators of significant intra-abdominal injury are present (Box 15.1), and the patient is stabilised, then there is time for further objective assessment. If the patient is unstable and an abdominal cause is not established clearly, then a balanced decision must be taken, aided by immediate bedside evaluation or imaging, as to whether surgical exploration is required.

In the initial management of abdominal trauma it is important to remember the following:

- Adequate analgesia will not impair your clinical assessment of the patient.
- Signs of peritonism or ongoing abdominal bleeding warrant surgical intervention.
- Blood transfusion does not stop the bleeding.

In addition to frank peritonism, other clinical signs that may prove useful include obvious or progressive abdominal distension. Care should also be taken to avoid being caught out by 'transient responders' – patients in whom haemodynamic compromise is stabilised initially with fluid resuscitation, only for instability to reoccur as blood pressure is restored due to on-going underlying haemorrhage.

● INVESTIGATIONS IN ABDOMINAL TRAUMA

Baseline investigations

All trauma cases, regardless of aetiology and mechanism, require baseline investigations in accordance with Advanced Trauma Life Support (ATLS) guidelines. Blood samples should be taken for full blood count, urea and electrolytes, clotting, and group and save/cross-match. Consider including a beta human chorionic gonadotrophin (β-HCG) in female patients of reproductive age.

Plain radiographs

A supine chest radiograph should be taken as part of the initial trauma series. Although reducing the ability to visualise free air under the diaphragm as per an erect chest radiograph, this may still be helpful in suggesting diaphragmatic rupture from a fundal bubble displaced into the chest, or lower rib fractures highlighting the potential for underlying liver, splenic or renal injury.

> ■ KEY POINT
> A supine chest radiograph should be taken as part of the initial trauma series.

Ultrasound

Ultrasound is a useful bedside adjunct in the rapid non-invasive assessment of the stable or unstable abdominal trauma patient. Ultrasound is particularly sensitive at revealing free fluid within the abdomen, although this has been shown to be related to the skill of the sonographer. Ultrasound is not useful in detecting intra-abdominal injuries that do not result in free fluid. In the trauma setting, handheld ultrasound machines can now be used by trained emergency department and surgical team members to quickly evaluate specific sites within the abdomen. The use of this focused assessment with sonography for trauma (FAST) is described in Chapter 14.

Diagnostic peritoneal lavage

Diagnostic peritoneal lavage (DPL) is a traditional method of evaluating the equivocal traumatised abdomen. It has been largely superseded by FAST (see above) and computed tomography (CT) where available. In the assessment of blunt trauma without indication for immediate laparotomy, DPL's principle of rapid, sensitive detection of free intra-abdominal fluid (whether blood, faeces or bile) still stands, with a 98 per cent sensitivity for detecting intra-abdominal bleeding. Its use in the assessment of penetrating trauma is less sensitive.

> ■ KEY POINT
> DPL has been largely superseded by FAST and CT.

Diagnostic peritoneal lavage is carried out as follows:

1 Place a urinary catheter and nasogastric tube.
2 Make a small midline abdominal incision under local anaesthetic, sufficient to allow introduction of a catheter.
3 Extend this through the linea alba and into the peritoneum.
4 Observe any free fluid on entering the abdominal cavity (positive criteria; Box 15.2).
5 If no free fluid is seen, pass catheter tubing into abdomen.
6 Infuse 1 L of normal saline.
7 Place back below the level of the patient and siphon fluid back out.
8 Observe for frank blood and bowel contents.
9 Send sample for laboratory analysis.

Diagnostic peritoneal lavage cannot detect which organ is injured or the degree of injury sustained; nor can it identify retroperitoneal injuries. Relative contraindications to DPL are pregnancy and patients who have undergone previous abdominal surgery, where adhesions render the technique much less sensitive. The presence of blood in the abdomen from other causes, such as pelvic injury, may give false positive results. Research indicates that many

---

Box 15.2 Positive peritoneal lavage criteria

■ Aspiration of frank blood
■ Aspiration of frank bowel contents
■ Lavage fluid in urinary catheter bag or chest drain (where present)
■ Aspirate red cell count > 100 000/mm^3
■ Aspirate white cell count > 500/mm^3
■ Aspirate amylase > 175 units/mL
■ Detection of bile, bacteria or faecal matter (laboratory examination required).

hospitals in the UK do not have on-site laboratory staff out of hours to process the aspirated samples rapidly.

Computed tomography

In a stable trauma patient, CT scanning remains the diagnostic modality of choice. However, great care is required in selecting patients for CT. Transporting the patient away from the resuscitation area to the scanner should not be undertaken in the presence of haemodynamic instability or without adequate monitoring, staff and facilities at hand in case the patient deteriorates.

> ■ KEY POINT
> In a stable trauma patient, CT scanning remains the diagnostic modality of choice.

The advantages of CT over other imaging methods are numerous. The use of contrast enhancement aids the diagnosis of solid organ injury, and this can be graded according to radiological criteria, greatly guiding management decisions. Free gas and air within the abdominal cavity are also readily identified. Computed tomography is not without its limitations, however, and its sensitivity for mesenteric, small bowel and diaphragmatic injuries is low.

If a CT scan is indicated, consider scanning head to toe in order to avoid unnecessary returns to the scanner.

Contrast studies

Contrast studies are of use in the diagnosis and evaluation of suspected bladder rupture or renal injury. Intravenous contrast urography allows appropriate imaging of the kidneys via CT. Cystography via instillation of contrast into the bladder through a urinary catheter followed by plain radiography can be sufficient to identify leakage into the abdominal cavity or surrounding structures.

Diagnostic laparoscopy

In the equivocal, stable patient, diagnostic laparoscopy is useful in identifying diaphragmatic injuries or where it is unclear whether a penetrating injury has broached the abdominal cavity. Otherwise, the use of diagnostic laparoscopy has not been established as beneficial in blunt abdominal trauma, as it offers no benefit over other imaging modalities in the diagnosis of retroperitoneal injury or assessment of small bowel injury. Diagnostic laparoscopy also carries considerable risks, as well as costs, with the requirement for anaesthetic and pneumoperitoneum (Zantut et al., 1997).

● PRINCIPLES OF ABDOMINAL TRAUMA MANAGEMENT

The overriding principles for the surgical management of acute abdominal trauma are to control bleeding and to limit contamination, whether from bowel contents, bile or otherwise.

Trauma laparotomy

If the decision is made for surgical intervention, then this should proceed as a 'trauma laparotomy'. Rapid transfer to the operating theatre is required, and resuscitation continues simultaneously rather than delaying definitive treatment. The safest place in the hospital to resuscitate such a patient is inside the operating theatre.

A generous midline incision should be made from xiphisternum to symphysis pubis. With suction and packs standing by, the abdominal cavity is entered, and bleeding is controlled by way of packing the four quadrants. These packs are removed in a stepwise fashion, such that the most likely area of haemorrhage is exposed last, and bleeding points are dealt with appropriately as they are encountered. In extremis, bleeding may be controlled by manual pressure on the abdominal aorta by reaching up under the diaphragm to the point it descends through the hiatus.

Following the control of bleeding, contamination within the cavity is controlled by suturing or stapling off the affected bowel. A systematic inspection of the entire abdominal cavity must then take place, looking for further injuries. Starting proximally as the gastrointestinal tract enters the abdomen, the bowel must be examined methodically from stomach, duodenum, small bowel, mesentery and finally colon into the pelvis. The liver and spleen are inspected, followed by retroperitoneal structures and finally the diaphragm.

Damage-control laparotomy

The concept of damage-control surgery, or abbreviated laparotomy, was developed in the American urban trauma centres in the 1980s. Although traditional teaching promoted the definitive repair of abdominal injuries at initial trauma laparotomy, damage-control surgery eschews this in favour of prioritising haemorrhage and contamination control. Further surgery is then deferred until the patient has been resuscitated adequately in an intensive care setting (Hirshberg and Walden, 1997).

The principle stems from observation that such trauma patients were frequently dying not from failure of the definitive surgery but from a 'lethal triad' of coagulopathy, acidosis and hypothermia. These were exacerbated by prolonged definitive operating, such that a survival advantage could be gained from curtailing this. Once lifesaving procedures are complete, damage-control surgery is halted and a temporary abdominal closure is fashioned. A planned 'second look' occurs after appropriate stabilisation has taken place, typically 24–48 h later. At this point, definitive surgery may take place.

Not all patients with abdominal trauma require damage-control techniques. Patient selection is important and includes those showing evidence of significant physiological derangement that has not been corrected with initial resuscitation.

Indications for damage-control surgery include the following:

- Acidosis: pH $\leq$ 7.2
- Hypothermia: core temperature $\leq$ 34 °C
- Coagulopathy: transfusion of $\geq$ 5000 mL or total fluid infusion $\geq$ 1200 mL
- Injuries that would otherwise require overly time-consuming surgery (> 90 min)
- Intra-abdominal tissue oedema preventing formal closure of the abdominal wall.

Conservative management

Non-operative intervention is an equally important strategy in dealing with abdominal trauma. A trauma laparotomy is not mandatory in all cases. Patient selection is vital, as the additional morbidity and mortality associated with negative findings are considerable. Particularly for solid viscus injuries, CT imaging in an otherwise stable patient is useful in guiding the need for intervention. If a decision is made to pursue non-operative management, then close, regular reassessment of the patient is required, preferably within a high dependency or intensive care environment.

Indications for trauma laparotomy include the following:

- Haemodynamically unstable patient with abdominal trauma
- Positive findings on objective evaluation necessitating surgical intervention (FAST or CT scan)
- Penetrating abdominal gunshot injury

- Stab wound to abdomen penetrating the peritoneum
- Evisceration of abdominal viscus.

● MANAGEMENT OF SPECIFIC ORGAN INJURIES

Diaphragmatic injuries

Although penetrating thoracoabdominal trauma is likely to involve diaphragmatic injury, similar injuries arising from blunt abdominal trauma are frequently missed. Subsequent critical cardiovascular and respiratory compromise may result from abdominal contents herniating into the chest. Smaller defects may not become apparent until months or years after the original trauma (gastric incarceration and bowel obstruction are well recognised complications). Diaphragmatic rupture is an important indicator of the severity of trauma, commonly associated with other intra-abdominal injuries. It is more common on the left side, due to the protective position of the liver on the right, and most cases are identified only at surgery. Computed tomography has a low sensitivity for detecting diaphragmatic injury, and suspicion of this, in the absence of other indicators for immediate surgery, is best confirmed by laparoscopy. Once identified, small injuries can be oversewn with interrupted, non-absorbable sutures, while larger injuries may require a prosthetic mesh to cover the defect.

> ■ KEY POINT
> Smaller defects may not become apparent until months or years after the original trauma.

Gastric injury

The stomach is generally well protected by the ribcage, such that penetrating injury is more likely than blunt trauma to cause damage. Diagnosis may not always be obvious; where suspected, aspiration of blood from a nasogastric tube may confirm suspicions in an otherwise stable patient. It is important to look for posterior wall injuries by opening the lesser sac through the gastrocolic omentum. Primary closure of the injury can usually be achieved in layers following local tissue debridement.

Duodenal injury

Injury to the duodenum may occur by blunt or penetrating trauma. Isolated injury is unusual, given the duodenum's close anatomical relations and retroperitoneal position within the abdomen. Diagnosis may be particularly delayed in the case of a posterior rupture into the retroperitoneum. Although CT scanning may reveal characteristic signs of localised air or extravasation of contrast, intraoperative evaluation at trauma laparotomy is required if surgery is indicated. Here, a Kocher's manoeuvre is used in order to mobilise the duodenum, thus allowing adequate inspection. Surgical management depends on the degree of injury sustained. The duodenum injury scale can be used to guide management decisions regarding the need for operative intervention. Primary suture and drainage following local tissue debridement may be possible, whereas more complex injuries frequently require specialist input when the patient is stabilised.

Pancreatic injury

The pancreas lies deep within the abdominal cavity and is well protected by surrounding structures, such that direct injury is uncommon. In common with duodenal injuries, diagnosis is not always obvious and may be delayed (Boffard and Brooks, 2000). Other than penetrating trauma, epigastric crush-type injuries can also occur, whereby the pancreas is compressed against the vertebral bodies posteriorly. Where there is suspicion of pancreatic trauma at laparotomy, such as visible haematoma around the pancreas, the organ must be evaluated thoroughly. An extended Kocher's manoeuvre with division of the gastrocolic omentum allows access for visualisation. Further mobilisation is required to inspect the organ posteriorly. Simple injuries without duct involvement can be managed by local tissue debridement and drainage, and on-table pancreatography has been supported by some surgeons in order to identify this. Distal pancreatectomy is used for other injuries in the tail and body, with ligation of the pancreatic duct. These more complex injuries may require resection, with specialist input when the patient is stabilised. Pancreatic injuries carry a significant morbidity, with pancreatic fistula being the most frequent complication. The pancreatic injury scale may be useful in guiding management. Complications of pancreatic injury include the following:

- Fistula formation
- Acute pancreatitis
- Pseudo-cyst formation
- Intra-abdominal abscess.

Small bowel injury

The small bowel is commonly injured in penetrating trauma. However, deceleration and shearing forces may also cause significant damage from blunt mechanisms. Indirect injury may occur from damage to the mesentery and subsequent interruption of blood supply. Although penetrating trauma triggers a trauma laparotomy at which the small bowel can be 'run' and inspected for damage, small bowel injuries associated with blunt trauma may be more difficult to diagnose. Computed tomography findings for hollow viscus injury lack sensitivity, and false negative rates of 15 per cent have been reported. Penetrating injuries may be debrided and closed with suture. More widespread damage to the bowel or mesentery may necessitate resection. In the damage-control setting, this is commonly controlled by simply stapling off the stumps of affected bowel, with later stoma formation or restoration of continuity.

Colonic injury

Colonic injury most frequently arises from penetrating injury. Management of colonic trauma has been controversial. Traditional repair with accompanying faecal diversion by way of a colostomy is falling out of favour due to its considerable associated morbidity; many surgeons now advocate primary repair without stoma (Basel *et al.*, 1998). Patient selection is important, as the anastomosis is liable to fail in critically injured patients with significant physiological compromise and in patients with widespread abdominal contamination. In this group, colostomy is still the preferred option. Severe injury to the right colon may be treated with right hemicolectomy. The right colon is mobilised by incising the peritoneum along the right paracolic gutter, safeguarding the right ureter, the right gonadal vessels and the second part of the duodenum. Septic complications are a common following colonic injury, with abscess formation resulting within the abdominal cavity.

Rectal injury

Damage to the rectum may be associated with blunt or penetrating injury to the abdomen, pelvis or thighs. Adequate assessment via digital rectal examination and the use of proctoscopy or sigmoidoscopy, where appropriate, is vital in order to avoid missed injuries. Primary repair is safe, providing adequate mobilisation can be achieved for intraperitoneal injury, or the wound is amenable to trans-anal repair. Where this fails or is judged not to be feasible, a proximal colostomy or loop ileostomy is required to divert faecal contents. In this situation, pre-sacral drainage should be considered in order to reduce infective complications; delayed repair may then be considered at a later stage.

Renal injury

Up to 10 per cent of patients with abdominal trauma have associated renal injury. The retroperitoneal position protects the kidneys to some degree from blunt abdominal trauma, with higher-grade injuries more frequently associated with penetrating trauma. Haematuria is the most common symptom, although this may be absent in the most severe injuries, such as renal avulsion. The majority of renal injuries are minor, and there is a trend towards conservative management based on radiological assessment. In patients with blunt injury and haematuria, contrast-enhanced CT or intravenous urography (IVU) should be performed to assess the extent of the injury. Penetrating wounds are more likely to require exploration. In either case, surgery is required for avulsion, major lacerations, devitalised tissue, and indication of ongoing renal bleeding. Extravasation of urine does not in itself always mandate surgery; this may resolve without surgical intervention. Nephrectomy should be the last resort. Care is required in patients with a solitary or non-functioning contralateral kidney; IVU is indicated if renal injury is suspected.

■ KEY POINT
Haematuria is the most common symptom, although this may be absent in the most severe injuries.

■ KEY POINT
Nephrectomy should be the last resort.

Bladder injury

Injuries to the bladder may arise from either blunt or penetrating abdominal trauma. A high degree of suspicion must be maintained, particularly in the presence of other pelvic injuries. Where a history is available, the patient may describe a combination of suprapubic pain, haematuria and an inability to micturate; however, these symptoms may be absent initially. A cystogram remains the investigation of choice, although it is important to exclude distal urethral injury before attempting this. Such an injury may be suggested by the presence of blood at the urethral meatus on examination. Anteroposterior and oblique views of the bladder are obtained both before and after instillation of contrast. Where extravasation of this is seen, injuries are considered in terms of intra- or extraperitoneal rupture. Extraperitoneal rupture may be treated conservatively with urinary catheterisation for about a week, during which time the majority of injuries will heal. Repeat cystograms may be used to confirm this. Intraperitoneal rupture requires surgical repair, with the defect closed in two layers, and continued postoperative urinary catheterisation.

Hepatic injury

The liver is the largest organ in the body. It receives 1500 mL/min of blood, which is equal to 25–30 per cent of cardiac output, through its dual blood supply (portal vein, hepatic artery).

The liver is commonly injured in penetrating trauma. Compressive or shear forces from blunt trauma may also cause significant injury. Bleeding with such trauma can be catastrophic and life-threatening. Non-operative treatment, where possible, is increasingly promoted. In a stable patient, contrast-enhanced CT allows characterisation of the damage and correlation to the American Association for Surgery of Trauma (AAST) liver injury scale (Moore *et al.*, 1995) (Figure 15.1). Low-grade blunt liver injury may be monitored in a high dependency setting, with careful observation of vital signs and haematocrit. Radiographic embolisation is an option in the treatment of these stable patients. More serious insult may result in a range of injuries from parenchymal bleeding through to avulsion of the hepatic veins from the inferior vena cava. In unstable patients and in patients with peritoneal signs, trauma laparotomy is required to arrest the bleeding. Initial packing of the liver is a useful emergency measure, particularly for low-pressure venous bleeding. These may then be left in place for a planned 're-look'. With bright-red arterial bleeding, Pringle's manoeuvre (application of digital pressure on the free border of the lesser omentum) may be utilised to temporarily occlude the hepatic artery, which may be the source of bleeding. If bleeding continues, then haemorrhage from the porta hepatis should be suspected. This is more difficult to control and atrial-caval shunt may be required to allow identification and repair of the site by direct suture. Massive haemobilia may be treated with radiological embolisation in acute situations. With direct haemorrhage from the liver itself, mobilisation of the involved lobe (by dividing the triangular and coronary ligaments) is needed before deciding on the treatment necessary to control this, such as selective vascular ligation. An omental pack, using a pedicle graft of omentum detached from the transverse colon, may be used as filler in treating liver lacerations. Hepatic resection (segmental or lobe) is rarely required, with high mortality reported in most series. Selective hepatic artery ligation can be used if the cause of bleeding is arterial and clamping of the extralobar hepatic artery causes cessation of bleeding.

> ■ KEY POINT
> Initial packing of the liver is a useful emergency measure, particularly for low-pressure venous bleeding.

Complications of liver injuries include the following:

- Rebleeding
- Coagulopathy
- Biloma/biliary fistula
- Hepatic sepsis
- Hepatic duct injury
- Budd–Chiari syndrome
- Haemobilia.

Splenic injury

The spleen is the most commonly injured organ in blunt abdominal trauma. A history of blunt abdominal trauma involving the upper abdomen and left flank should always prompt consideration of spleen injury. In the stable patient, imaging should be obtained in order to evaluate the potential injury, which may then be correlated to the AAST splenic injury scale (Moore *et al.*, 1995) (Figures 15.2 and 15.3). Although non-operative management has proved very successful in paediatric trauma cases, trauma laparotomy and splenectomy are the mainstay of treatment for ongoing bleeding and instability associated with splenic injury in adults. Temporary control of haemorrhage can be achieved by occluding the splenic vasculature at the pedicle, with subsequent mobilisation and identification of the bleeding point. When undertaking this manoeuvre, it is important to identify and protect the underlying tail of the pancreas in order to prevent injury and subsequent pancreatic fistula. Superficial injuries to the capsule may be managed with simple suture. More complex damage requires a partial or complete

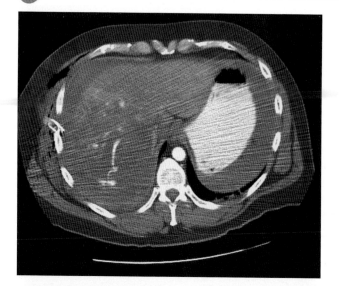

Figure 15.1 ● Hepatic injury. Active arterial extravasation of contrast from the right lobe of the liver.

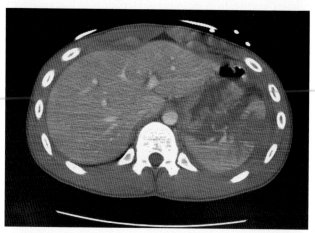

Figure 15.2 ● Splenic injury. Grade 5 splenic laceration with active bleeding.

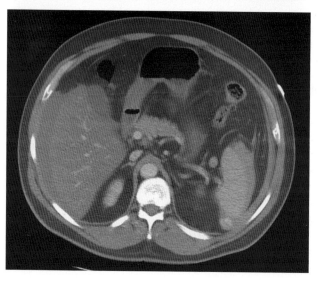

Figure 15.3 ● Splenic laceration, with a large amount of contrast extravasation, suggesting rapid bleeding.

splenectomy. During splenectomy, care must be taken in dissecting the splenic flexure in order to prevent colonic injury. Gastric fistula is a less frequent but equally important complication that may arise during ligation of the short gastric vessels or from surgical trauma during the splenectomy.

> ■ KEY POINT
> The spleen is the most commonly injured organ in blunt abdominal trauma.

Given the important immune role of the spleen in protecting against sepsis from encapsulated organs, it is vital that local protocol is followed with regard to appropriate vaccinations and prophylactic antibiotics.

● COMPLICATIONS OF ABDOMINAL TRAUMA

Raised intra-abdominal pressure resulting from tissue oedema, sepsis or ileus may give rise to abdominal compartment syndrome (Burch *et al.*, 1996). Normal abdominal pressure is less than 10 cmH$_2$O. As this rises, a pattern of physiological compromise develops, including reduced intra-abdominal visceral perfusion, reduced renal perfusion, decreased cardiac return from pressure on the inferior vena cava, and respiratory embarrassment from raised intra-thoracic pressure. Direct abdominal closure should be avoided in patients at risk of developing raised intra-abdominal pressure, by means of temporary closure using a 'Bogota bag' (an empty saline bag cut open) or an 'Opsite sandwich' (an abdominal pack wrapped in Opsite® to cover the open defect, and held in place with a further laying of Opsite).

Diagnosis depends on a familiarity with the risk factors and knowledge of the disparate clinical signs. Diaphragmatic splinting may lead to compromised ventilation, and decreased pre-load in combination with an increased afterload will lead to a fall in cardiac output. In the patient at risk of increased abdominal pressure, measurement can be estimated by measuring intravesical pressure via a Foley catheter and a pressure transducer. Reduction in urinary output is a late sign, reflecting decreasing renal perfusion.

● SUMMARY

- Traumatic abdominal injuries can be missed: a high index of suspicion is required for all trauma patients, including those in whom no initial symptoms or signs are present.
- The mechanism of injury should guide your investigations. In stable patients for whom immediate surgical intervention is not required, further objective evaluation is still required.
- Diagnostic adjuncts have limitations with respect to different organ injuries, and it is important to be aware of these. Ultimately, the clinical picture may necessitate laparotomy as the definitive investigation.
- Trauma patients frequently die not for want of definitive surgical repair of their injuries but from the 'lethal triad' of acidosis, coagulopathy and hypothermia that develops while lengthy procedures are undertaken. Damage-control laparotomy should be considered in these patients.

● QUESTIONS

1 In your initial assessment of a patient with abdominal trauma, what indicates or contraindicates the need for further objective assessment of the injuries?
2 What are the main imaging and diagnostic adjuncts available to assess abdominal trauma? What are their sensitivities with respect to different organ injuries?

3 Describe when and how you would undertake a trauma laparotomy. What do you understand by the term 'damage-control laparotomy', and when would you undertake one?

4 How would you manage abdominal haemorrhage associated with liver trauma? What complications might arise?

5 In the postoperative management of the surgical trauma patient, what symptoms may suggest the onset of abdominal compartment syndrome? What treatment would you offer? How might the syndrome be avoided?

● REFERENCES

Basel K, Borgstrom D, Weigelt J (1998). Management of penetrating colonic trauma. *Surgery* **123**: 157–64.

Boffard KD, Brooks AJ (2000). Pancreatic trauma: injuries to the pancreas and pancreatic duct. *Eur J Surg* **166**: 4–12.

Burch JM, Moore EE, Moore FA, Franciose R (1996). The abdominal compartment syndrome. *Surg Clin North Am* **76**: 833–42.

Hirshberg A, Walden R (1997). Damage control for abdominal trauma. *Surg Clin North Am* **77**: 813–20.

Moore E, Cogbill T, Jurkovich M, *et al.* (1995). Organ injury scaling: spleen and liver (1994 revision). *J Trauma* **38**: 323.

Zantut LF, Ivatury RR, Smith RS, *et al.* (1997). Diagnostic and therapeutic laparoscopy for penetrating abdominal trauma: a multicenter experience. *J Trauma* **42**: 825–9.

● FURTHER READING

Boffard KD (2007). *Manual of Definitive Surgical Trauma Care*, 2nd edn. London: Arnold.

Dondelinger RF (ed.) (2003). *Imaging and Intervention in Abdominal Trauma*. Berlin: Springer-Verlag.

Flint LM, Meredith JW, Schwab CW, Trunkey DD, Rue L (2007). *Trauma: Contemporary Principles and Therapy*. Philadelphia, PA: Lippincott Williams & Wilkins.

Monson J, Duthie G, O'Malley K (1999). *Surgical Emergencies*. Oxford: Blackwell Science.

Trauma.org. Care of the injured. www.trauma.org.

16 Management of acute abdomen

Assad Aghahoseini and David J Alexander

INTRODUCTION

The subject of the acute abdomen cannot be covered comprehensively in a single chapter, so we concentrate on the thought processes required in the early stages of assessment of the acute abdomen. We give some selective references and suggestions for further reading. We focus on the common and mention the rare.

DEFINITION

There is no universally accepted definition of 'acute abdomen'. We refer to 'acute abdomen' as a clinical scenario in which a patient presents acutely with an intra-abdominal pathology manifesting with abdominal pain or obstruction, which warrants urgent investigation and treatment, often including parenteral fluid and analgesia and sometimes surgery.

This may also present as an acute exacerbation of a chronic condition.

ART OF CLINICAL DIAGNOSIS

History

Careful attention to history obtained from the patient or family pays dividends in successful management and allowing the development of self-experience. Muscular young men with classical histories for acute appendicitis, but with minimal signs, might be inappropriately observed, as they are not thought to be tender enough to *justify* surgery. Experience will allow for the possibility that such a patient might harbour a severely inflamed or necrotic appendix, even in the presence of a normal white cell count (WCC), C-reactive protein (CRP) or temperature. The clues are often there and should be looked for, even in retrospect.

Colic versus inflammation

'What did you do when you got the pain?' is a useful question in distinguishing between colic (for which there are three main causes – biliary, renal and intestinal obstruction; uterine is a fourth cause) and peritoneal inflammation (where it might hurt to move, walk, or simply drive over speed bumps in a car). Is the patient rolling around trying to get comfortable, perhaps on all-fours? Locating the pain broadly to the upper abdomen, radiating through to the back or right scapular region, as opposed to loin to groin, can help in differentiating biliary from renal causes – but not always. Abdominal examination is usually unhelpful, apart from exclusion of other pathologies; however, other items in the history (dark urine, pale stools, jaundice) will suggest biliary cause, while microscopic haematuria will point towards the renal tract. Colic is often extremely painful but settles quickly with analgesia, with or without antispasmodics. Resulting abdominal examination reveals a soft abdomen, unless the patient has been vomiting or retching and has developed abdominal wall tenderness as a result. This is important to differentiate as patients can be commenced inappropriately on antibiotics on the basis of minor upper abdominal tenderness, but with a clear history of colic, for a presumed diagnosis of acute cholecystitis. Antibiotics are indicated, however, in this instance if a diagnosis of acute cholangitis is made.

> ■ KEY POINT
> A useful question to distinguish between colic and peritoneal inflammation is 'What did you do when you got the pain?'

Biliary colic can cause central chest pain and result in admission to the coronary care unit, where cardiac investigations prove normal. It is not unusual for realisation to occur some time later, when ultrasound is then requested. Equally, however, myocardial pain may also present with isolated upper abdominal pain.

Bowel obstruction

Suspected bowel obstruction, as a reason for emergency admission, is a common scenario. Careful history can often differentiate likely causes, such as malignant or adhesive obstruction, or alternative diagnoses. Adhesive small bowel obstruction is often related to previous abdominal surgery, but it can occur in the absence of an abdominal scar. This is important, as the diagnosis of small bowel obstruction might not be considered in a younger patient (in whom a malignant cause is highly unlikely); the consequences of delay in diagnosis can be catastrophic if a trapped loop of bowel is allowed to become critically ischaemic. Such a loop might be full of fluid and not obvious on plain film, and so a high index of suspicion is required. Severe abdominal colic, perhaps out of proportion to the clinical signs, should alert the physician, as might localising tenderness or an associated pyrexia. It is important to look for these clinical signs in patients with presumed adhesive small bowel obstruction managed conservatively, as again ischaemia might have developed in the trapped bowel.

Malignant causes are more common in older patients. A recent preceding history of an unexplained change in bowel habit, along with recent absolute constipation and abdominal distension, may be supportive. Severe constipation may present with similar clinical signs; however, plain X-ray will demonstrate faecal loading throughout the colon and not the cut-off sign of obstructed large bowel. Vomiting is a common feature in small bowel obstruction; it may also occur in large bowel obstruction, particularly if the ileocaecal valve (ICV) is incompetent. Such valvular incompetence in large bowel obstruction is protective, as a so-called 'closed loop' obstruction (when the valve is competent) is a surgical emergency; otherwise, caecal perforation might occur as decompression into the small bowel is prevented. An acute history of abdominal distension in a patient with Parkinson's disease or taking psychiatric medication might suggest colonic volvulus (usually sigmoid). The diagnosis can be confirmed by the typical 'coffee bean' appearance on plain abdominal film and is treated by flatus tube per rectum.

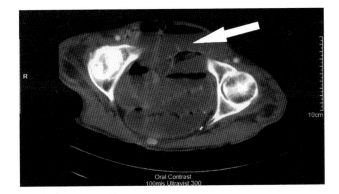

Figure 16.1 ● Small bowel obstruction due to obturator hernia. The arrow shows dilated fluid-filled loops of small bowel.

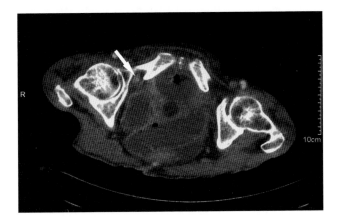

Figure 16.2 ● Knuckle of bowel (arrow) protruding through the obturator foramen, with associated dilated loops of small bowel in the pelvis of the same patient as in Figure 16.1.

Pseudo-obstruction is encountered regularly during the surgical acute take. The presentation is very similar to that of bowel obstruction in terms of symptoms and signs, but with one main difference: there is no mechanical cause. History of comorbidity, recent sepsis, pneumonia, myocardial infarction, immobility, renal failure, uraemic state or electrolyte derangement may suggest this possibility. Internal hernias are less common causes of small bowel obstruction (Figures 16.1 and 16.2).

Signs and symptoms of intestinal obstruction (Table 16.1) depend on:

- the level of obstruction;
- whether obstruction is complete or subacute;
- the competence of the ileocaecal valve (ICV).

Table 16.2 shows the distribution of pathology in patients presenting with acute abdominal pain in a study by Irvin (1989). More than one-third of patients were diagnosed with non-specific abdominal pain, while the following diagnoses each contributed 1 per cent or less: peptic ulcer, ruptured abdominal aortic aneurysm, inflammatory bowel disease, and mesenteric ischaemia.

Table 16.1 Signs and symptoms of intestinal obstruction

Level	Symptoms	Signs	X-ray features
Pylorus/D1	Early: upper abdominal distension, non-bilious vomiting Late: constipation	Dehydrated, succussion splash	Gastric dilation
Duodenal beyond D2	Early: upper abdominal distension, bilious vomiting Late: constipation	Dehydrated, succussion splash	Gastric and duodenal dilation
Small bowel and caecum	Early: distension, foregut pain, faecal vomiting Late: constipation	Distended tympanic abdomen, usually non-tender[a]; tinkling bowel sounds	Dilated loops of small bowels up to the level of obstruction[b]
Large bowel, ICV incompetent	Early: constipation, distension Late: faecal vomiting	Distended tympanic abdomen Reduced bowel sounds is a late sign	Dilated loops of small and large bowel
Large bowel, ICV competent	Constipation, increasing abdominal pain, distension, often no vomiting	Flank distension, can be peritonitic[c], reduced bowel sounds	Dilated loops of large bowels up to caecum

ICV, ileocaecal valve.
[a]Tenderness may suggest ischaemia. [b]This may not be apparent due to fluid-filled loops of small bowel, which gives a featureless appearance. [c]Features of intestinal obstruction in presence of right iliac fossa tenderness requires urgent surgery in order to prevent caecal perforation.

Table 16.2 Acute presentations of acute abdominal pain in a study by Irvin (1989)

Cause of acute abdominal pain	%
Non-specific abdominal pain	35
Appendicitis	17
Obstruction	15
Urinary disease	6
Biliary disease	5
Diverticular disease	4
Trauma	3
Malignancy	3
Perforated ulcer	3
Pancreatitis	2

Musculoskeletal pain

Differentiating intra-abdominal from musculoskeletal causes can be difficult. If the patient can localise the discomfort with a finger, then this should arouse suspicion of a myofascial cause or nerve entrapment. Exacerbation by abdominal muscle contraction, such as when trying to sit up, might support this suspicion. A history of localised pain, swelling and bruising, perhaps following a bout of coughing, might enable you to clinically distinguish between rectus sheath haematoma and incarcerated abdominal wall hernia; only the latter requires emergency surgery.

Examination

It is beyond the scope of this chapter to describe the details of abdominal examination, but a word on specific signs is warranted. Deep palpation, particularly performed roughly, will elicit tenderness in the right upper quadrant, irrespective of whether an inflamed gallbladder exists. This is not a positive Murphy's sign (when the patient catches their breath on deep inspiration on subtle pressure in the right upper quadrant) and hence per se does not necessarily warrant a course of antibiotics for the patient. Gentle percussion of the left iliac fossa in order to assess right iliac fossa peritonism (Rovsing's sign) is a useful clinical sign in acute appendicitis but does not require extravagant pressure. Gentle abdominal percussion, especially in children, can replace the traditional evaluation of rebound tenderness, which can be painful. It is important to exclude a silent, irreducible and often non-tender femoral hernia, particularly in elderly women, as a cause for small bowel obstruction. The hernia has often not been noticed or assumed to be significant by the patient, but if present it will usually be the cause and will often contain bowel.

Rectal examination is often an essential part of assessment in the acute abdomen. It may be useful in children, particularly in excluding pelvic appendicitis, as long as a great deal of care and tact is exercised. A cavernous rectum with fluid faeces is consistent with pseudo-obstruction, while a collapsed empty rectum may indicate mechanical obstruction.

Preliminary investigation

The majority of acutely admitted patients are over-investigated and exposed to risk as a result. Suspected acute appendicitis is an excellent example: this is largely a clinical diagnosis in the majority of cases. The results of a WCC will not discourage surgery if they are normal in the presence of classical symptoms and signs; equally, a raised white cell count could have many other causes apart from appendicitis. If the patient is young and does not appear anaemic, then a haemoglobin (Hb) assessment is unnecessary, as is urea and electrolytes (U&E), if there is no reason to expect possible abnormality, such as diuretic use. Local protocols agreed with anaesthetic colleagues will be in place, generally in order to minimise effect on the patient and to respect precious resources. Plain X-rays are usually not required in suspected appendicitis, but they may be helpful in older patients and in patients with atypical history. Perforated peptic ulcer can present with predominantly right iliac fossa tenderness as a result of collection in the paracolic gutter and therefore mimic appendicitis – this is an example of migratory (not referred) pain. Using an erect chest X-ray to try to rule out free gas if present, and because of an atypical history, is an example of selective and patient-specific investigation, as opposed to a blanket approach, which is easier and requires little thought.

Urinalysis is quick, cheap and often instructive. A pregnancy test must be done in women of childbearing age with lower abdominal pain in order to exclude ectopic pregnancy. In most patients with generalised abdominal pain, it is helpful to take plain films of abdomen and erect chest, despite plain abdominal film being reported to affect the management in less than 10 per cent of patients. In patients with lower abdominal pain, it is reasonable to perform haematological (Hb, WCC) and biochemical (U&E) profiles. In patients with upper abdominal pain, we would add serum amylase and liver function tests and consider doing an electrocardiogram

(ECG) in order to exclude myocardial infarction. Basal pneumonia can present with pain and signs solely within the abdomen; one might hope for clues in the history, but a chest X-ray may also help. C-reactive protein is probably overused in the acute setting. In certain conditions (e.g. acute pancreatitis), CRP has been shown to be an accurate predictor of severity of disease and is helpful in following progress, providing an early marker of intra-abdominal deterioration such as superadded infection. A normal CRP level in a patient with unexplained and perhaps apparently severe abdominal pain, but whom you want to manage conservatively, can provide some reassurance. Table 16.3 provides a summary of the more common investigations and their uses and limitations in acute abdomen.

Table 16.3 Investigations in acute abdomen

Investigation	Value	Limitations/cautions
FBC	Anaemia, leucocytosis, thrombocytosis	Non-specific
U&E	Renal function, dehydration	In chronic renal failure; urea elevated in upper gastrointestinal bleed
LFT	CBD stone; hepatitis	Lag between onset of pain and biochemical changes; may need repeat in 24 h
Amylase	3× normal: pancreatitis; < 3× normal: consider AAA, SB ischaemia, perforation	Not organ-specific; short half-life; lipase more specific
Urinalysis and PDT	Nitrites = UTI; renal calculi; pregnancy	Reactive haematuria in appendicitis; PDT can be negative in ectopic pregnancy
CRP	Severity of acute pancreatitis; serial measurements in sepsis and IBD	Non-specific; relatively expensive
CXR erect	Free gas in perforation; lower lobe pneumonia	False negative rate of 10%
AXR	SBO; aneurysm; pneumobilia	Changes management in 10% of patients; beware of fluid-filled loops in cases of SBO
Ultrasound scan	Superior to CT scan in assessing gallbladder and biliary tree; appendicitis	Operator-dependent; miss up to 25% of gallstones in acute setting; poor pick-up rate of distal CBD stones
CT scan	Widespread metastatic disease; pancreatitis; small bowel pathology	Radiation; limited access; can be done too soon, especially in trauma
ECG	MI/severe angina	Ischaemic changes may be subtle; may need troponin T level
ABG	Acute pancreatitis; bowel ischaemia; coexisting respiratory disease	Check for collateral circulation with Allen's test; acidotic patient with normal pH

AAA, abdominal aortic aneurysm; ABG, arterial blood gases; AXR, abdominal X-ray; CBD, common bile duct; CRP, C-reactive protein; CT, computed tomography; CXR, chest X-ray; ECG, electrocardiogram; FBC, full blood count; IBD, inflammatory bowel disease; LFT, liver function tests; MI, myocardial infarction; PDT, pregnancy detection test; SB, small bowel; SBO, small bowel obstruction; U&E, urea and electrolytes; UTI, urinary tract infection.

Table 16.4 Comparison of radiation doses for some common investigations

Investigation	Effective dose (mSv)[*]	Equivalent of natural background radiation
Chest X-ray	0.1	10 days
CT of abdomen	10	3 years
CT colonography	5	20 months
Intravenous pyelogram (IVP)	1.6	6 months

CT, computed tomography.
[*]The millisievert (mSv) is one of the units used to measure the dose of radiation. Other units include the roentgen and the rad.
Data from Radiological Society of North America.

Safety of radiological investigation

A request for investigations should be with a specific question in mind in order to avoid harming the patient and wasting resources. Table 16.4 provides a rough guide to the relative risk of radiation for some common investigations. The effective radiation dose of a computed tomography (CT) scan of the abdomen is 100 times that of a chest X-ray.

● AETIOLOGY OF ACUTE ABDOMEN

The aetiology of the acute abdomen can be broadly categorised into three groups:

- Surgical
- Gynaecological
- Urological.

Surgical causes can be further subdivided as follows:

- *Inflammatory:*
  - Gastritis
  - Gastroenteritis
  - Biliary sepsis, cholecystitis, ascending cholangitis
  - Pancreatitis
  - Meckel's disease
  - Appendicitis
  - Inflammatory bowel disease (IBD): ulcerative colitis, Crohn's disease
  - Diverticulitis
  - Inflammatory mass/abscess: appendicular, diverticular, Crohn's disease
  - Peritonitis and perforation:
    - Peptic ulcer: gastric/duodenal
    - Large bowel: diverticular, malignant, faecal, mechanical obstruction and closed loop, e.g. caecal perforation as a result of distal obstruction and competent ileocaecal valve.
- *Vascular:*
  - Rupture: aneurysm of aorta, iliacs and visceral arteries
  - Thromboembolic: ischaemia, infarct of bowels and solid organs

- *Obstruction and colic:*
  - Intrinsic: bolus, calculi, bezoar, faeces, neoplastic, inflammation, intussusception
  - Extrinsic: neoplastic, inflammatory
  - Hernia: abdominal wall, internal
  - Adhesions: congenital, iatrogenic.

  Gynaecological causes can be subdivided thus:

- Ectopic pregnancy
- Ovarian cysts: rupture, haemorrhage, torsion, infarction
- Pelvic inflammatory disease, Fitz–Hugh–Curtis syndrome
- Endometriosis
- Retrograde menstruation.

  Urological causes include:

- renal colic;
- ruptured bladder;
- infection of renal tract.

Urological causes of acute abdomen

Renal colic does not always present with the classic loin-to-groin pain, associated microscopic haematuria is absent in 5 per cent of patients, and the patient may have lower abdominal tenderness on examination – all of which may cause confusion. It is important to avoid diagnosing renal colic in a patient with abdominal and back pain without considering, and perhaps formally excluding, a leaking abdominal aortic aneurysm. Plain X-ray might alert you to widened aortic calcification. Aortic aneurysm generally presents in the seventh decade and above; however, because the management of renal colic is usually conservative and based on analgesia, a missed diagnosis of aortic rupture is disastrous. Rupture of a normal-sized aorta can occur as a result of primary infection and in younger age groups, but thankfully it is rare. Be wary of the diagnosis of renal colic in an elderly patient with no similar past history.

Gynaecological causes of acute abdomen

The diagnoses to exclude are ruptured ectopic pregnancy (pregnancy test is normally positive), pelvic inflammatory disease (Curtis–Fitz–Hugh syndrome results from spreading inflammation towards the right upper quadrant, where symptomatic perihepatic adhesions result) or ruptured ovarian cyst. Differentiating particularly between the latter two causes and appendicitis may be difficult clinically, but the history is often crucial. The absence of initial periumbilical colic with presentation in mid-cycle might suggest ruptured cyst, while bilateral pelvic clinical signs with cervical excitation and vaginal discharge may point to pelvic infection; however, the diagnosis may not be clear and may only be confirmed in time. Peritoneal irritation from retrograde menstruation can occur. Negative appendicectomy rates of around 15 per cent are reported widely, are deemed acceptable and are testament to the difficulties surrounding diagnosis in this area.

● EARLY MANAGEMENT OF ACUTE ABDOMEN

Following careful history, examination and preliminary investigation, it should be possible to decide upon a shortlist of differential diagnoses. Further investigations and treatment depend upon these differential diagnoses, but there are a few important basic generic requirements to early management.

Resuscitation

The patient may be in obvious need of urgent resuscitation, with a tachycardia, hypotension and oliguria. You should respond with wide-bore venous access and appropriate intravenous fluids, urinary catheter insertion in order to help assess the effect, and antibiotics if a septic cause is suspected. There is no place for central venous access in the initial stages of resuscitation. Lack of immediate response may require high dependency or intensive care, perhaps including inotropic or respiratory support with arterial and central venous access. Unless the patient is actively bleeding, it is rare for emergency surgery before resuscitation to be indicated or effective. It is important to be sensitive to patients who are not obviously shocked on presentation but in whom the diagnosis (e.g. perforated viscus) or the history (e.g. prolonged vomiting, loose stool) might predict the development of sepsis or hypovolaemia. Active early management in such patients, allowing for the difficulties in patients with cardiac failure, may prevent progression to the 'urgent' scenario, which is not always reversible. A patient with bowel obstruction who has been vomiting for days will be depleted of many litres of fluid – that lost, along with that not taken.

Hypotension is a late sign of circulatory shock. Resuscitation should start promptly in its anticipation rather than be delayed until its arrival.

■ KEY POINT
Hypotension is a late sign of circulatory shock. Resuscitation should start promptly in its anticipation rather than be delayed until its arrival.

Pain relief

Despite pain being the usual presenting symptom, we are often slow to remember to provide the necessary analgesia. It is much easier to make a careful and effective clinical assessment if the patient is comfortable. If you examine sensitively, signs are not masked by analgesia (Ranji *et al.*, 2006). An exception is the difficult scenario in assessing the postoperative patient who is likely to be sore or who might have had an epidural for pain relief.

Communication with the patient and family

It is important to make sure that you return to the patient and their family after viewing X-rays and other test results in order to explain your differential diagnosis and plan. This requires discipline, particularly on busy acute rounds.

Further specific investigations

Futher investigations should be targeted, may be unnecessary and should contribute to the patient's management.

The importance of a CT scan in cases of acute abdomen has evolved, probably as out-of-hours access has increased over recent years. Apart from its diagnostic role (including in trauma), CT scanning may help to avoid unnecessary laparotomy. Differentiation between a diverticular and an appendix cause for lower abdominal peritonitis is helpful, as might be the demonstration of widespread metastatic disease, which might avoid the dreaded 'open-and-close' laparotomy.

A water-soluble contrast enema is useful in excluding pseudo-obstruction as a cause of large bowel obstruction. Depending on local circumstances and experience, CT scanning might be used instead. There are advantages to CT scanning (e.g. views of the rest of the abdomen, alternative diagnoses), but it is possible for CT scanning to miss small cicatrising colonic tumours – although a clear cut-off in colonic width may suggest occlusive disease.

Ultrasound in presumed biliary disease will often confirm gallstones, give information on the bile duct, and perhaps suggest associated fluid collections or gallbladder wall thickness. The mere presence of gallstones does not prove their malicious intent. Alternative diagnoses, including liver abscess, can be made. Ultrasound has been reported to add value in a number of gastrointestinal emergencies (Puylaert, 2003; Vasavada, 2004), but it is operator-dependent and has been superseded by cross-sectional imaging. The exception to this in general surgical practice is in the evaluation of the gallbladder for stones. Here, ultrasound is superior to CT but may miss stones, in acute assessment, in the large and distended patient.

There is variable enthusiasm for diagnostic laparoscopy, but it can be useful in diagnosis and as a therapeutic tool to wash out the pelvis if an ovarian cyst has ruptured or to complete appendicectomy. Diagnostic laparoscopy should perhaps not replace careful history, examination and observation.

Indications for early surgery

Haemorrhage

The main diagnosis is leaking abdominal aortic aneurysm (AAA). Other, rarer causes include spontaneous splenic rupture, visceral artery aneurysm and ruptured pancreatic pseudo-aneurysm (all of which the authors have encountered in their practice).

The presentation of leaking AAA is variable, but in most cases it is a clinical diagnosis. Attempts at confirming the diagnosis may delay treatment and prove fatal. Sudden severe back pain followed by collapse, with a definite record of hypotension and palpable abdominal mass in a patient over 60 years of age should be regarded as leaking AAA, unless a credible alternative exists, and deserves excluding. Most patients require immediate surgery in parallel to resuscitation. Avoid overzealous blood and fluid resuscitation in patients with active bleeding, as these efforts disrupt the body's attempt to control the bleeding and may lead to further blood loss. This is the main principle behind hypotensive resuscitation during which the blood and other fluids are administered in a controlled way, with regular monitoring of blood pressure (BP); the aim is to keep the systolic pressure below 100 mmHg in order to allow adequate tissue perfusion of vital organs.

> ■ KEY POINT
> The presentation of leaking AAA is variable, but in most cases it is a clinical diagnosis.

Spontaneous retroperitoneal and rectus sheath haematomas may present with a similar clinical picture to leaking AAA, including circulatory collapse. These patients may be on warfarin and may be over-anticoagulated. A CT scan is helpful in making the diagnosis (Figure 16.3), as the mainstay of treatment is supportive, including the reversal of anticoagulation.

Perforated viscus

The source may be suggested by the patient's age, preceding history and general state. This may be important because, although perforated peptic ulcer is usually dealt with surgically, there is a clinical scenario in which an often elderly patient, with severe coexisting morbidity, presents with abdominal pain, localised upper abdominal peritonitis and free gas on plain X-ray and in whom conservative management (nil by mouth, intravenous fluids, nasogastric drainage, antibiotics) presents the only likely successful conclusion (Figure 16.4). A recent history of a change in bowel habit, however, may point more to a colonic perforation, which is extremely unlikely to be managed conservatively with success. Faecal peritonitis is usually associated

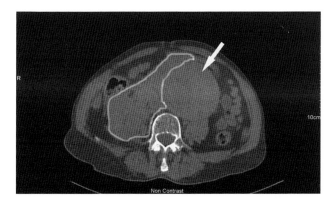

Figure 16.3 ● Non-contrast computed tomography (CT) scan, demonstrating an aortic aneurysm with calcification in its wall (arrow) and associated retroperitoneal haematoma (bordered area), in keeping with acute rupture.

Figure 16.4 ● A large volume of free gas is demonstrated under both diaphragms, indicating pneumoperitoneum. The patient had a history of right pneumonectomy for primary lung cancer.

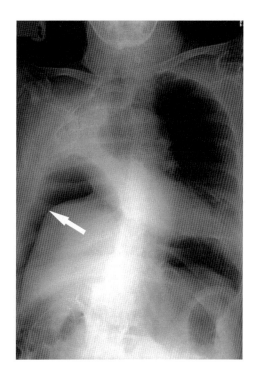

with a greater systemic inflammatory response. Diverticular perforation is a common cause of peritonitis; however, stercoral perforation can also occur. There is normally time to prepare and optimise the patient before surgery.

Adhesive small bowel obstruction

This is usually managed conservatively; however, localised tenderness, particularly if associated with a pyrexia and rising tachycardia, may suggest ischaemic bowel. A picture of metabolic acidosis may further support this diagnosis. Failure to act in timely fashion may result in perforation, which increases the risks of morbidity and mortality or the loss of what may be a considerable length of small bowel.

Peritonitis

Peritonitis may be associated with an in-dwelling peritoneal dialysis catheter. It is not always a definite indication for surgery, but in general terms a diagnosis of peritonitis usually equates with a need for laparotomy. An associated preceding history consistent with, or indeed documented, disseminated malignant disease might stay the surgical hand and avoid the open-and-shut laparotomy, and so immediate investigation (e.g. CT) might be helpful. It is important to exclude acute pancreatitis before embarking on laparotomy for apparent peritonitis. Serum amylase can be raised in alternative diagnoses, such as perforated ulcer, dissected aneurysm and even torted ovarian cyst; however, a serum amylase level three times or more the upper limit of normal is diagnostic of acute pancreatitis. Most surgeons avoid laparotomy for lower abdominal peritonitis if the diagnosis is sigmoid diverticulitis, as this can be managed conservatively with success – and may be another indication for CT before surgery. The inflamed sigmoid loop might have flopped towards the right iliac fossa and suggest acute appendicitis, and the scenario of grid-iron exploration and conversion to laparotomy is still a common one. This is preferably avoided, not only because it is untidy but also because, having operated and found an inflamed sigmoid colon associated with pus, one is usually forced to consider resection (which might require a stoma) for a condition that might have settled conservatively.

Intestinal ischaemia

Colonic ischaemia usually presents subacutely and may be missed, although the history of bloody diarrhoea, associated with often predominantly left-sided abdominal pain, should arouse suspicion. This will normally settle conservatively while the differential diagnoses of infection and inflammatory bowel disease are excluded. The only suggestion of likely diagnosis might be a stricture at the splenic flexure on subsequent barium enema. An alternative scenario is of sigmoid colonic ischaemia occurring a few days after aortic aneurysm repair, which requires laparotomy and colonic resection. This diagnosis can be confirmed by preoperative flexible sigmoidoscopy. Small bowel ischaemia might be related to internal hernia or adhesions, be of embolic cause and associated with atrial fibrillation, or, rarely, be related to a vasculitic illness (Passam *et al.*, 2004). Venous small bowel ischaemia is more insidious in onset. Embolic disease to the superior mesenteric artery often results in extensive, irreversible disease and coexists with a patient in extremis; however, mesenteric embolectomy is occasionally successful. In general, abdominal pain disproportionate to the clinical signs in an elderly patient with dysrhythmia should alert the clinician to the possibility of small bowel ischaemia. Elevated serum lactate and significant acidosis can support such diagnosis.

Aetiology of abdominal visceral ischaemia includes the following:

- Embolic due to cardiac disease:
  - Intraventricular thrombosis following myocardial infarction
  - Dysrhythmia
  - Valvular disease with vegetation
- Thrombotic, i.e. atheroma of visceral arteries
- Shock:
  - Cardiogenic
  - Hypovolaemia
  - Sepsis
- Inotropic drugs
- Blood disorders, e.g. hypercoagulability, thrombophilia
- Connective tissue disorder, e.g. vasculitis
- Abdominal compartment syndrome.

Bowel obstruction

Large bowel obstruction with caecal distension and tenderness, particularly with a competent ileocaecal valve that prevents decompression back up the small bowel, requires urgent surgery. Preoperative exclusion of pseudo-obstruction (which is more common in patients admitted with other pathologies such as chest infection and pelvic trauma, and rarely in patients admitted directly on the surgical take) by either gastrograffin enema or CT scan is advisable. Clues to the possible diagnosis of pseudo-obstruction include metabolic derangements (e.g. dehydration, electrolyte imbalance (particularly potassium), hypoxia) and the possibility of retroperitoneal problems (e.g. haematoma, pelvic or spinal injury, following hip surgery). Certain drugs and current chest infection may be associated with pseudo-obstruction. The choice of surgical procedure depends on a number of factors, including the level and nature of the obstruction. Rectal cancer unusually presents with obstruction; because of the role of preoperative radiotherapy, it may be best to simply de-function the obstruction and plan definitive treatment after full staging, as for elective presentation. Surgery otherwise involves resection of the obstruction, with or without primary anastomosis. Caecal tenderness may reflect impending perforation, hence the urgency, as faecal peritonitis significantly increases the postoperative mortality of what is already a high-risk procedure. At operation, the ischaemic caecum with multiple serosal tears might not be salvageable, necessitating a more complete colonic resection.

Aetiology of small bowel obstruction includes the following:

- Adhesions:
  - Iatrogenic
  - Congenital
- Hernia:
  - Abdominal wall
- Intra-abdominal:
  - Obturator
  - Inter-loop
- Inflammatory, i.e. Crohn's stricture
- Volvulus
- Neoplasia
- Intussusception
- Gallstone
- Ischaemia
- Bezoar.

Aetiology of large bowel obstruction includes the following:

- Carcinoma
- Diverticular stricture
- Faecal impaction
- Volvulus:
  - Sigmoid
  - Caecum
- Hernia, parastomal
- Gynaecological malignancy
- Endometriosis
- Pseudo-obstruction due to:
  - Sepsis
  - Renal failure

- Electrolytes derangement
- Pneumonia.

LATER MANAGEMENT OF SPECIFIC CONDITIONS

Acute diverticulitis

Acute diverticulitis (Table 16.5) is common. It presents with predominantly left iliac fossa or lower abdominal pain and tenderness, and it is usually associated with fever. The incidence of diverticular disease increases with age, but it may be present in young patients and may have already been documented in your patient. Response to antibiotic therapy is often within 24–48 h, and the patient may be allowed home with plans for colonic investigation when all has settled, usually at least 6 weeks later. Occasionally a perforated carcinoma mimics diverticulitis and responds to conservative treatment, hence the need for further investigation. The patient may not settle quickly and urgent CT will be required both to confirm diagnosis and to seek associated complications. An abscess is often amenable to ultrasound or CT-guided drainage and allows continued successful conservative management. Unless the patient presents with peritonitis, it is unusual for urgent laparotomy to be required. The current opinion in the management of diverticular peritonitis includes the use of laparoscopy and wash out instead of bowel resection.

There has been a move towards greater elective surgery in patients who have had one or more episodes of acute diverticulitis. Age and comorbidity are important contributors to the decision. This is colonic resection, with all of its risks, for benign disease, however, and therefore the decision to operate is more difficult than when presented with cancer. A diagnosis of colonic fistula to the bladder or vagina related to complicated diverticular disease usually results in the need for colonic resection.

Gallstones

There are four main acute presentations of gallstones:

- *Acute cholecystitis:*
  - The long-held wisdom that cholecystectomy is particularly difficult within 3 days or more of the start of an attack, and for up to six weeks or so, has not been challenged.
  - For clinical and logistical reasons, there has been a move towards performing acute cholecystectomy soon after presentation. This is likely to shorten patient stay and obviate the need for a return for elective surgery (and reduce further attacks in the meantime).
  - The rate of recurrent biliary complications while waiting for laparoscopic cholecystectomy was 5.9 per cent among our patients (Thornton *et al.*, 2002), but it has been reported to be as high as 20 per cent (Schiphorst *et al.*, 2008).
  - Liver function tests may be abnormal as a result of an inflammatory gall bladder mass, but a common bile duct (CBD) stone may need to be excluded. Acute cholecystectomy is a challenging procedure with a higher risk of conversion rate and CBD injury than elective surgery.
- *Biliary colic:*
  - This is usually due to impacted stone in the neck of the gallbladder or cystic duct or stone in the CBD.
  - Ultrasound has low sensitivity for detection of distal CBD stones, but it may show dilated CBD or intrahepatic ducts.
  - In the presence of dilated CBD (> 6 mm) and deranged liver tests, endoscopic retrograde cholangiopancreatography (ERCP) or magnetic resonance cholangiopancreatography (MRCP) is indicated to ascertain CBD clearance before any definitive treatment for the gallstones. Laparoscopic cholecystectomy and exploration of the CBD is an alternative approach.

Table 16.5 Clinical presentations of acute diverticulitis

Description	Uncomplicated diverticulitis	Diverticular phlegmon	Diverticular abscess	Diverticular perforation
Pathology	Inflammation confined to affected loop of bowel	Inflammatory mass due to extension to adjacent loops	Localised perforation resulting in paracolic or pelvic abscess	Perforation with subsequent release of pus/faeces
Signs and symptoms	Abdominal pain ± pyrexia; LIF tenderness; no peritonitis	Abdominal pain, pyrexia, localised peritonitis, LIF or pelvic mass		Septic, circulatory shock, generalised peritonitis
Early management	Basic investigations, IV fluid, IV antibiotics	CT scan, IV antibiotics, ?laparotomy*	CT scan, percutaneous drainage, ?laparotomy	Free gas on chest X-ray, resuscitation, Hartman's
Later management	If the first attack, consider barium enema in 6 weeks	If no surgery during acute phase, consider resection and primary anastomosis; if Hartman's, consider reversal		Consider reversal of Hartman's

CT, computed tomography; IV, intravenous; LIF, left iliac fossa.

*A nationwide study into the adverse outcomes following treatment of complicated diverticular disease has shown that Hartmann's procedure is associated with higher levels of morbidity and adverse outcomes compared with primary resection and anastomosis. The latter option should be considered in patients with favourable clinical picture, i.e. young patient with minimal intra-abdominal contamination and comorbidity (Constantinidis et al., 2006).

- The true incidence of CBD stones is not known, but there is some indirect evidence about the scale of this problem; in one study, 17 per cent of all the patients who had undergone laparoscopic cholecystectomy and on-table cholangiogram had CBD stones (Rhodes *et al.*, 1998).
- *Ascending cholangitis:*
  - This is a life-threatening combination of bacterial infection and obstructed biliary system.
  - Usually presents with Charcot's triad of fever/rigors, jaundice and right upper quadrant pain.
  - Raynaud's pentad of the above three signs plus hypotension and mental confusion are signs of more advanced disease.
  - Patients are usually systemically unwell as a result of sepsis, dehydration and acute renal failure.
  - Antibiotics and fluid resuscitation are needed.
  - Urgent ERCP will allow removal of the offending stones or placement of a stent, which will drain the infected bile and may be the definitive treatment in elderly or infirm patients.
  - The bacteriology of cholangitis is usually polymicrobial. The predominant organisms in order of their prevalence are: *Escherichia coli*, *Klebsiella* spp., *Bacteroides* spp. and anaerobes. This means that anaerobic cover needs to be included in the antimicrobial regime in biliary sepsis, especially for patients with potentially impaired immunity, e.g. diabetic patients and patients on steroids, immunosuppressants and chemotherapy.
- *Acute pancreatitis:* gallstones remains the most common cause of acute pancreatitis, which pursues a severe course in 20 per cent of cases.

Aetiology of acute pancreatitis includes the following:

- Gallstones and excess alcohol intake (80 per cent)
- Idiopathic (10 per cent)
- Other rare causes:
  - Hyperlipidaemia
  - Hypercalcaemia
  - Trauma
  - Iatrogenic (ERCP)
  - Drugs:
    - Sodium valproate
    - Tetracycline
    - Thiazide
    - Furosemide.

Greater awareness of the need for early, careful fluid management, particularly in severe acute pancreatitis, has reduced the mortality from early multiorgan failure. There is a reduced role for surgical management of subsequent pseudo-cysts, as most recede spontaneously given time, and endoscopic drainage has proven to be a more conservative option for a persistent cyst. Meta-analyses have suggested a place for appropriate (that penetrate into pancreatic juice, e.g. third-generation cephalosporins) antibiotics (Sharma and Howden, 2001). Early enteral nutrition (nasojejunal or nasogastric) probably reduces the incidence of complications such as infected pancreatic necrosis and abscess (UK Working Party on Acute Pancreatitis, 2005). Retroperitoneal sepsis without drainage is incompatible with survival; however, a discrete infected collection or abscess may be solved by percutaneous drainage. Pancreatic necrosis (Figure 16.5) is managed conservatively, but superadded infection not amenable to drainage requires often radical and morbid surgery. Laparoscopic debridement is the current practice in some specialist centres. Definitive surgery for the stones is ideal as soon as the patient has recovered from the attack (UK Working Party on Acute Pancreatitis, 2005).

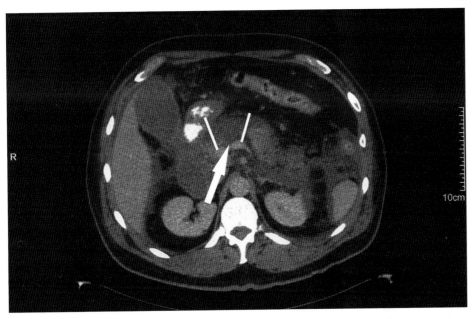

Figure 16.5 ● Portal venous-phase computed tomography (CT), demonstrating normal enhancement of a fragment of the pancreatic body and of the tail. The intervening pancreatic neck is not enhancing, in keeping with necrosis here (area between lines, indicated by arrow).

The following are recommendations from the UK guidelines for the management of acute pancreatitis:

- Aetiology should be established in 80 per cent of cases, even if it involves repeat investigations. Only 20 per cent of cases can be classified as idiopathic.
- Diagnosis is made through raised serum amylase. If amylase is normal and pancreatitis is suspected, then serum lipase or CT scanning can be used for diagnosis.
- Early severity scoring is clinically relevant and based on Atlanta criteria. This should be done at the time of admission and 48 h after admission.
- A severe attack is characterised by the Atlanta criteria:
  - Clinical impression of severity and organ dysfunction
  - Body mass index > 30
  - Severity score system:
    - APACHE II > 8
    - Glasgow > 3
  - CRP > 150 mg/L as an independent factor.
- All cases of severe pancreatitis should be cared for in high dependency/intensive care setting.
- Patients with severe attacks and persisting organ failure require dynamic contrast-enhanced CT scan 6–10 days from the onset, in order to assess the extend of necrosis using the Balthazar CT severity index.
- The use of prophylactic antibiotics and enteral feeding remain controversial.

- Aetiology assessment and treatment:
  - Early ERCP in the first 72 h in severe cases caused by gallstone.
  - Definitive treatment of gallstone during the same hospital admission or in the following 2 weeks after discharge.
- In cases of infected necrosis of pancreas, active intervention is needed:
  - Percutaneous radiological drainage may be effective in cases of abscess and liquefied collection.
  - Surgical debridement of pancreatic bed is needed to remove solid necrotic tissue and to establish an irrigation system.
- Cases of severe pancreatitis with necrosis need to be referred to the specialist team.

The Glasgow criteria constitute an uncomplicated system for the assessment of the severity of pancreatitis in the first 48 h after admission. The original scale included nine criteria; the modified Glasgow scale has eight criteria (Table 16.6).

Table 16.6 Modified Glasgow criteria and scoring system for acute pancreatitis

Criteria	Scoring
Age (years)	> 55 = 1
	< 55 = 0
Serum albumin (g/L)	< 32 = 1
	> 32 = 0
Pao$_2$ on air (mmHg)	< 60 = 1
	> 60 = 0
Serum calcium (mmol/L)	< 2.0 = 1
	> 2.0 = 0
Blood glucose (mmol/L)	> 10 = 1
	< 10 = 0
Serum LDH (units/L)	> 600 = 1
	< 600 = 0
Blood urea (mmol/L)	> 16 = 1
	< 16 = 0
White cell count (mm^{-3})	> 15 000 = 1
	< 15 000 = 0

LDH, lactate dehydrogenase.
Minimum score is 0 and maximum score is 8. Scores above 3 may indicate severe pancreatitis.
Use the mnemonic PANCREAS to memorise the criteria:
Pao$_2$
Age
Neutrophils (white cells)
Calcium
Raised urea
Enzymes
Albumin
Sugar
Modified from Institute for Algorithmic Medicine, Houston, TX, USA.

Balthazar computed tomography severity index for acute pancreatitis

The Balthazar system is based on the radiological appearance of the pancreas during an acute attack and is used to assess severity and predict prognosis. The system (Table 16.7) is based on the two main features of:

- extent of inflammatory reaction;
- degree of necrosis.

A combined score of 7–10 is associated with a 17 per cent mortality rate (Table 16.8).

Pancreatic pseudo-cyst can complicate an attack of moderate to severe acute pancreatitis. The cyst, lined by a pseudo-epithelium, contains fluid rich in amylase and other pancreatic enzymes (e.g. lipase). The cyst usually develops over a few weeks following the acute attack and therefore differs from inflammatory/infective collections, which can develop in the early stages of pancreatitis. There is usually a correlation between the cyst size and level of symptoms: the latter is the most important factor in deciding on active treatment.

Table 16.7 Balthazar system for grading the severity of pancreatitis

Severity		Grade	Score
Inflammation	Normal pancreas	A	0
	Diffuse pancreatic enlargement	B	1
	Inflammation of pancreas and peripancreatic fat	C	2
	Single fluid collection or phlegmon	D	3
	Two or more fluid collections or phlegmons	E	4
Necrosis	No necrosis		0
	Necrosis of one-third		2
	Necrosis of one-half		4
	Necrosis of > one-half		6

Modified from Institute for Algorithmic Medicine, Houston, TX, USA.

Table 16.8 Balthazar system for grading the predicted mortality and complication rate of pancreatitis

Severity index	Mortality (%)	Complications (%)
0–1	0	0
2–3	3	8
4–6	6	35
7–10	17	92

Modified from Institute for Algorithmic Medicine, Houston, TX, USA.

Most pseudo-cysts are self-resolving. Large and symptomatic cysts causing pain or extrinsic gastric compression require active treatment. Percutaneous drainage, useful for draining infective collections, has no real place in the elective treatment of pseudo-cysts. The recurrence rate is high and persistent pancreaticocutaneous fistula can result.

The two main approaches to treatment are endoscopic and surgical.

The endoscopic technique can be either:

- transmural, through the wall of stomach or duodenum, guided by the extrinsic bulge, or endoluminal ultrasound, if the cyst is relatively small;
- transpapillary, which, although technically more difficult, can result in better functional outcome and with fewer side effects.

The success rate of the endoscopic approach is 85–90 per cent, and the complication rate is 15–20 per cent.

With the surgical approach, the principal aim is to establish an internal drainage system for the cyst in the form of a cystogastrostomy or cystojejunostomy. The success rate is over 90 per cent, but the complication rate (including recurrence) can be over 20 per cent, which may reflect the added complexities in selected patients not suitable for an endoscopic approach.

Studies have shown comparable efficacy in the laparoscopic approach compared with the open approach, with the added benefits of the minimally invasive approach and with a conversion rate of just over 10 per cent (Hauters *et al.*, 2004).

Appendicitis

Acute appendicitis is a common presentation during an acute surgical take. The diagnosis is essentially clinical but can be difficult at times. It is by no means an admission of failure if the diagnosis of appendicitis and its potential complications is made by CT scan, especially in older patients. Magnetic resonance imaging (MRI) can be used in young patients with suspected appendicitis (Figures 16.6 and 16.7).

Patients occasionally present with appendicular mass or abscess. These are the sequelae of missed diagnosis and late presentation. The treatment is usually conservative, with intravenous fluid and antibiotics for the mass and percutaneous drainage for the abscess. If ineffective, surgery may be required.

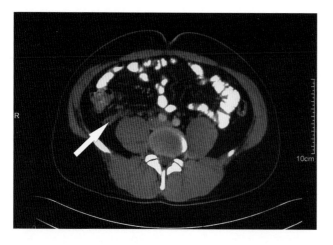

Figure 16.6 ● Computed tomography scan (CT), demonstrating wall thickening and mild distension of the appendix, with a little inflammatory stranding in the adjacent meso-appendix (arrow).

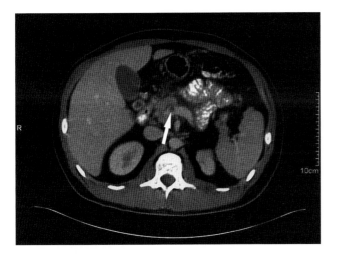

Figure 16.7 ● The same patient as in Figure 16.3. There is a filling defect in the proximal superior mesenteric vein, in keeping with non-occlusive thrombus, in this case secondary to acute appendicitis (indicated by arrow).

Interval appendicectomy remains controversial (Willemsen *et al.*, 2002; Corfield, 2007). Three issues need to be addressed before a decision is made:

● Recurrence of appendicitis: the quoted figure from large studies is 11 per cent.
● Complication rate of interval appendicectomy is about 23 per cent.
● Caecal and appendicular malignancy may be missed. Colonoscopy is a far better way to exclude the former, while the latter usually remain symptomatic.

On the basis of these issues, there is no justification for routine interval appendicectomy. These patients need surgical follow-up in an outpatient clinic a few weeks later for reassessment and possible interventions on the basis of their symptoms (Figure 16.8).

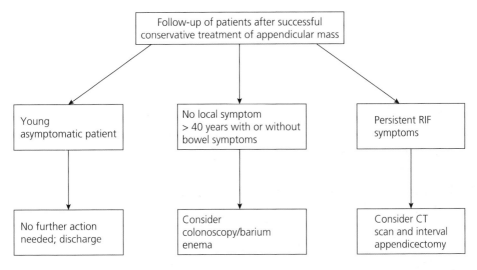

Figure 16.8 ● Algorithm for further follow-up of patients with appendicular mass following successful conservative management.

CT, computed tomography; RIF, right iliac fossa.

> ■ KEY POINT
> There is no justification for routine interval appendicectomy.

● ACUTE ABDOMEN IN PREGNANCY

Any surgical or medical emergency can complicate pregnancy. History remains particularly important in suspected acute appendicitis, as the presence of an enlarged uterus and distended lower abdomen alters the surface marking relative to the position of the appendix. Accepting the normal variance of inflammatory markers during pregnancy, serial deterioration may help influence the decision. Referral of the pregnant woman with right-sided abdominal pain is common; acute appendicitis is unusual but does occur, and delayed diagnosis can have serious implications for both mother and fetus. Pain from the enlarging uterus itself is not uncommon, and urinary tract infections are common. Gallstones are common and may develop during pregnancy. A tendency for the sigmoid colon to undergo volvulus has been described during pregnancy. Acute abdominal pain may result from complications of the pregnancy itself, such as fibroid degeneration, ovarian cyst torsion, placental abruption, ectopic pregnancy, and of course preterm and normal labour. Magnetic resonance imaging of the pregnant patient with acute abdominal pain provides an effective and safe tool (Brown *et al.*, 2005; Pedrosa *et al.*, 2006).

Peculiarities to managing the acute abdomen in pregnancy include the following:

- Two patients are assessed simultaneously. The health and clinical condition of the fetus should not be overlooked. The fetus needs to be evaluated and monitored.
- The acute symptoms need to be differentiated from the normal aches and pains of pregnancy.
- The effect of the gravid uterus on findings during examination include the following:
  - Displacement of mobile internal organs, especially the appendix – by the end of the third trimester, the appendix is located near the gallbladder.
  - Lifting of the anterior abdominal wall separating the peritoneum from the inflamed appendix, which can mask signs of peritonitis.
- A mild leukocytosis (up to 16 000 mm^{-3}) can be regarded as normal in pregnancy. Ultrasound scanning is the safest mode of imaging. Magnetic resonance imaging has been shown to be useful and safe in the diagnosis of appendicitis if there is clinical uncertainty.
- There is a higher incidence of the following conditions during pregnancy:
  - Acute pyelonephritis
  - Acute cystitis
  - Acute cholecystitis
  - Rupture of rectus abdominis muscle.
- The safest time for surgery, as far as the health of the fetus is concerned, is the second trimester. Laparoscopic cholecystectomy can be done safely during pregnancy but ideally should be left until postpartum if possible.
- In the case of appendicitis, surgery needs to be done as soon as possible after diagnosis. The risk of perforation in the pregnant patient is higher than in non-gravid patients.
- The risk of premature delivery following appendicectomy is around 2 per cent, with the risk of discovering normal appendix. This risk should be weighed against the risk of abortion in cases of peritonitis associated with late diagnosis of some 20–40 per cent.
- Do not forget the pregnancy-related causes of acute abdomen:
  - Ruptured ectopic pregnancy
  - Septic abortion and peritonitis
  - Premature labour

- Placenta abruption
- Degeneration or torsion of pedunculated fibroid.

● ACUTE ABDOMEN IN CHILDHOOD

We will not discuss neonatal conditions here, but we will briefly mention some childhood presentations of acute abdomen.

Acute appendicitis

Acute appendicitis is unusual in young infants. However, right iliac fossa pain and tenderness is a common presentation in childhood, and the preceding history may be atypical, leading to late diagnosis. A common differential diagnosis in this age group is mesenteric adenitis, often associated with a recent history of viral illness or sore throat – in which case, appendicitis is unlikely. This allows for a period of observation; however, continuing tenderness may force the surgical hand, when either an inflamed appendix is removed (lymphoid hyperplasia can result in obstructive appendicitis) or a diagnosis of mesenteric adenitis is made. The appendix is removed and a search is made to exclude Meckel's diverticulum. Meckel's diverticulum is a remnant of the primitive yolk sac that occurs in 2 per cent of the population; it can be an asymptomatic finding (in which case, it is left alone) or it may become inflamed, perforate or bleed as a result of ulceration of ectopic gastric mucosa.

Beware missing torsion of the testis, which can present as lower abdominal pain/?appendicitis. The child may not complain of testicular pain in the early stages.

Henoch–Schonlein purpura

This is a potential cause of acute abdomen, particularly in children, and is a sequel of beta-haemolytic streptococcal tonsillar infection. The purpura can affect the subserosa, leading to haematoma and rectal bleeding as well as affecting the joints and renal tract.

● UNUSUAL CAUSES OF ACUTE ABDOMEN

For information on the following unusual causes, see the list of further reading:

- Porphyria
- Diabetic ketoacidosis
- Addisonian crisis
- Small bowel ulceration
- Syphilis
- Lead poisoning
- Sickle cell crisis
- Acute leukaemia
- Parathyroid disease
- Narcotic withdrawal
- Mesenteric cystic lymphangioma
- Small intestinal angiosarcoma
- Retrograde menstruation
- Eosinophilic gastroenteritis (Charalabopoulos *et al.*, 2004)
- Spinal epidural abscess (Bremer and Darouiche, 2004).

● SUMMARY

Having read this chapter you should be familiar with the following concepts:

- Definition of acute abdomen
- Principles of management of any acute abdomen, regardless of aetiology
- Investigations used in the initial stages and the information that can be obtained from them
- The system used to assess the severity of pancreatitis and the significance of a patient's severity score
- Hypotensive resuscitation in the management of a patient with a ruptured AAA or gastrointestinal bleeding
- Acute presentations of diverticular disease, and the treatment options in their management
- Role of laparoscopy in the management of acute abdomen.

● QUESTIONS

1 What is an acute abdomen?
2 What are the principles in the management of any acute abdomen, regardless of aetiology?
3 What investigations are used in the initial stages? What information can be obtained from them?
4 What system is used to assess the severity of pancreatitis? What is the significance of the patient's severity score?
5 What is hypotensive resuscitation? How does it affect the management of patients with ruptured abdominal aortic aneurysm or gastrointestinal tract bleeding?
6 What are the acute presentations of diverticular disease? What are the treatment options in their management?
7 What is the role of laparoscopy in management of acute abdomen?

● ACKNOWLEDGEMENTS

The authors would like to express their gratitude to Dr D Petty, consultant radiologist at York hospital, for his contribution to this chapter by providing the radiological images and captions.

● REFERENCES

Bremer AA, Darouiche RO (2004). Spinal epidural abscess presenting as intra-abdominal pathology: a case report and literature review. *J Emerg Med* **26**: 51–6.

Brown MA, Birchard KR, Semelka RC (2005). Magnetic resonance evaluation of pregnant patients with acute abdominal pain. *Semin Ultrasound CT MR* **26**: 206–11.

Charalabopoulos A, Charalabopoulos K, Avuzuklidou M, *et al.* (2004). Eosinophilic gastroenteritis: presentation of two patients with unusual affect of terminal ileum and caecum with manifestations of acute abdomen and literature review. *Int J Clin Pract* **58**: 413–16.

Constantinidis A, Tekkis PP, Senapati A, Association of Coloproctology of Great Britain and Ireland (2006). Prospective multicentre evaluation of adverse outcomes following treatment for complicated diverticular disease. *Br J Surg* **93**: 1503–13.

Corfield L (2007). Interval appendicectomy after appendiceal mass or abscess in adults: what is 'best practice'? *Surg Today* **37**: 1–4.

Hauters P, Weerts J, Navez B, *et al.* (2004). Laparoscopic treatment of pancreatic pseudocysts. *Surg Endosc* **18**: 1645–8.

Irvin TT (1989). Abdominal pain: a surgical audit of 1190 emergency admissions. *Br J Surg* **76**: 1121–5.

Passam FH, Diamantis ID, Perisinaki G, *et al.* (2004). Intestinal ischemia as the first manifestation of vasculitis. *Semin Arthritis Rheum* **34**: 431–41.

Pedrosa I, Levine D, Eyvazzadeh AD, *et al.* (2006). MR imaging evaluation of acute appendicitis in pregnancy. *Radiology* **238**: 891–9.

Puylaert JBCM (2003).Ultrasonography of the acute abdomen: gastrointestinal conditions. *Radiol Clin North Am* **41**: 1227–42.

Ranji SR, Goldman LE, Simel DL, Shojania KG (2006). Do opiates affect the clinical evaluation of patients with acute abdominal pain? *J Am Med Assoc* **296**: 1764–74.

Rhodes M, Sussman L, Cohen L, *et al.* (1998). Randomised trial of laparoscopic exploration of CBD versus pos operative ERCP for CBD stones. *Lancet* **351**: 159–61.

Schiphorst AH, Besselink MG, Boerma D, *et al.* (2008). Timing of cholecystectomy after endoscopic sphincterotomy for common bile duct stones. *Surg Endosc* 13 Feb [Epub ahead of print].

Sharma VK, Howden CW (2001). Prophylactic antibiotic administration reduces sepsis and mortality in acute necrotizing pancreatitis: a meta-analysis. *Pancreas* **22**: 28–31.

Thornton DJ, Robertson A, Alexander DJ. (2002). Laparoscopic cholecystectomy without routine operative cholangiography does not result in significant problems related to retained stones. *Surg Endosc* **16**: 592–5.

UK Working Party on Acute Pancreatitis (2005). UK guidelines for the management of acute pancreatitis. *Gut* **54**: 1–9.

Vasavada P (2004). Ultrasound evaluation of acute abdominal emergencies in infants and children. *Radiol Clin North Am* **42**: 445–56.

Willemsen PJ, Hoorntje LE, Eddes E-H, Ploeg RJ (2002). The need for interval appendectomy after resolution of an appendiceal mass questioned. *Dig Surg* **19**: 216–22.

● FURTHER READING

British Society of Gastroenterology (1998). United Kingdom guidelines for the management of acute pancreatitis. *Gut* **42** (suppl.): S1–13.

Paterson-Brown S (ed.) (1997). *Emergency Surgery and Critical Care*. London: WB Saunders.

Smith GCS, Paterson-Brown S (2002). The acute abdomen and intestinal obstruction. In: Garden OJ, Bradbury AW, Forsythe JLR (eds). *Principles and Practice of Surgery*, 4th edn. Edinburgh: Churchill Livingstone.

UK Working Party on Acute Pancreatitis (2005). UK guidelines for the management of acute pancreatitis. *Gut* **54**: 1–9.

Chronic critical limb ischaemia and the diabetic foot

Timothy R Wilson and Munther I Aldoori

- Chronic critical limb ischaemia
- Diabetic foot
- Summary
- Questions
- References
- Further reading

● CHRONIC CRITICAL LIMB ISCHAEMIA

Definition

Chronic critical limb ischaemia is defined by the presence of rest pain or tissue loss (ulceration or gangrene) in association with an ankle pressure of less than 50 mmHg or an ankle brachial pressure index (ABPI) of less than 0.5.

Epidemiology

The incidence of critical limb ischaemia in the UK is 50–100 per 100 000 per annum. The cost to the UK health service is estimated at £200 million per annum.

The risk factors for developing critical limb ischaemia are the same as those for general vascular disease, including smoking, diabetes, hyperlipidaemia and hypertension. Table 17.1 lists some of the important risk factors for the development of critical limb ischaemia, along with their relative risks.

Clinical assessment

Patients with critical ischaemia present with rest pain and/or trophic changes of the foot.

Rest pain

Rest pain specifically describes the state when the resting foot is not receiving sufficient blood flow to supply the skin. Consequently, pain is felt in the distal foot and is often described as burning in nature. Classically, pain occurs in bed at night due to a combination of the horizontal position of the leg, drop in blood pressure and increased metabolic requirements of the foot's skin due to venodilation with warming under the bedclothes. Pain is relieved by hanging

Table 17.1 Risk factors for development of chronic limb ischaemia

Risk factor	Relative risk
Diabetes	4
Tobacco smoking	3
Abnormal lipid profile	2
Age > 65 years	2
ABPI < 0.7	2

ABPI, ankle brachial pressure index.

the foot out of bed, which, in addition to assuming a vertical posture, results in vasoconstriction. Calf pains at rest may be misinterpreted as vascular rest pain by inexperienced clinicians. This is illogical, as the calf cannot be starved of blood flow if the skin of the foot is spared. Such pains are frequently due to nocturnal cramps and may be treated effectively with quinine.

> ■ KEY POINT
> Calf pains at rest may be misinterpreted as vascular rest pain by inexperienced clinicians.

Trophic changes

Two types of tissue loss occur in patients with chronic critical limb ischaemia: gangrene and ulceration.

Gangrene

Gangrene most commonly affects the toes and heels. Without the presence of infection, gangrenous tissue will mummify and demarcate, as shown clearly in Figure 17.1. This is termed 'dry gangrene' and eventually results in auto-amputation if the stump receives sufficient blood flow. The presence of infection in gangrenous tissue results in 'wet gangrene'. This requires surgical debridement or amputation to prevent worsening sepsis (Figure 17.2).

Figure 17.1 ● Dry gangrene of the toes.

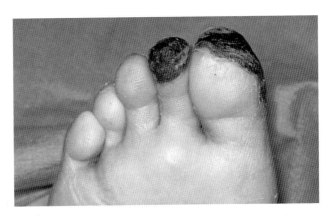

Figure 17.2 ● Wet gangrene.

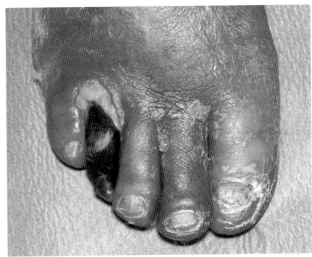

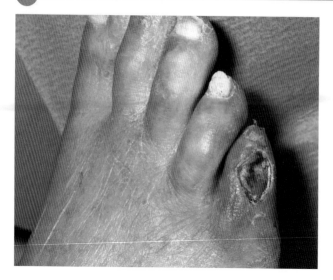

Figure 17.3 ● Arterial ulcer at the margin of the foot.

Ulcers

Ischaemic ulcers most commonly affect the tips of the toes, the margins of the foot (e.g. lateral to fifth metatarsophalangeal joint) where the circulation is poorest, and also at the lateral malleolus (Figure 17.3). Ulceration in diabetic patients may have a neuropathic component; this is discussed more fully in the section relating to diabetic foot (see page 242).

Vascular history

The schedule of a vascular history should be similar for both patients with chronic limb ischaemia and those with claudication. A suggested approach is summarised in Table 17.2. The initial focus of the history should relate to the peripheral vascular symptoms. Many arterio-pathic patients complaining of rest pain will give a preceding history of claudication, although this may not be evident in patients who live sedentary lives or in diabetic patients. Similarly, ulcers and gangrene often arise without prior history of pain, particularly in the presence of dia-betic neuropathy. Since atherosclerosis affects the circulation globally, the presence of cardio-vascular and cerebrovascular symptoms should also be elicited. Social history is also important, particularly with regard to the impact that the patient's symptoms are having on their life. This may be instrumental in planning treatment, particularly for claudicant patients.

Vascular examination

Although the main focus of the vascular examination for patients with critical ischaemia is the lower limb, it is important to adopt a systematic approach. Other important clinical signs may be elicited that may affect the patient's future management. A suggested approach to general cardiovascular examination is outlined in Box 17.1. When inspecting the feet, it is important to check for tissue loss between the toes and at the heels.

Investigation of vascular disease

Revascularisation is normally possible in 70 per cent of patients with critical limb ischaemia. Therefore, unless amputation is the preferable option, all patients with critical ischaemia should undergo vascular imaging. The advantages, disadvantages and contraindications of the four most commonly used modalities are presented in Table 17.3. The choice of imaging modality often depends on local services and expertise, but where contraindications exist, one

Table 17.2 Taking a vascular history

History	Specific points to cover
Peripheral vascular symptoms	Claudication Rest pain Tissue loss
Past vascular history	Previous vascular imaging Previous attempts at revascularisation Outcomes and complications
Other vascular symptoms	Angina or myocardial infarction Palpitations and atrial fibrillation Amaurosis fugax, TIAs or strokes
Risk factors	Smoking Hypertension Diabetes Abnormal lipids Family history (especially in young patients)
Other past medical history	
Drug history and allergies	Antiplatelets Beta-blockers Statins
Social history	Impact of patient's symptoms

TIA, transient ischaemic attack.

Table 17.3 Advantages and disadvantages of vascular imaging modalities

Modality	Advantages	Disadvantages
Angiography	Established gold standard	Nephrotoxic Allergic reactions Access site complications Radiation
CT angiography	Very quick 3D reconstruction possible	Nephrotoxic Allergic reactions Radiation
MR angiography	No radiation Less nephrotoxic 3D reconstruction possible	Contraindications (e.g. pacemaker, implants) Claustrophobic
Arterial duplex	Safe No contraindications Functional information	Time-consuming Operator-dependent

CT, computed tomography; 3D, three-dimensional; MR, magnetic resonance.

Box 17.1 Cardiovascular examination

Upper limb, head and neck

Hands
- Nicotine staining
- Clubbing
- Palmer erythema
- Muscle wasting
- Signs of subclavian embolisation.

Radial pulse
- Check for rate, volume, rhythm and character.
- Compare both sides – decreased volume or absent pulse may suggest subclavian steal.
- Look for radial femoral delay present in coarctation of aorta (and aortic dissection).

Subclavian steal syndrome
- Proximal subclavian stenosis causes retrograde flow of blood in the vertebral artery when exercising the arm, resulting in dizziness and intermittent claudication of the upper limb.
- More common on the left side.
- Systolic blood pressure is typically 20 mmHg lower in affected arm.
- Examine patient for brachial and axillary aneurysms, which may cause similar symptoms.
- Confirm diagnosis with duplex scan, looking for retrograde vertebral artery flow during exercise of arm.

Blood pressure
Compare in both arms (see above).

Blood pressure control
The treatment threshold for hypertension depends on the degree of associated cardiovascular risk:

Presence of risk factors	Systolic threshold (mmHg)	Diastolic threshold (mmHg)
No diabetes (but other risk factors)	140	90
Diabetes	130	85

Head and neck
- Check eyes for arcus senilis, jaundice and xanthelasma.
- Look for facial weakness that might represent stroke.
- Look for scar of carotid endarterectomy along anterior border of sternocleidomastoid.
- Look for raised jugular venous pulsation (JVP).
- Palpate carotid and subclavian arteries for aneurysms or carotid body tumour (rare).
- Check for lymphadenopathy.
- Auscultate for subclavian, common carotid and carotid bifurcation bruits (the carotid bifurcation is located deep to the anterior border of the sternocleidomastoid, between the thyroid cartilage and the angle of the jaw).

continued

Nerve damage in carotid endarterectomy

Nerve	Deficit
Superficial branches of cervical plexus	Loss of sensation in neck/angle of jaw
Great auricular nerve	Loss of sensation in earlobe
Marginal mandibular (from facial nerve)	Ipsilateral mouth-drop (weak orbicularis oris)
Recurrent laryngeal nerve (vagus)	Hoarse voice
Hypoglossal nerve	Contralateral deviation of tongue
Glossopharyngeal nerve*	Loss of sensation of ipsilateral oropharynx

*Only at risk if the posterior belly of diagastric is divided

Bruits
- Caused by turbulent blood flow vibrating the wall of the vessel.
- Audible only with greater than 40% and less than 85% stenosis.
- Should be distinguished from heart murmurs (aortic stenosis radiates to the carotid and subclavian arteries).
- Carotid bruits are present in 5% of people over 55 years of age and usually signify generalised disease.
- Carotid bruits are not specific and may signify common, internal or external carotid stenosis.

Thorax and abdomen
Chest and heart
- Inspect for mid sternotomy or other chest scars.
- Auscultate heart for murmurs.
- Auscultate chest.

Sternotomy scar
- Mid-sternotomy is commonly used for coronary artery bypass grafting and for cardiac valve replacement.
- Evidence of vein harvesting from the legs with sternotomy suggests bypass surgery.
- Metal valve replacements usually produce an audible clicking noise at the bedside.

Common murmurs
- *Aortic stenosis:* ejection systolic at right sternal margin radiating to neck.
- *Mitral stenosis:* soft mid-diastolic at apex heard better on expiration.
- *Mitral regurgitation:* pan-systolic at apex radiating to axilla.

Abdomen
- Observe for scars or extra-anatomical grafts (axillo-bifemoral, iliofemoral, femoral-femoral).
- Look for an epigastric pulsation at level of patient due to abdominal aortic aneurysm (AAA).
- Palpate for AAA between umbilicus and xiphisternum and wait for pulsation.
- Auscultate the same site for an aortic bruit, which signifies aorto-occlusive disease.
- Auscultate for renal bruits halfway between the umbilicus and the xiphisternum either side of the mid-line.

Surface anatomy of abdominal aorta
- Coeliac axis arises at lower border of T12.
- Superior mesenteric artery arises at L1.

continued

- Renal arteries arise at L2.
- Inferior mesenteric artery arises at L3.
- Aorta divides at L4.

Aortic pulsation and abdominal aortic aneurysm
- An expansile pulse of an AAA should push fingers out laterally and must be differentiated from a transmitted pulse, which pushes fingers upwards only.
- A transmitted pulse results from a mass overlying the aorta, such as lymphoid, gastric or transverse colon neoplasia.
- A normal aortic pulsation can be felt in thin individuals.
- The normal size of the aorta is 1.5–3 cm and is larger in males.
- 10% of people with an abdominal aortic aneurysm have a popliteal aneurysm.

Lower limb

Inspection
- Scars from previous operations:
  - Groin scar only suggests femoral embolectomy or endarterectomy
  - Scar along majority of thigh (with bridges) suggests vein graft
  - Scar at groin and knee suggests synthetic graft
- Colour of legs/feet and recent or unilateral hairlessness
- Deformity and muscle wasting
- Trophic changes:
  - Check specifically between toes and at heels
  - See pp. 243–4 for description of vascular and neuropathic ulcers
- Buerger's test:
  - Lift leg and look for development of pallor and venous guttering
  - Hang legs in dependent position and look for the rubor of reactive hyperaemia.

Palpation
- Feel temperature of feet/lower leg.
- Check capillary refill.

Palpation of pulses
- Feel for femoral, popliteal and pedal pulses.
- Easily palpable popliteal pulses may suggest popliteal aneurysms.
- Auscultate femoral artery for bruits, which can sometimes be felt as a thrill.

Popliteal aneurysms
- Popliteal aneurysms are bilateral in 50% of cases.
- Distal ischaemia in the presence of a contralateral popliteal aneurysm should raise the possibility of a thrombosed ipsilateral popliteal aneurysm.
- 30% of people with a popliteal aneurysm will have an abdominal aortic aneurysm.
- Suspected popliteal aneurysms should be confirmed by ultrasound, and the aorta and iliac arteries should also be investigated.

Ankle brachial pressure index
- May be recorded at dorsalis pedis, posterior tibial or peroneal arteries.
- 0.9–1.0 is normal.
- 0.5–0.9 is typically obtained with intermittent claudication.
- < 0.5 is typically obtained with critical ischaemia.
- (> 1.0 may be seen in diabetic patients with calcified vessels).

modality may afford a clear benefit. It is important to check a patient's renal function before imaging, as the intravenous contrast used for plain angiography, computed tomography (CT) angiography and, to a lesser extent, magnetic resonance angiography is nephrotoxic. Where possible, metformin should be stopped for 2 days before and 2 days after angiography. In such patients, and in patients with a degree of renal impairment, patients should ideally be kept well dehydrated before, during and after the procedure.

■ KEY POINT
Revascularisation is normally possible in 70 per cent of patients with critical limb ischaemia.

Management of chronic critical ischaemia

Pain relief

Rest pain may be particularly debilitating. While further investigations are being planned, consideration should be given to pain control. Opiate analgesia is often required, and it may be necessary to admit the patient for analgesia while they are being investigated.

Revascularisation

In critical limb ischaemia, disease is often multilevel and complicated. Revascularisation should be attempted where possible. Successful revascularisation requires sufficient inflow and outflow, and careful preoperative investigation is mandatory. There is often no clear optimum solution for revascularisation; endovascular intervention, surgery or a combination of both may be required. As patients with critical limb ischaemia are often old and frail, surgeons often look towards endovascular intervention for a solution to revascularisation. However, it is important to recognise the limitations and complications of such therapy. The Transatlantic Inter-Society Consensus (TASC) guidelines for the use of angioplasty are helpful in this regard.

Indications for angioplasty
For the purposes of assessing suitability for angioplasty, vascular disease is assessed according to four TASC categories. Table 17.4 provides a description of each of these categories, alongside the appropriate morphology for iliac and femoral-popliteal vascular lesions.

Complications of angioplasty
The potential complications of angioplasty/stenting include groin haematoma (4%), false aneurysm formation (0.5%), arterial-venous fistula (0.1%), distal embolisation with tissue damage (5%), vessel occlusion (3%) ruptured vessel (0.5%) and need for emergency surgery (3%).

Treatment options for aorto-iliac disease
Figure 17.4 demonstrates possible surgical and endovascular procedures that may be used for critical limb ischaemia involving proximal vessels. The 5-year patency rates of these procedures are compared in Table 17.5. Aorto-bifemoral grafting has the best long-term outcome of all the procedures, but it is associated with significantly higher morbidity and mortality. For this reason, it is an inappropriate choice for the many patients with critical limb ischaemia who usually have significant comorbidity. Endovascular and extra-anatomical bypass procedures carry less risk and have similar 5-year patency rates – in the region of 70 per cent. The addition of stenting (Figure 17.5) improves the 5-year patency of aorto-iliac angioplasty to around 80 per cent. Axillo-femoral grafts should be taken to both femoral arteries, as the long-term patency of a unilateral bypass is much poorer.

Table 17.4 Transatlantic Inter-Society Consensus (TASC) classification for suitability of vascular lesions for angioplasty

Category	Suitability for PTA	Iliac morphology	Femoral-popliteal morphology
A	Treatment of choice High chance of technical success Symptoms relieved	Single non-calcified stenoses < 3 cm	Single stenosis/occlusion < 3 cm (not at origin SFA or distal PA)
B	Well suited Good chance of technical success Symptoms usually relieved	Single non-calcified stenosis of 3–5 cm Calcified stenosis < 3 cm	Stenosis/occlusion 3–10 cm (not distal PA) Heavily calcified stenosis < 3 cm Multiple stenoses < 3 cm
C	Amenable to PTA with moderate chance of technical success Usually reserved for when surgery is too risky for patient	Stenoses 5–10 cm Occlusions < 5 cm	Single stenoses 3–10 cm including distal PA Multiple heavily calcified stenoses 3–5 cm Stenosis/occlusions > 10 cm
D	Extensive disease with poor chance of success, but where surgery is not possible	Stenoses > 10 cm Occlusions > 5 cm Extensive bilateral disease	Complete CFA or SFA occlusion

CFA, common femoral artery; PA, popliteal artery; PTA, percutaneous transluminal angioplasty; SFA, superficial femoral artery.
For more details refer to the TASC II management guidelines – see Further Reading.

Table 17.5 Five-year patency rates of proximal vascular procedures

Procedure	5-year patency rate (range)		
	Critical ischaemia	Claudication	Not specified
Aorto-bifemoral	87% (80–88)	91% (90–94)	–
Femoral-femoral cross-over	–	–	75% (55–02)
Axillo-bifemoral	–	–	71% (50–76)
Axillo-unifemoral	–	–	51% (44–79)
Angioplasty (alone)	–	–	71% (64–75)
Angioplasty and stenting	–	–	77% (72–81)

All data from Norgen *et al.* (2007).

Treatment options for femoral disease
Table 17.6 compares the 5-year patency rates for common femoral procedures. Angioplasty is ideally suited to short proximal stenoses, but it is less effective with longer segments of more distal disease. There is little evidence that stenting improves patency rates of stenoses below the inguinal ligament. Further angioplasty can be undertaken safely in many patients following re-stenosis. For the treatment of claudication, patency rates for above-knee, vein and synthetic

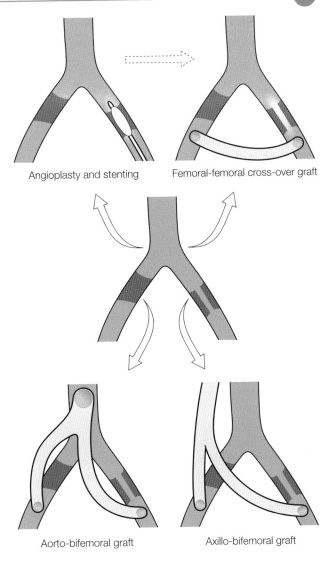

Figure 17.4 ● Surgical and endovascular options for revascularisation of supra-inguinal arterial disease.

Angioplasty and stenting

Femoral-femoral cross-over graft

Aorto-bifemoral graft

Axillo-bifemoral graft

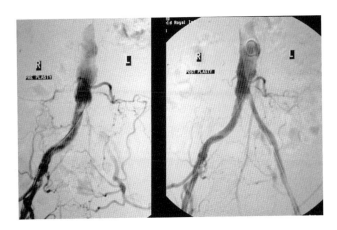

Figure 17.5 ● Iliac artery occlusion before and after treatment with angioplasty and stenting.

Table 17.6 Five-year patency rates for procedures involving femoral disease

Procedure	5-year patency rates (range)		
	Critical ischaemia	Claudication	Not specified
Vein graft to any level	66%	80%	–
Above-knee PTFE graft	47%	75%	–
Below-knee PTFE graft	33%	65%	–
Angioplasty for stenosis	–	–	55% (52–62)
Angioplasty for occlusion	–	–	42% (33–51)

PTFE, polytetrafluoroethylene.
All data from Norgen *et al.* (2007).

polytetrafluoroethylene (PTFE) grafts are similar. However, vein appears to be superior to PTFE when used for above-knee grafts in patients with critical ischaemia. For below-knee grafts, PTFE has unacceptably poor long-term results and should be avoided where possible. The potential for serious infective complications with synthetic grafts should always be borne in mind, particularly where patients have pre-existing soft-tissue infection.

> ■ KEY POINT
> Angioplasty is ideally suited to short proximal stenoses but is less effective with longer segments of more distal disease.

Treatment options for distal disease
Angioplasty can be used with some effect in the popliteal artery, but it is generally considered unsuitable for cural vessels. Femoral to cural bypass is often the only option to revascularise many patients with critical limb ischaemia. Success depends on adequate outflow, and the patency of the pedal arch should be determined prior to considering surgery. Vein is vastly superior to prosthetic material over long distances (see Table 17.5). Venous mapping is helpful in assessing the quality of veins before surgery.

Managing tissue loss

Ulcers
Healing of ulcers depends on restoration of sufficient blood flow and eradication of infection. In the presence of deep-seated infection, debridement may be necessary. A more detailed review of ulcer management is given below in the section on the diabetic foot.

Gangrenous digits
If pain is controlled adequately, dry gangrene can be left to separate naturally; this usually guarantees better healing. Surgical amputation runs the risk of wounds not healing, but it may be appropriate as part of a revascularisation procedure or in patients with intractable pain. Wet gangrene signifies infection and should be debrided.

Foot salvage
In patients with more extensive tissue loss and in those with infected tissue, surgery to salvage the foot should be considered after successful revascularisation. The aim of such surgery is to eradicate all dead and infected tissue while preserving as much function as possible. Figure 17.6 shows the extent of surgery required for different levels of disease.

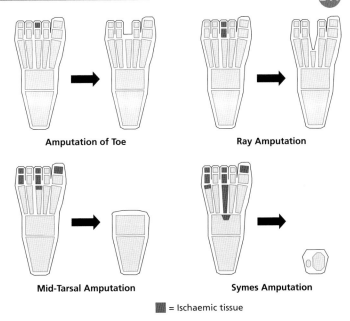

Figure 17.6 ● Levels of amputation required in foot salvage surgery.

Amputation of Toe

Ray Amputation

Mid-Tarsal Amputation

Symes Amputation

▓ = Ischaemic tissue

Pharmacological treatment

Where revascularisation is not possible, clinicians have examined the role of pharmacological agents in preserving limbs.

Prostanoids inhibit platelet activation and may benefit up to 40 per cent of patients with critical limb ischaemia in whom revascularisation is not possible. In some studies, prostanoids have been shown to reduce the risk of amputation and increase ulcer healing. The most widely known prostanoid is ileoprost (prostaglandin I2); it is given as a daily infusion, but it is often poorly tolerated due to its side-effect profile, which includes hypotension, flushing and headaches.

There is no evidence that vasodilators (e.g. nifedipine, nitrates), vasoactive drugs (e.g. naftidrofuryl, pentoxifylline), antiplatelets (e.g. aspirin) or anticoagulants (e.g. heparin) improve symptoms or outcomes in critical limb ischaemia. However, antiplatelets have a cardio- and cerebral protective benefit.

Management of risk factors

As part of the definitive management of critical limb ischaemia, it will be necessary to address the patient's cardiac risk factors. This process includes the following:

- Advice and support for smoking cessation
- Screening for and maintaining tight control of diabetes
- Prescribing statins for cholesterol over 5 mmol/L
- Screening for and maintaining tight control of hypertension
- Prescribing antiplatelet agents.

Amputation

Amputation is frequently the result of failed revascularisation or persistent sepsis despite revascularisation. In the following instances, however, a primary amputation should be considered:

- Overwhelming and life-threatening infection
- Loss of the foot
- Uncontrollable rest pain without possibility of revascularisation
- Critically ischaemic limbs in non-ambulatory patients, particularly those with contractures.

> ■ KEY POINT
> In some instances a primary amputation should be considered.

The aims of amputation should be primary wound healing at the distal-most level. Below-knee amputation may still allow some older and frailer patients to ambulate. Such patients are unlikely to mobilise with above-knee amputation. In non-ambulatory patients, consideration should be given to a through-knee (Gritty–Stokes) amputation if a below-knee amputation is not possible, since this preserves limb length and facilitates easier transfer.

Prognosis

The prognosis for critical limb ischaemia is poor. Within 1 year of onset, 25 per cent of patients will have died and 25 per cent will have undergone major amputation. Many of the remaining patients will still have rest pain or ulceration.

> KEY POINT
> The prognosis for critical limb ischaemia is poor: within 1 year of onset, 25 per cent of patients will have died and 25 per cent will have undergone major amputation.

● DIABETIC FOOT

Definition

Diabetic foot does not refer to a single clinical entity; rather, it covers a collection of foot pathologies affecting people with diabetes. The three main elements of diabetic foot comprise:

- Peripheral neuropathy
- Peripheral vascular disease
- Infection.

Epidemiology

Due to its imprecise definition, the prevalence of diabetic foot is not easy to establish. Studies suggest that the annual incidence of foot ulcers in diabetic people is around 2–4 per cent. The prevalence of diabetic foot among diabetic people may be estimated to be around 10 per cent.

The health and financial costs of diabetic foot are significant. Diabetic foot carries a 15-fold increased risk of amputation. The cost of diabetic foot ulceration was estimated by one Swedish study to be US$18 000, rising to US$34 000 if an amputation was required.

Classification and pathophysiology

Although the aetiological factors resulting in diabetic foot disease tend to be multifactorial, three patterns of disease are commonly recognised:

- Neuropathic (50%)
- Ischaemic (15%)
- Neuroischaemic (35%).

Neuropathic disease

Peripheral neuropathy is common in diabetes and may affect up to 50 per cent of diabetic people over the age of 60 years. All types of nerve fibre – sensory, motor, autonomic – can be affected. In many patients the onset of peripheral neuropathy goes unnoticed, but it can produce a wide manifestation of symptoms, including neuropathic pain, hyperaesthesia, paraesthesia and allodynia. The typical clinical finding is that of loss of sensation in a stocking distribution.

> ■ KEY POINT
> Peripheral neuropathy is common in diabetes and may affect up to 50 per cent of diabetic people over the age of 60 years.

Around one-third of patients with diabetic neuropathy develop ulceration. Figure 17.7 summarises the pathway by which neuropathy leads to ulceration. The main factors are as follows:

- *Loss of sensation resulting in foot trauma*: this may be a single event, such as standing on a nail, but it is often be repetitive, for example rubbing from ill-fitting shoes. Arthritic patients have similar deformities to diabetic patients, but because the former experience pain they are forced to rest the foot and modify their activities; in consequence, they are less prone to ulcer formation.
- *Loss of motor fibres to the intrinsic muscles of the foot*: this results in imbalance between the long flexors and extensors, leading to clawing of the toes, subluxation of the metatarsophalangeal joints and development of a high plantar arch. The net effect of this deformity is to reduce the load-bearing surface of the foot, resulting in the sole of the foot being exposed to higher pressures. Deformity also increases the likelihood of repetitive injury from shoes.
- *Callus formation*: in response to high pressure, the skin of the foot is prone to hyperkeratinisation or callus formation. This exacerbates the problem by reducing the elasticity of the skin and increasing the shearing forces between the skin and the underlying bone.

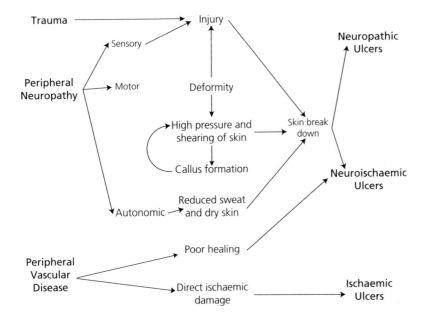

Figure 17.7 ● Pathways resulting in diabetic foot ulceration.

- *Autonomic neuropathy resulting in dry skin:* loss of autonomic fibres leads to reduced sweating, causing cracking, and may play a role in the breakdown of the skin resulting in ulcers. Autonomic neuropathy also results in loss of sympathetic tone at the arteriolar level, causing arteriole-venous shunting and a paradoxically red and warm foot. In addition, there may be an increase in hydrostatic capillary pressure, resulting in neuropathic oedema.

Clinical appearance

Examples of typical neuropathic ulcers can be seen in Figures 17.8 and 17.9. Neuropathic ulcers tend to occur in the weight-bearing areas of the foot that are subject to excess plantar pressure, as shown in Figure 17.10. Alternatively, ulceration may occur at the site of any

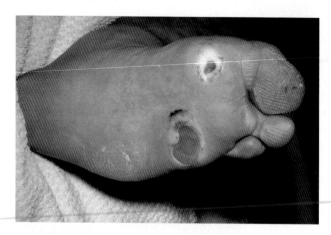

Figure 17.8 • Typical neuropathic ulcers with callus (note also previous digital amputation and Charcot's deformity).

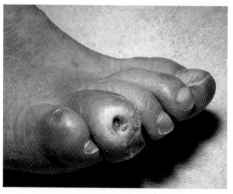

Figure 17.9 • Neuropathic ulcer on the dorsum of the fourth toe due to trauma from shoe.

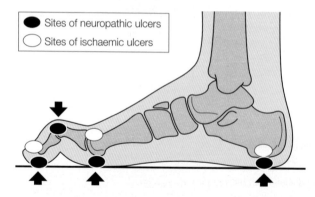

● Sites of neuropathic ulcers
○ Sites of ischaemic ulcers

Figure 17.10 • Areas of the foot susceptible to neuropathic and ischaemic ulceration.

trauma, which often includes the dorsal surface of clawed toes (Figure 17.9). Callus is often present and the ulcers are typically painless due to the presence of neuropathy. The feet will show evidence of peripheral neuropathy, including loss of sensation. In the presence of autonomic neuropathy, the feet may also be warm and pink due to shunting. This finding does not exclude the presence of peripheral vascular disease, which may also be present in patients with neuroischaemic ulcers. A thorough vascular examination, including ABPIs, is necessary in all diabetic patients presenting with ulcers.

Ischaemic disease

As mentioned previously, ischaemic disease may complicate neuropathic ulceration by impairing wound healing, thereby resulting in neuroischaemic ulceration. However, peripheral vascular disease may result in ulceration and gangrene in diabetic patients without evidence of peripheral neuropathy. The pathophysiology of ischaemic ulceration is the same in diabetic and non-diabetic patients, with insufficient blood flow to maintain the integrity of the skin. Nevertheless, diabetic claudicant patients have a two-fold increased risk of developing rest pain and a six-fold increased risk of developing gangrene in comparison with non-diabetic claudicant patients. Part of this difference may be explained by the increased propensity for small-vessel (infra-popliteal) disease in diabetics. Ischaemic disease is discussed more extensively in the first half of this chapter.

Clinical appearance

Ischaemic ulceration (see Figure 17.3) tends to affect the margins of the foot, typically the distal toes, but also the heel and the medial aspect of the first metatarsophalangeal joint (see Figure 17.10). Ulcers may be associated with marked rest pain, depending on the degree of concurrent neuropathy. The ulcers are without callus. The ischaemic foot is normally pale and hairless. Venous guttering may be present with a positive Buerger's test. Foot pulses are normally absent and the ABPIs are normally less than 0.9, unless the vessels are non-compressible, in which case the ABPIs are abnormally high. The presence of dry gangrene usually signifies an ischaemic problem. Wet gangrene may occur in neuropathic feet secondary to infection. The main differences between neuropathic and ischaemic ulcers are given in Table 17.7.

Infection

Although diabetic foot ulceration will initially develop without microbial involvement, there is a high propensity for septic complications, and these may evolve rapidly. The spectrum of infection encompasses cellulitis, abscess formation and osteomyelitis. Deeper tissue infections can spread quickly in the fascial planes of the foot and may cause thrombosis of blood vessels,

Table 17.7 Differences between neuropathic and ischaemic ulcers

Neuropathic	Ischaemic
Painless	Painful
Plantar surfaces	Toes and margins of foot
Callus	No callus
No sensation but pulses present	No pulses but sensation present
Good venous filling	Venous guttering
Warm, red foot	Cold, pale, hairless foot

resulting in gangrene, even in the absence of vascular disease. Frequently, infections are caused by more than one bacterium, which may include *Staphylococcus*, *Streptococcus*, Gram-negative organisms and anaerobes. The presence of infection confers a greatly increased risk of amputation.

> ■ KEY POINT
> Diabetic foot infections are frequently caused by more than one bacterium.

Charcot's neuroarthropathy

Within the context of the diabetic foot, Charcot's neuroarthropathy concerns neuropathic mediated destruction of joints within the foot. It affects one in ten diabetic patients with evidence of peripheral neuropathy. The pathogenesis is not elucidated fully. Autonomic neuropathy is thought to result in increased blood flow to the bone, which leads to activation of osteoclasts and rarefaction of the bone. Such joints become susceptible to easy trauma, which goes unrecognised by the neuropathic patient and continued weight-bearing precipitates further damage. As a consequence, patients often present late.

Patients typically present with a markedly swollen, hot foot and may also have a recent history of trauma. This acute phase is frequently described as painless, but patients often experience some degree of pain and discomfort despite their peripheral neuropathy. Once the acute phase subsides, patients are normally left with some degree of deformity. The most common joint to be affected is the tarsometatarsal joint, which results in subluxation of the mid-foot causing the classic rocker-bottom foot deformity (Figure 17.11). The resulting deformity has implications for the development of ulceration due to altered pressures on the foot and local trauma to the skin. Diagnosis may be made with serial radiographs, which show severe destruction of joints with atrophic and hypertrophic changes. Pathological fractures may also be seen. Magnetic resonance imaging (MRI) and isotope scanning may be useful for excluding infection during the initial presentation, although it is not always possible to differentiate between Charcot's neuroarthropathy and infection with either modality. Ultrasound can be helpful in excluding a soft-tissue collection.

> ■ KEY POINT
> Charcot's neuroarthropathy most commonly affects the tarsometatarsal joint.

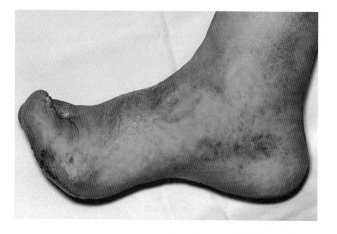

Figure 17.11 ● The typical 'rocker bottom' deformity of tarsometatarsal Charcot's neuroarthropathy.

In the acute phase, treatment is directed towards resting the foot and promoting the quiescent stable phase. In the early presentation, bed-rest may be necessary and the patient should not weight-bear. With time, protected ambulation may be introduced using casts or braces. There is some evidence that bisphosphonates may be of benefit in reducing the activation of osteoclasts and reducing the sequelae of the disease. The acute phase may take 3 months to subside. Once the acute phase has subsided, patients normally require specialised footwear in order to avoid damage to the skin and subsequent ulceration. In selected patients, where conservative measures have failed to prevent such problems, corrective surgery may be considered in the absence of peripheral vascular disease.

Prevention of ulceration

The vast majority of foot ulceration affecting diabetic patients is entirely preventable. Prevention relies on the identification of at-risk patients and the involvement of a multidisciplinary team comprising diabetologists, podiatrists, vascular surgeons, providers of appliances and orthopaedic surgeons.

Identification and assessment of at-risk patients

The three biggest causative factors for ulceration are loss of sensation, excessive plantar pressure and trauma. Other risk factors include previous history of ulceration, a history of diabetes for more than 10 years, poor diabetic control (haemoglobin A1c (HbA1c) > 9.0) and low visual acuity.

> ■ KEY POINT
> The three biggest causative factors for ulceration are loss of sensation, excessive plantar pressure and trauma.

Assessment of the at-risk patient should include the following:

- Screening for sensory neuropathy using standardised monofilament (the Semmes–Weinstein monofilament exerts a standard 10-g force when it touches the skin and bends for 1 s; inability to feel this force is indicative of sensory neuropathy)
- Examination for foot deformities
- Assessment of skin integrity and quality
- ABPIs
- Angiography if ABPIs are equivocal.

Prevention strategies

Patient education
There is some evidence that patient education may reduce the risk of ulceration. Patients should be advised to check their own feet or see a podiatrist regularly.

Diabetic control
Due to the deleterious long-term consequences of poor glycaemic control, the patient's diabetic control and medication should be reviewed regularly. Other risk factors for vascular disease should also be corrected, including cessation of smoking.

Podiatry
The role of the podiatrist is important in ulcer presentation, and regular podiatry input has been shown to reduce deep ulceration, septic complications and hospitalisation. In addition to picking up early signs of problems, podiatrists can de-roof calluses, reducing pressure on the skin, and may help to pad deformities in order to reduce pressure and prevent local trauma.

Vascular surgery

The role of the vascular surgeon in ulcer prevention is debatable. Vascular procedures have a definite role in ulcer healing but are not typically used in asymptomatic patients due to the risk of failure with subsequent precipitation of symptoms. Nevertheless, vascular surgeons are pivotal in the management in established disease and should be consulted early.

Orthopaedic surgery

Orthopaedic surgery to correct deformity and to reduce the risk of ulceration may be appropriate in selected patients. However, there is little evidence to support this approach. Corrective surgery should not be undertaken in patients with significant vascular disease where wound healing could be problematic.

Shoes and appliances

Patents with diabetic feet have specialist footwear requirements. Shock-absorbing insoles and extra-depth shoes should be considered for any diabetic patients with loss of sensation in the feet. With significant deformity or ulcers, custom-moulded shoes and rocker outsoles can also be of benefit. These adaptations reduce weight-bearing pressure and shear forces affecting the feet.

Management of ulceration

Figure 17.12 provides an overview of diabetic ulcer management. Significant infection and critical ischaemia pose the greatest risks to the diabetic foot. Patients with significant sepsis require urgent hospitalisation for treatment. Critical ischaemia requires urgent investigation and may also require the patient to be hospitalised. Other forms of ulceration can usually be managed in the outpatient setting.

Infection in the diabetic foot

Colonisation of diabetic ulcers is common and should not be treated with antibiotics in the absence of established clinical signs of infection due to the risk of selecting resistant bacteria. Acute deep-seated infection mandates prompt treatment, which in most cases requires

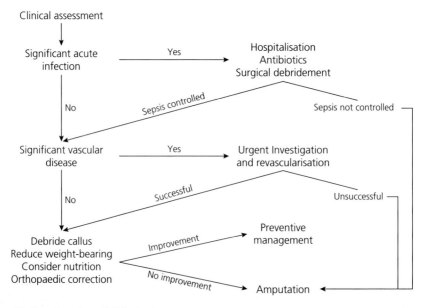

Figure 17.12 ● Overview of diabetic ulcer management.

hospitalisation. Any acute infection treated in the community should be reviewed regularly to look for signs of deterioration. In addition to baseline blood tests (with inflammatory markers) and blood cultures if indicated, all patients should have a plain radiograph of the foot in order to exclude the presence of soft-tissue gas and to look for evidence of osteomyelitis. Ultrasound may be used to rule out soft-tissue collections, and a bone scan may be used to detect osteomyelitis. Alternatively, MRI can be used to look for all forms of sepsis. The principles of treatment include tight diabetic control (with a sliding scale if necessary), appropriate antibiotics and surgical debridement of necrotic tissue.

■ KEY POINT

Colonisation of diabetic ulcers is common and should not be treated with antibiotics in the absence of established clinical signs of infection.

Where possible, tissue should be sent for culture before starting antibiotics. Cultures from the surface of ulcers rarely identify the pathogen involved in acute infection, and deeper tissue samples (especially following debridement) are often more helpful in this regard. Empirical intravenous antibiotics should be commenced immediately and should cover Gram-negative organisms and anaerobes as well as *Staphylococcus* and *Streptococcus*. Cefuroxime and metronidazole or amoxicillin, flucloxacillin and metronidazole are popular regimens. Clindamycin has a wide spectrum of activity that includes anaerobes; it also has excellent bone penetration. However, it is rarely used as a first-line agent because of the risk of causing *Clostridium difficile* colitis.

Pus requires formal drainage, and necrotic tissue in an infected foot should be surgically excised. The surgical principles of debridement are simple: remove all dead tissue including bone, do not leave bone exposed, and leave the wound (or at least part of it) open in order to allow drainage. In the presence of significant vascular disease, consideration should be given to revascularisation of the foot in order to facilitate healing following the eradication of infection.

Chronic infections and discharging sinuses in the foot are often due to osteomyelitis. About 70 per cent of cases of osteomyelitis can be diagnosed radiographically, but bone scans and MRI may be needed to make a diagnosis. The latter may be helpful in differentiating osteomyelitis from Charcot's neuroarthropathy.

Management of critical ischaemia

Diabetic ulcers in the presence of critical ischaemia are unlikely to heal without revascularisation. Patients with significant rest pain may require hospitalisation for symptom control, but if the patient is well and has no signs of sepsis they can be investigated urgently in the outpatient setting if imaging is readily available. Clinical assessment should include correction of risk factors, including smoking, hypertension and lipid dysfunction. Patients should be on antiplatelet therapy where possible. Angiotensin-converting enzyme (ACE) inhibitors have been shown to be cardioprotective in diabetic patients and should be given as first-line treatment for hypertension where there is no contraindication, particularly chronic renal failure. The management of critical ischaemia is outlined more fully in the first part of this chapter.

Management of non-infected neuropathic ulcers

The first step in the management of uncomplicated neuropathic ulcers is to de-roof callus and drain haematomas. As well as exposing the ulcer, this has been shown to significantly reduce weight-bearing forces. Consideration should then be given to resting the foot in order to eliminate the weight-bearing on the ulcer. This can be attained by bed-rest, but this is costly and has other health implications, including risk of venous thrombosis. Ambulatory resting of the foot can be achieved through the use of Scotchcast® boots, rocker cast shoes or modified shoes, which help spread weight to other parts of the foot. In ulcers that are slow to heal, further investigation should be undertaken to exclude arterial disease. Assessment should also be made of the patient's nutritional status.

Prognosis

The majority of diabetic ulcers are entirely preventable. However, non-traumatic lower-limb amputations are up to 30 times more common in diabetic patients. The 5-year survival following amputation is less than 60 per cent – worse than for most malignancies.

● SUMMARY

- Chronic critical limb ischaemia is defined by the presence of rest pain, ulceration or gangrene in association with an ankle pressure of less than 50 mmHg (ABPI < 0.5).
- Revascularisation should be considered in all patients with chronic critical limb ischaemia. Percutaneous endovascular revascularisation may be preferable to surgery in many patients due to a lower associated morbidity, but the long-term outcomes of such procedures are usually less successful.
- The diabetic foot is not a single disease entity but a number of pathologies (principally ischaemia, peripheral neuropathy and sepsis) that place the foot at risk.
- Diabetic ulcers are classified as neuropathic, ischaemic or neuroischaemic. Neuropathic ulcers are caused by a combination of sensory, motor and autonomic neuropathy. Ischaemic ulcers are due to macrovascular disease. Neuroischaemic ulcers are the result of concurrent neuropathy and vascular disease.
- The management of the diabetic foot should be multidisciplinary and preventive, with regular foot checks, patient advice and judicious use of foot appliances forming the basis of care.
- The approach for acute deterioration of the diabetic foot should comprise control of sepsis, restoration of perfusion (where possible) and management of ulcers. Early amputation may be necessary to control disease.

● QUESTIONS

1 How is critical limb ischaemia defined?
2 Discuss the complications of angioplasty.
3 What therapeutic options are available to treat a patient with proximal iliac disease who presents with a critically ischaemic limb?
4 Explain what is meant by the term 'diabetic foot', and outline the different pathologies involved.
5 How do ischaemic and neuropathic foot ulcers differ clinically?
6 Outline the multidisciplinary approach to managing the diabetic foot.

● REFERENCES

Norgen L, Hiatt WR, Dormandy JA, et al. (2007). Inter-society consensus for the management of peripheral arterial disease (TASC II). Eur J Vasc Endovasc Surg 33 (suppl. 1): S1–75.

● FURTHER READING

Beard JD (2000). Chronic lower limb ischaemia: ABC of arterial and venous disease. Br Med J 320: 854–7.
Norgen L, Hiatt WR, Dormandy JA, et al. (2007). Inter-society consensus for the management of peripheral arterial disease (TASC II). Eur J Vasc Endovasc Surg 33 (suppl. 1): S1–75.
Singh N, Armstrong DG, Lipsky BA (2005). Preventing foot ulcers in patients with diabetes. J Am Med Assoc 293: 217–28.
Watkins PJ (2000). The diabetic foot: ABC of arterial and venous disease. Br Med J 326: 977–9.

Laparoscopic surgery

Peter Sedman

● INTRODUCTION

This chapter outlines the basic principles of laparoscopic abdominal surgery and illustrates these principles as they apply to cholecystectomy. The topics covered include access and port placement, physiology, energy sources and the management of complications.

● BACKGROUND

In 1991 Sir Alfred Cuschieri suggested that 70 per cent of all abdominal operations would be performed laparoscopically by the turn of the century. This prediction was greeted with scepticism but, although the time frame may have been wrong, the ultimate figure looks increasingly likely to be achieved within our working lives. All abdominal operations (with the exception of transplants and caesarean sections) have now been performed laparoscopically, thus proving they are technical feasible.

The increase in the complexity of these laparoscopic operations has been made possible because of:

- increased technical skills and confidence;
- improved optical lenses;
- the availability of stack systems with high-definition resolution;
- the development of integrated laparoscopic theatre suites;
- the emergence of robotic assistants;
- developments in haemostasis, both chemical- and energy-based, resulting in reduced blood loss;
- the rapid rise in the use of alternative energy sources to monopolar diathermy.

Much of the development of laparoscopic surgery has been driven by patient demand because of the improved cosmesis and shortened postoperative convalescence associated with the absence of conventional wounds. Pressure to minimise or avoid hospital stays, and to minimise postoperative hospital-acquired infections, has been a major driver for doctors and managers. Operative times are generally similar now for most operations, whether open or laparoscopic, but some new challenges exist for the laparoscopic surgeon with regard to access, and especially in the previously operated abdomen. In laparoscopic surgery, it is gaining access that is perhaps the most dangerous part of the operation in inexperienced hands.

> ■ KEY POINT
> Much of the development of laparoscopic surgery has been driven by patient demand for improved cosmesis and shortened postoperative convalescence.

Operations in which the laparoscopic approach is preferred include the following:

- Cholecystectomy
- Hiatus hernia repair and anti-reflux surgery (Nissen's)
- Adrenalectomy
- Closure of simple perforated duodenal ulcer
- Splenectomy
- Anderson–Hynes pyeloplasty.

Operations in which the laparoscopic approach is firmly established and preferred by many surgeons include the following:

- Surgery for morbid obesity (lap band and Roux-en-Y bypass)
- Appendicectomy
- Inguinal hernia repair
- Colorectal cancer resections
- Nephrectomy
- Exploration of common bile duct (CBD).

Promising operations in which the benefit of laparoscopy remains to be proven include the following:

- Oesophagogastrectomy
- Umbilical hernia repair
- Incisional hernia repair
- Prostatectomy.

● GENERAL CONSIDERATIONS OF LAPAROSCOPIC OPERATIONS

Fundamentally, laparoscopic operations differ from their open counterparts in several key areas:

- Principles of access
- Physiology of the pneumoperitoneum
- Energy sources
- Recognising complications
- Preoperative preparations.

Principles of access

Primary trocar

The single potentially most dangerous part of the laparoscopic operation is the establishment of the primary port. Horror stories abound regarding major vascular and bowel injury due to primary trocar injury. It is beyond the scope of this chapter to discuss these in detail, and attendance at a skills course to practise the various methods is recommended.

■ KEY POINT

The most dangerous part of the laparoscopic operation is the establishment of the primary port. Major vascular and bowel injury may occur due to primary trocar injury.

There are three principal accepted ways to create pneumoperitoneum and establish the first port. It is essential that the surgeon becomes familiar with one technique and practises safe principles when using it. Adopting one method safely is more important than the choice of technique. The main choices are:

- Veress needle, pneumoperitoneum and closed primary trocar entry
- Open (Hasson) cannula entry
- Optical trocar entry.

Meta-analyses have suggested that the closed (Veress) technique is associated with a slightly higher incidence of vascular injury than the open (Hasson) technique. In contrast, the latter may be associated with gas leaks, making the operation much more difficult, and can be very difficult to perform, especially in obese patients. The incidence of bowel injury is the same for both approaches, at 1 in 1000 cases, and must be a consideration. Optical trocar devices are a more recent development and are increasing in popularity.

The design of the trocar is important. A wide variety are available. Sharp-bladed trocars are dwindling rapidly in popularity due to the risk of organ penetration, and a vogue for more blunt instruments, especially pencil-point trocars, is emerging.

■ KEY POINT
A vogue for more blunt instruments, especially pencil-point trocars, is emerging.

Secondary trocars

Since secondary trocars are placed under direct laparoscopic vision, they are generally safer to introduce than the primary trocar. However, the trick with the placement of secondary trocars is getting them in the correct sites for ergonomic control during the operation. Poor port placement can make the rest of the operation difficult, and good setup can make the difference between a stress-free operation and a struggle.

Optimum setup

Optimum setup can always be calculated from first principles:

- Consider the site of the primary trocar and of the target organ, and set up the patient, the surgical team and the stack appropriately, such that, for the surgeon, the ergonomics of the laparoscopic operation match as closely as possible the open equivalent. In the example of a gallbladder operation shown in Figure 18.1, the surgeon's head is in line with the line of the laparoscope and the stack. For a hiatal hernia repair, the surgeon would stand between the patient's legs, and the stack would be situated above the patient's head.
- Place secondary trocars for left- and right-hand instruments where they lie comfortably, such that the instruments subtend the target at 90 degrees (Figure 18.2), as the hands do for open surgery. Remember also that intra-abdominal movement of laparoscopic instruments is a fulcrum effect, with the abdominal wall being the fulcrum, and ideally this should lie approximately in the midshaft of the instrument.
- When the primary and secondary instruments are in place, the ports for retracting instruments may be sited outwith the operative field of view (Figure 18.3).

Physiology of the pneumoperitoneum

Carbon dioxide (CO_2) pneumoperitoneum has definite physiological consequences for the patient. These can be considered as chemical effects and physical effects, and they have potential consequences, especially for the patient with poor cardiac reserve, in whom laparoscopy can lead to heart failure. Remember also that, if the patient is unfit for general anaesthetic,

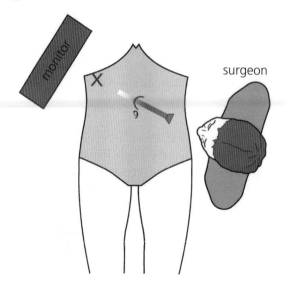

Figure 18.1 ● Alignment of surgeon, laparoscope, target organ and monitor.

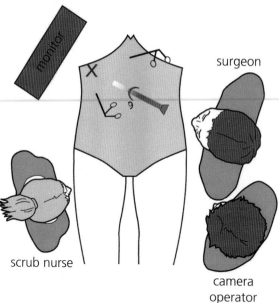

Figure 18.2 ● Introduction of left- and right-hand working ports.

muscle relaxant or open surgery, then the patient is also unfit for laparoscopy. There is always the potential need to convert to open surgery midway through any laparoscopic operation.

> ■ KEY POINT
> If the patient is unfit for general anaesthetic, muscle relaxant or open surgery, then the patient is also unfit for laparoscopy.

Physical effects of pneumoperitoneum

Positive intraperitoneal pressure is required to maintain the working space of the abdominal cavity, and maximal muscle relaxation and therefore general anaesthesia is necessary for all complex laparoscopic procedures.

Figure 18.3 ● Place retraction ports anywhere outside the operative triangle, i.e. in the dark shaded areas.

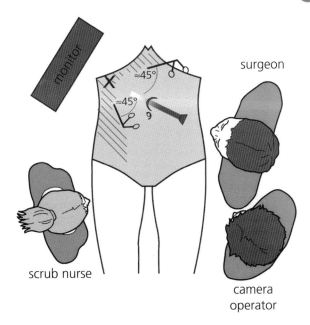

surgeon

monitor

≈45°

≈45°

scrub nurse

camera operator

The physiological consequences of a pneumoperitoneum are, however, in part pressure-sensitive: the lower the inflation pressure, the less pronounced the physiological consequences will be. These effects include the following:

● Splinting of the diaphragm
● Vagal stimulation, leading to pronounced bradycardia (especially in fit young people with good muscle tone and rapid insufflation at the start of the operation)
● Compression of the inferior vena cava, leading to decreased venous return (especially in head-up tilt) and venous stasis
● Pressure on the adrenals, leading to catecholamine surge.

With modern insufflators, most operations can be performed with inflation pressures in the region of 8–11 mmHg. When operating with pressures above 15 mmHg, the pressure effects become marked; above 20 mmHg, measurable changes occur.

> ■ KEY POINT
> When operating with inflation pressures above 15 mmHg, pressure effects are marked; above 20 mmHg, measurable changes occur.

Chemical effects of pneumoperitoneum

Carbon dioxide dissolves in peritoneal fluid to form carbonic acid, which is readily soluble. In effect, the peritoneal cavity acts as a giant alveolus through which CO_2 respiratory exchange may occur with blood. This may, therefore, cause respiratory acidosis, leading to myocardial irritability and myocardial depression. The effects of these may be reduced if the anaesthetist hyperventilates the patient, thereby 'blowing off' the CO_2.

For prolonged procedures above 2 h, there is the potential for CO_2 to be deposited in the tissues, especially bone and muscle, which may manifest as a late CO_2 narcosis in the immediate postoperative period. Re-ventilation may be required occasionally.

Alternative gases have been postulated, but none has proved sufficiently good to replace CO_2.

Energy sources

Monopolar diathermy

Laser diathermy was used in early laparoscopy, but the variable depth of beam penetration caused collateral damage and has been abandoned.

Monopolar diathermy has been the mainstay of open surgery for many decades, but within the closed abdomen it has limitations and the potential for harm. Various problems are described, and an understanding of these is essential for safe use. Monopolar diathermy may still be used for laparoscopic surgery, but its use is targeted, sparing and restricted to areas where there will be no pedicle effect.

Argon-beam diathermy is available in some centres for laparoscopic use and may be useful. It results in a form of controlled spray coagulation using monopolar cautery through the argon gas beam. Its availability is not universal.

Bipolar diathermy

Bipolar diathermy is more accepted and versatile. The past decade has seen significant improvements in this technology, to the extent that vessels up to 7 mm in diameter may be safely coagulated by bipolar diathermy. 'Intelligent' bipolar machines calculate tissue impedance and 'know' when coagulation is complete and when the vessel may be cut. Pulsed delivery of the current may further improve the efficacy of this approach.

Ultrasonic dissection

The energy required to cause cutting or coagulation of tissue need not be delivered solely in electrical form as above but instead may be provided as kinetic energy at ultrasound frequencies. These instruments are often referred to as 'harmonic scalpels', although strictly speaking this is a trademark of the most widely used type.

Chemical coagulation

Some circumstances do not lend themselves easily to mechanical or electrical cautery. An excellent example of this is the liver or splenic surface, where there is no tissue to pick up.

Much excitement now surrounds the topical application of thrombin or fibrin as a chemical coagulant glue. Using a special disposable applicator, thrombin or fibrin may be applied on to the bleeding tissues with almost instant effect, and the need to convert to open surgery because of bleeding has become a rarity.

Recognising complications

The most obvious benefit from laparoscopic surgery is the truly remarkable postoperative convalescence normally seen by the patients. Wound infections and chest infections are uncommon, and most patients can mobilise reasonably freely on the first postoperative day. A daily improvement is the norm. If the patient does not improve steadily at home, then they are advised to seek attention because a late bile duct leak after cholecystectomy may present in this way.

> ■ KEY POINT
> If the patient does not improve steadily at home, then they are advised to seek attention because a late bile duct leak after cholecystectomy may present in this way.

Similarly, if the patient is not comfortable in hospital, then alarm bells should ring, especially in the presence of an unexplained tachycardia. In the obese patient, tachycardia above 100 beats/min may be the *only* sign that something is wrong. Isolated shoulder tip pain occurs in up to 15 per cent of patients after upper abdominal laparoscopy and may simply be due to diaphragmatic stretching or irritation; if so, it will settle within 36 h.

> ■ KEY POINT
> If the patient is not comfortable in hospital, then alarm bells should ring, especially in the presence of an unexplained tachycardia.

Investigating possible complications

After considering the possible differential diagnoses in light of the history and examination, and with the benefit of relevant blood test results, the most reliable test may be a computed tomography (CT) scan. Ultrasound scanning may be easy to obtain but is not the most reliable in this situation, unless it is to show free fluid, as CT scanning gives more detail. It is important to remember that free gas in the peritoneal cavity beyond 36 h is abnormal. If such gas is present, then it is air from the bowel and not retained CO_2, which is reabsorbed transperitoneally within a few hours of the end of surgery.

> ■ KEY POINT
> The most reliable test for investigating complications is a CT scan.

In the presence of abnormal findings, or in the absence of available tests, the safest course of action is to re-laparoscope without delay and to treat the findings. A negative re-laparoscopy delays discharge by 1 day and is preferable to a counterproductive 'wait and see' policy. Indeed, most laparoscopic bariatric surgeons will re-laparoscope on the first postoperative day solely on the finding of a sustained tachycardia above 100 beats/min rather than seek other investigations.

> ■ KEY POINT
> In the presence of abnormal findings, or in the absence of available tests, the safest course of action is to re-laparoscope without delay and to treat the findings.

● LAPAROSCOPIC CHOLECYSTECTOMY

The indications for surgery are primarily:

- for the relief of symptoms from gallstones (5% failure rate);
- as prophylaxis against future pancreatitis following an episode of gallstone pancreatitis.

There are no good alternatives. Asymptomatic gallstones may reasonably be left untreated, but dissolution therapy and shockwave lithotripsy have been abandoned because they are relatively ineffective and leave the gallbladder in situ. Recurrent stone formation is therefore common. In elderly patients it is reasonable to treat CBD stones by endoscopic retrograde cholangiopancreatography (ERCP) and sphincterotomy and to leave any asymptomatic gallbladder stones alone.

Major complications

Major complications of laparoscopic cholecystectomy include the following:

- Risk of trocar injury
- Bleeding
- Bile leakage (1%)
- Bile duct injury (0.2%) or damage to surrounding structures (rare)
- Risk of deep vein thrombosis (DVT)/pulmonary embolism.

Conversion to open surgery

Conversion to open surgery is not a complication but the decision of a responsible surgeon who cannot proceed safely with the laparoscope. Conversion rates vary considerably from unit to unit, depending on the experience of the surgeon and the quality of the equipment available. A conversion rate for elective cholecystectomy of 2 per cent is reasonable and for acute cholecystectomy of 5 per cent. Conversion should therefore be discussed, but in the context of a possible additional procedure rather than as a complication.

Bile duct considerations

It is important to consider the possibility of bile duct stones in the following situations:

- Dilated CBD on ultrasound scan (> 0.5 cm)
- CBD stone seen on ultrasound scan
- History of obstructive jaundice
- History of pancreatitis
- Abnormal liver function test.

Methods of investigating the common bile duct

- *Preoperative ERCP*: the procedural morbidity (0.01%) and mortality (0.1%) and development of alternative investigations have made diagnostic ERCP redundant. ERCP should be reserved for therapeutic use only, when it is known that there are bile duct stones or when bile duct decompression is needed.
- *Preoperative spiral CT cholangiogram*: an intravenous contrast dye is injected and allowed to concentrate in the bile for 1–2 h before high-definition spiral CT scan images are acquired. This method is diagnostic only. Excellent picture quality is possible with minimal scanning times, but the method is unsuitable if the bilirubin level is above 50, as inadequate biliary concentration occurs.
- *Magnetic resonance cholangiopancreatography (MRCP)*: impressive non-invasive views of the CBD are possible, irrespective of the level of bilirubin, as contrast is not required. This is an alternative to spiral CT.

On-table cholangiogram

Some authors recommend this as a routine undertaking during cholecystectomy, but this is controversial. Most surgeons adopt a selective policy based on the criteria above for the higher probability of CBD stones. If on-table cholangiogram reveals stones, then they must be dealt with by one of the following:

- Laparoscopic exploration of the CBD, which is technically challenging and time-consuming

- Conversion to open surgery and exploration, thereby losing the advantages of laparoscopy and increasing postoperative morbidity
- Postoperative ERCP (risk of failure 5%, needing redo (probably open) surgery).

It may be concluded that it is preferable to deal with CBD stones preoperatively when suspected, unless laparoscopic exploration of the CBD is available.

Common bile duct injuries in laparoscopic cholecystectomy

Perhaps the most notorious complication of laparoscopic cholecystectomy is CBD injury. This is a potentially life-threatening complication and is guaranteed to achieve notoriety for the surgeon. In the early days of laparoscopic cholecystectomy, CBD injuries were much more common than had been the case with open cholecystectomy, but recognition of the mistakes in laparoscopic dissection leading to CBD injuries has enabled strategies to be devised in order to avoid them. Following are some important points regarding CBD injuries in laparoscopic cholecystectomy:

- They occur in the hands of experienced and inexperienced surgeons alike.
- They occur almost as frequently in the 'easy gallbladder' as in difficult cases.
- Less than 50 per cent are recognised at the time of surgery.
- Reliance on an operative cholangiogram to identify anatomy is unreliable as it is often done only *after* the damage has been done.
- Injury to the CBD may be associated with extensive injury to the hepatic artery and portal vein.
- The severity of CBD injury ranges from minor bile leaks to extensive excision of the CBD.
- It is widely considered medicolegally indefensible and has to date not been defended successfully in court.

Patient factors undoubtedly may make life difficult, but it is the surgeon who damages the duct – and usually because of errors in dissection. However, there are steps that the surgeon can take in order to minimise the risk.

Patient factors include pathological fibrosis in Calot's triangle, abnormal anatomy and, in some cases, excessive laxity of the tissues. Any one of these factors increases the risk of the surgeon injuring the bile duct, but only if the surgeon dissects in the wrong place. The error usually made is erroneously starting dissection to the left of the common bile duct, mistaking it for the cystic duct. The tendency to do this has been made more likely in the laparoscopic era because of the position of the surgeon on the patient's left and retracting Calot's triangle laterally. The classical injury sustained in laparoscopic cholecystectomy is therefore excision of the upper part of the CBD, the lower part of the common hepatic duct and the right hepatic artery.

In the difficult gallbladder, Calot's triangle may be fused and fibrotic. In extreme cases, Hartmann's pouch may be fused to the common duct so densely that the resulting extrinsic compression causes jaundice (Mirizzi's syndrome). In some cases, the CBD may be so wide that it is mistaken for the gallbladder (choledochal cyst, gallbladder agenesis with ductal dilation). Difficulties in identifying the anatomy can arise here despite the most careful of approaches, and in these circumstances the surgeon should consider 'fundus first' dissection, subtotal cholecystectomy or even conversion to open surgery.

In as many cases, however, the tissues are normal, very flexible and almost hyperelastic. In these latter cases, problems can arise with retraction of Hartmann's pouch causing inadvertent and unrecognised tenting-up of the CBD. If this tenting-up causes the CBD to overly the hepatic duct in the line of laparoscopic view, then the potential mistake is to divide the lower CBD, believing it to be the cystic duct, and only later in the dissection to find the common hepatic duct behind, by which stage a significant length of the bile duct has been dissected out and/or excised. The surgeon has been lured into a false sense of security – this mistake befalls both experienced and inexperienced surgeons.

Uncontrolled bleeding in the region of Calot's triangle will lead to problems if clips or cautery are applied indiscriminately. It is a useful (and achievable) principle never to use monopolar diathermy in Calot's triangle or anywhere near the CBD.

Occasionally, bile leaks occur as a result of clips falling off the cystic duct or as a result of sub-hepatic ducts (of Lushka) leaking postoperatively. Unlike anatomical misidentification, there is usually no tissue loss and these usually become apparent postoperatively and may often be managed conservatively.

Abnormal anatomy may trap the unwary. Biliary anatomy is notoriously variable, and numerous textbooks detail these variants. Correct interpretation of a routine cholangiogram is the only reliable way of spotting the variants intraoperatively, but one surgical principle, when applied correctly, renders knowledge of these variants to almost intellectual interest only.

■ KEY POINT

When dissecting in Calot's triangle, divide no structure until the junction of the gallbladder and the cystic duct has been demonstrated clearly.

Traditional 'open' teaching suggested the cystic duct–CBD junction as the important landmark. This is wrong advice for the laparoscopic surgeon. The ideal is not to see the CBD at all. Leaving a long cystic duct is acceptable and in fact is desirable, as it confirms the above principle has been followed.

Fifty per cent of CBD injuries are unrecognised at the time of surgery and appear postoperatively as bile leaks, peritonitis or jaundice. Whenever bile duct injury is suspected, treatment and investigation should start without delay. The priority in the event of biliary peritonitis and a bile leak is to establish effective drainage of bile from the peritoneal cavity either by percutaneous drainage or by repeat laparoscopy. Good-sized drains to the affected area usually suffice, and these drains control the immediate clinical danger while investigation is pursued. The anatomical injury needs to be diagnosed promptly; this may be done by MRCP, spiral CT, percutaneous transhepatic cholangiography (PTC) or ERCP (or a combination of these). Percutaneous transhepatic cholangiography and drainage may be required for obstructive jaundice.

With the clinical problem under control and the anatomical injury established, longer-term treatment can be planned. With the exception of minor bile leaks from the liver bed (duct of Lushka leaks) or leaks from the cystic duct, management should be discussed with the local hepatobiliary unit. Minor injuries may be treated conservatively and usually settle within a week or so; this is sometimes aided by stenting of the ampulla by ERCP to decompress the biliary tree and speed fistula closure.

More major injuries, especially those with major duct disruption, are the province of the specialist and may involve hepaticojejunostomy or more major reconstructions.

If a duct injury is recognised at surgery, then the above algorithm is still relevant. In addition, cholangiography should be performed; occasionally, conversion and primary repair with a T-tube is an additional option if the defect in the CBD is very small. Description of the options for major reconstructions is outside the scope of this chapter.

Preoperative preparations

At the preoperative assessment stage:

- Gain consent.
- Take blood tests, especially clotting, group and stage, blood chemistry profile and full blood count (FBC).

- Recognise special needs or considerations.

  Immediately preoperatively:

- Standard fast for 6 h.
- Advise patient to pass urine immediately preoperatively in order to reduce the risk of bladder injury.
- Administer subcutaneous heparin if prescribed.

  Prophylaxis should be employed for all patients with one or more risk factors.

■ KEY POINT

Preoperative prophylaxis should be employed for all patients with one or more risk factors.

Operative setup

The administration of a general anaesthetic with muscle relaxation is mandatory. The facility for intraoperative head-up tilt is essential; the operating table should accommodate this. Side-to-side tilt is desirable and, if intraoperative cholangiography is needed, the operating table and the patient's position on it must be able to accommodate this.

Port positioning

Rather than slavishly using other people's port positions, it is more useful to use the principles of port placement discussed above and to apply them to cholecystectomy.

For most patients the umbilicus is a convenient site for the primary trocar. This is the thinnest point on the anterior abdominal wall, where the skin linea alba and peritoneum are fused as a single layer, and it gives the widest exposure to the abdominal cavity for diagnostic laparoscopy. However, for upper abdominal surgery, the xiphoid is a more useful reference point, especially in the obese patient (Figure 18.4), and a distance approximately 10 cm infe-

Figure 18.4 ● Do not always use the umbilicus as the site for the primary trocar!

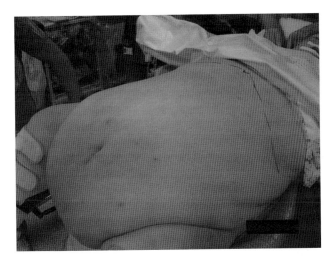

rior to the xiphoid is appropriate. This allows excellent exposure of the hiatus for fundoplication and of Calot's triangle without the transverse colon obscuring the view.

The next consideration is for the surgeon to be comfortable. To achieve this, the surgeon should be able to stand behind the line of the camera with the monitor in direct visual line (see Figure 18.1). In the future, modern flat screens will allow the monitor to be placed just above the patient's torso, making it even more ergonomic for the surgeon.

Once the primary trocar is in situ, secondary ports may be placed under direct vision. These should be sited so that the instruments through them approach the target organ at 60–90 degrees. This most accurately reproduces the open surgery situation, whereby one's hands work best together when at right-angles to each other. Remember that laparoscopic instruments work on a fulcrum through the anterior abdominal wall and that this fulcrum is best placed at the midpoint of the instruments.

Once the surgeon is happy with the camera position and operating ports, then additional trocars for retraction may be placed at any point outside this operative triangle, such that the instruments do not impede each other.

Technique of laparoscopic cholecystectomy

The initial experience with the laparoscopic version of cholecystectomy was notable because of the sudden increase in the incidence of bile duct injury, and much analysis was undertaken to understand why. The two overriding factors for this were found to be the result of:

- specific anatomy;
- the use of diathermy.

Anatomy

The important landmark in laparoscopic cholecystectomy is the junction of the gallbladder and the cystic duct. This should always be defined. The syndrome of the 'long cystic duct' has been dismissed, and it is now acceptable – indeed, desirable – to leave the cystic duct as long as possible. This often necessitates the dissection of the proximal half of the gallbladder from the liver bed before any other structures are divided. This ensures the confident exposure of the junction between Hartmann's pouch and the cystic duct, and only then may it be clipped adjacent to the gallbladder. Any uncertainty is best dealt with by subtotal cholecystectomy rather than risk a bile duct injury, which is associated with an average 10-year decrease in life expectancy. If this junction is seen, then detailed knowledge of bile duct anatomical variation becomes less important because these variations are mostly circumvented.

> ■ KEY POINT
>
> The important landmark in laparoscopic cholecystectomy is the junction of the gallbladder and the cystic duct.

Use of diathermy

As discussed above, monopolar diathermy has potential problems in the confined abdomen. This is particularly true in dissection of Calot's triangle, where monopolar diathermy has been credited with injuries to the duodenum (immediate and delayed) and to the CBD by lateral pedicle spread. It is good practice to undertake the whole of the dissection of Calot's triangle without diathermy. Careful use of monopolar diathermy in the liver bed is acceptable.

The incidence of bile duct injury has fallen dramatically in the past 5 years, *but beware!* It may happen to junior and experienced surgeons alike and is equally common in the 'easy' gallbladder as in the difficult one. Always exercise caution when dividing the cystic duct. Know your anatomy before cutting anything.

THE FUTURE

The breathtaking speed of the introduction of minimal-access surgery in specialist centres has no precedent in surgical evolution, and laparoscopic surgeons in their fifties have had to learn all these techniques anew. It is unlikely to stop there, and trainees today will lead these new developments in whichever direction innovation leads. Already we have the prospect of 'scarless surgery', with operations being performed using flexible endoscopes through natural body cavities (e.g. transvaginal cholecystectomy, transgastric appendicectomy). These and remote robotic surgery are being actively pursued, and it is a question of watch this space, critically appraise new techniques and be prepared to change. Rarely can a career have been so exciting!

SUMMARY

This chapter has outlined the basic principles of laparoscopic abdominal surgery and illustrated these principles as they apply to cholecystectomy. The topics covered include access and port placement, physiology, energy sources and the management of complications.

QUESTIONS

1 Discuss some of the problems of access in laparoscopic surgery and some of the techniques available to minimise these.
2 What are the energy sources available for dissection and haemostasis at the laparoscopic surgeon's disposal? Describe some of the advantages and disadvantages of each.
3 Discuss the physiological effects of carbon dioxide pneumoperitoneum. How may these effects be reduced? Which patients are most at risk from these effects?
4 Advocate the argument for the routine use of operative cholangiography in laparoscopic cholecystectomy.
5 Advocate the argument for the selective use of operative cholangiography in laparoscopic cholecystectomy.

FURTHER READING

Association of Laparoscopic Surgeons of Great Britain and Ireland. www.alsgbi.org.
Bordeaux Institute of Laparoscopic Surgery. www.e-laparoscopy.com.

Valuable resource with excellent video-clips of advanced laparoscopic procedures.

Neugebauer EA, European Association for Endoscopic Surgery (2006). *EAES Guidelines for Endoscopic Surgery: Twelve Years Evidence-Based Surgery in Europe*. Berlin: Springer.

A valuable collection of evidence for the practice of laparoscopy, complied and analysed by the members of the European Association of Endoscopic Surgery (EAES).

Perissat J, Huibregtse K, Keane FBV, Russell RCG, Neoptolemos JP (1994). Management of bile duct stones in the era of laparoscopic cholecystectomy. *Br J Surg* **81**: 1364–6.

A comprehensive review of the natural history of bile duct stones and rationale for management approaches.

Scott-Conner CEH, Society of American Gastrointestinal Endoscopic Surgeons (2006). *The SAGES Manual: Fundamentals of Laparoscopy, Thoracoscopy, and GI Endoscopy*, 2nd edn. New York: Springer.

Introductory guidelines compiled by members of the Society of American Gastrointestinal Endoscopic Surgeons (SAGES), designed to guide the beginner in the techniques of laparoscopy and endoscopy.

Society of American Gastrointestinal and Endoscopic Surgeons. www.sages.org.
World Electronic Book of Surgery. www.websurg.com.

Large collection of educational programmes in laparoscopic surgery. Excellent, free, extensively accessed resource for laparoscopic surgeons.

Management of surgery in obese patients

Amer Aldouri and S Dexter

● INTRODUCTION

Obesity is a growing health problem in Western countries. It is associated with a significant increase in morbidity and a reduced life expectancy. Although medical management can be successful in reducing weight, the greatest and longest-term reduction in weight is achieved by bariatric surgery.

● EPIDEMIOLOGY OF OBESITY

Obesity is growing in epidemic proportions. Westernised countries such as the USA, Australia and the UK lead the way, but obesity is starting to become a significant problem in East Asia, as affluence and a Western diet become more established.

In the UK the prevalence of obesity has tripled in women between 1980 and 2004 (from 8% to 23%) and quadrupled in men (from 6% to 23%). Nearly 2.5 per cent of the adult population is morbidly obese, with a body mass index (BMI) of more than 40.

● AETIOLOGY OF OBESITY

The aetiology of obesity is complex and has much to do with the free availability of calorie- and fat-rich foodstuffs, combined with the sedentary lifestyle of the late twentieth and early twenty-first century. These very recent changes overwhelm body-weight regulatory mechanisms that have evolved over thousands of years of relative food scarcity.

Genetic factors influence but are not solely responsible for the obese phenotype. Twin studies confirm a strong genetic predisposition to obesity, although individual gene abnormalities are unusual as a cause of obesity.

Obesity syndromes are rare. The most common (1 in 25 000) and best known is Prader–Willi syndrome, characterised by short stature, mental retardation, hypogonadism, small hands and feet, and upper body obesity. The genetic abnormality is usually a deletion on the long arm of chromosome 15.

Metabolic causes of obesity are rare. Hypothyroidism commonly coexists with obesity, but treatment results in only, at most, modest weight loss, which is rarely of any impact in the morbid obese population. Cushing's syndrome causes progressive central obesity and, although rare, should be distinguished from simple obesity by the relatively short history and the various symptoms and physical signs; these include myopathy, depression, bruising, thin skin, striae, and a paucity of subcutaneous fat, despite the degree of central obesity.

● DEFINITION OF OBESITY

Obesity is defined as a BMI of more than 30. Body mass index is calculated thus:

$$BMI = weight/height^2$$

where weight is measured in kilograms and height in metres.

Overweight and obesity are defined by the BMI (Table 19.1).

Table 19.1 Definition of obesity according to body mass index (BMI)

BMI (kg/m^2)	Description
≤ 20	Underweight
20–25	Desirable
25–30	Overweight
> 30	Obese
> 40	Morbid (clinically severe) obesity
> 50	Super-obesity

● HEALTH RISKS OF MORBID OBESITY

The risk of mortality is related to BMI. The lowest risk of death lies within the BMI range of 20–25. A significant increase in the mortality ratio starts to emerge as the BMI increases above 27 or 28; at a BMI of 40, mortality is two to three times higher than at a BMI of 20–25.

> ■ KEY POINT
> The risk of mortality is related to BMI.

The mortality risk is elevated because obesity predisposes to a variety of morbid conditions, including the following:

- Diabetes mellitus: risk increases 4.5 per cent per kilogram of weight gained
- Arterial hypertension
- Coronary heart disease:
  - Myocardial infarction
  - Heart failure
  - Cardiomyopathy
- Obstructive sleep apnoea
- Gallstones

- Liver steatosis:
  - Non-alcoholic steatohepatitis
  - Cirrhosis
- High cholesterol/lipids
- Menstrual/ reproductive disorders:
  - Polycystic ovary syndrome
  - Infertility
  - Obstetric complications
- Stress incontinence
- Gastro-oesophageal reflux
- Stroke
- Cancer
- Arthritis
- Psychological disorders.

INDICATIONS FOR OBESITY SURGERY

Surgery is indicated for certain patients with morbid obesity with a BMI of 40 or greater, and for patients with a BMI of greater than 35 with obesity-related comorbidity such as type 2 diabetes mellitus, obstructive sleep apnoea or hypertension. The following criteria for obesity surgery have been proposed by bodies such as the International Federation of Surgery for Obesity (IFSO), the National Institutes of Health (NIH) in the USA and the National Institute for Health and Clinical Excellence (NICE) in the UK:

- BMI ≥ 40
- BMI 35–40 with obesity-related comorbidity
- Age 18–65 years[*]
- Obesity for more than 5 years
- Failed non-surgical attempts at weight loss
- Fit enough for surgery
- No specific clinical or psychological contraindications
- Patient understands risks of surgery
- Patient is committed to long-term follow-up.

[*]No longer applied in the latest NICE guidance.

The patient should have undergone meaningful attempts at non-surgical weight reduction over an extended period (at least 5 years) and ideally should have attended a hospital-based weight-management programme. The patient should not be addicted to alcohol or recreational drugs. The patient should understand the risks and implications of weight-loss surgery and be committed to long-term follow-up.

Psychiatric disease is not a contraindication to weight-loss surgery, and indeed depression is common among morbidly obese patients. Significant psychiatric disease, however, should be assessed in the context of the patient's ability to understand the surgery and to maintain compliance for dietary measures and nutritional supplements.

Age limits have been applied previously, but they have been lifted in the most recent NICE guidance. Patients at both ends of the age spectrum can benefit from surgery. Elderly patients have been shown to achieve a significant benefit in quality of life, even if they are unlikely to gain many extra years of life after surgery. Weight-loss surgery in children remains controversial, but it may be indicated in obese children beyond skeletal maturity. Children require a higher level of assessment from both an individual and a family perspective, and they should be treated by a specialist childhood obesity team before surgery is considered.

MULTIDISCIPLINARY TEAMWORKING

The treatment of obesity is not simply surgical, and the surgical treatment of obesity is not simple. The causes of obesity are multifactorial and the consequences of obesity affect patients psychologically and physically. Successful treatment of obesity requires a multidisciplinary approach. The team should include a dietician, a physician, a surgeon, an anaesthetist and ideally a specialist nurse. In addition, the patient needs access to a clinical psychologist/psychiatrist. Perioperative support is enhanced by access to a patient support group.

> ■ KEY POINT
> The treatment of obesity is not simply surgical, and the surgical treatment of obesity is not simple.

RISK MANAGEMENT IN OBESE SURGICAL PATIENTS

Morbidly obese patients are commonly at higher than average risk for anaesthesia and surgery because of both obesity and systemic comorbidity. Diabetes, hypertension and hypoventilation/sleep apnoea are common findings in patients undergoing obesity surgery. Preoperative assessment and management should aim to optimise these and any other conditions before the patient is subjected to an elective weight-reduction operation. This may require the institution of antihypertensive therapy, diabetic assessment, and referral to a sleep specialist and the use of continuous positive airway pressure (CPAP), for example.

The patient should be encouraged to take responsibility for reducing their own operative risks by such measures as stopping smoking for at least 6 weeks before surgery, maintaining physical activity as much as possible and adhering closely to any preoperative dietary advice.

Further measures designed to reduce the risk of perioperative complications include antithrombotic prophylaxis (fractionated heparin, intermittent calf compression), antibiotic prophylaxis and good pain control. Laparoscopic surgery is associated with lower morbidity than open surgery and is increasingly taking precedence for weight-loss procedures.

A preoperative low-fat, low-carbohydrate diet for 7–10 days reduces the size and friability of the steatotic liver, and improves access and safety, particularly for laparoscopic surgery.

SURGICAL OPERATIONS FOR OBESITY

Operations for obesity emerged in the early 1960s. Weight loss was induced by malabsorption through operations such as the jejunoileal bypass (JIB). By anastomosing the proximal jejunum to the distal ileum, much of the small bowel was taken out of circuit, resulting in a very short length of bowel for nutrient absorption (Figure 19.1). It became apparent that the excluded jejunum became a site for bacterial overgrowth, resulting in numerous major nutritional deficiencies, oxalate renal stones and liver failure. Adaptations to reduce the blind loop effect included isolating the excess small bowel by using an end-to-end rather than an end-to-side jejunoileal anastomosis, and draining the isolated small bowel into the stomach (Figure 19.2) (Cleator and Gourlay, 1988). Despite such alterations, the JIB has now been outlawed, although elements of the procedure form the basis for the modern malabsorptive operations.

Around the same time, Mason (1979) appreciated that patients lost weight after partial gastrectomy for ulcer disease and devised an operation that partitioned rather than resected the

Figure 19.1 ● Jejunoileal bypass.

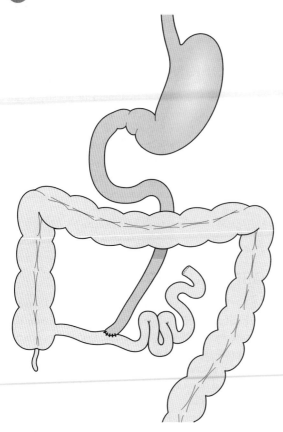

stomach. This was drained by a loop gastrojejunostomy and became the first gastric bypass (GBP; Figure 19.3). Numerous developments have followed since, resulting in the modern gastric bypass, which is the most common procedure employed worldwide for obesity. In addition, Mason continued to develop various restrictive gastroplasties in order to try to avoid the use of a small bowel anastomosis.

Large numbers of bariatric procedures have been described, but only a handful of procedures make up the vast majority of operations carried out worldwide today; only these few procedures are described in this chapter. They can be divided into gastric restrictive procedures and hybrid operations. Hybrid procedures include both gastric restrictive and malabsorptive elements, but they tend to be either restriction- or malabsorption-predominant.

Purely restrictive operations

Vertical banded gastroplasty

Vertical banded gastroplasty (VBG) involves the fashioning of a vertical gastric pouch of around 20 mL volume with a synthetic band or ring wrapped around the pouch outlet (Figure 19.4). The site of passage of the ring is created using a circular stapler through the stomach, and the pouch is then fashioned with a vertical staple line from this point to the angle of His. Trials have demonstrated inferior results of VBG compared with GBP. In addition, VBG is associated with complications, including pouch dilation, gastro-gastric fistula, mesh erosion, vomiting, reflux disease and mild vitamin deficiency. The procedure is rarely undertaken now as it has been superseded by adjustable gastric banding (AGB).

Figure 19.2 ● Cleator jejunoileal bypass.

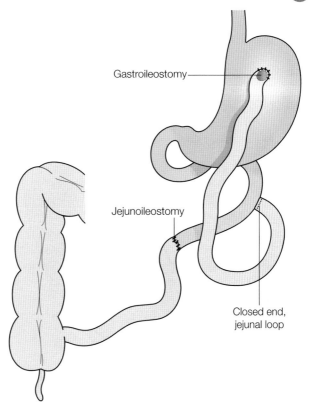

Gastroileostomy

Jejunoileostomy

Closed end, jejunal loop

Figure 19.3 ● Mason loop gastric bypass.

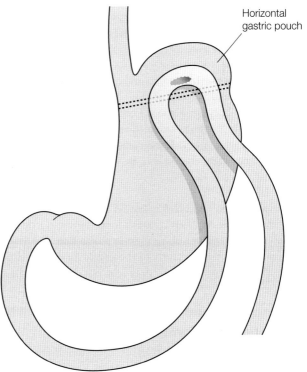

Horizontal gastric pouch

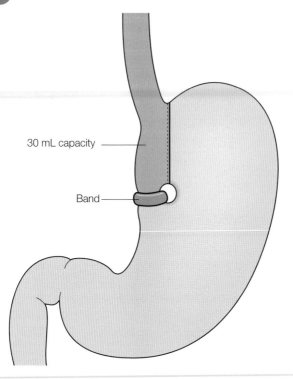

Figure 19.4 ● Vertical banded gastroplasty.

30 mL capacity

Band

Adjustable gastric banding

Adjustable gastric banding involves insertion of a rigid band with an inflatable silicone ring on the inside, which is connected to a reservoir or port placed on the abdominal wall or sternum. The band is positioned so as to create a small gastric pouch (volume almost 20 mL) with an adjustable outlet (Figure 19.5). The stoma is adjusted postoperatively by filling the reservoir; it is adjusted to the point where food passage is restricted and slows emptying of the pouch. Outcomes vary after gastric banding and can be as much to do with patient support as the technical aspects of band placement. The best results come from units with a dedicated follow-up service with full patient support. Poor follow-up is associated with poor weight loss. Complications are rare at the time of surgery, but late complications include band slippage, band erosion and oesophageal dilation. These complications are not time-dependent and result in a continued incidence of reoperation and, in some cases, band removal.

Sleeve gastrectomy

Sleeve gastrectomy involves resection of the body of the stomach over a bougie pushed up along the lesser curve. This creates a long, narrow, restricted gastric tube and removes the gastric fundus, greatly diminishing ghrelin production (Figure 19.6). Ghrelin is an orexigenic hormone produced predominantly in the gastric fundus; by removing its major source, appetite is reduced. Weight loss is usually dramatic, but dilation of the gastric tube over time can lead to weight gain. This is less common with the use of a narrow tube of 32–34Ch. Complications include staple line leakage, stenosis of the tube and gastro-oesophageal reflux.

Restriction-predominant operations

Roux-en-Y gastric bypass (RYGB) is a restriction-predominant procedure that includes creation of proximal gastric pouch of less than 30 mL with a Roux limb at least 75 cm long and an

Figure 19.5 ● (a) Laparoscopic adjustable gastric band. (b) Band with anterior tunnel.

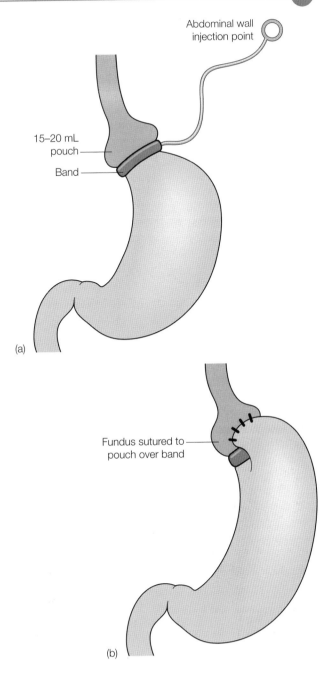

anastomotic stoma of 1 cm in diameter (Figure 19.7). RYGB produces better weight loss than the purely restrictive operations but it has a different profile of significant complications including marginal ulcer, stomal stenosis, anaemia (iron deficiency, vitamin B12 deficiency and folic acid deficiency), trace element deficiency (e.g. magnesium, calcium, zinc) and occasionally fat soluble vitamin deficiency.

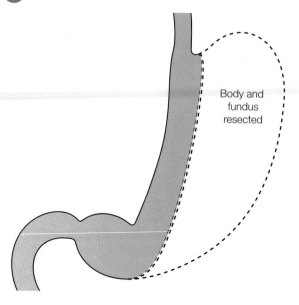

Figure 19.6 • Sleeve gastrectomy.

Body and fundus resected

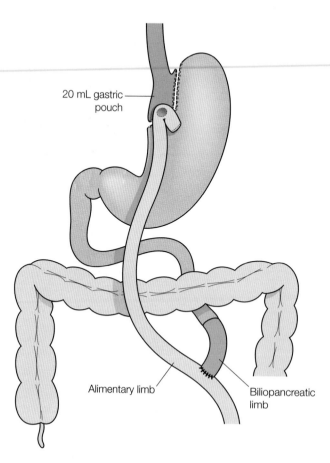

Figure 19.7 • Roux-en-Y gastric bypass.

20 mL gastric pouch

Alimentary limb

Biliopancreatic limb

Figure 19.8 ● Biliopancreatic diversity.

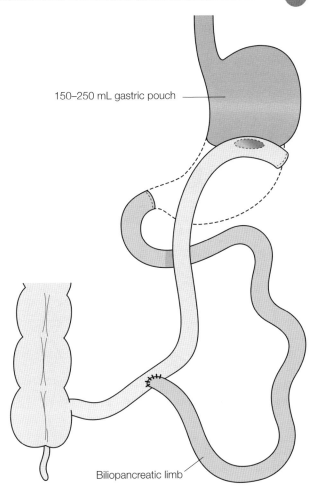

150–250 mL gastric pouch

Biliopancreatic limb

Malabsorption-predominant operations

Biliopancreatic diversion

Biliopancreatic diversion (BPD) is a malabsorption-predominant procedure that involves transection of the ileum 250 cm proximal to the ileocaecal junction. The distal ileal limb is anastomosed to a proximal stomach pouch created by subtotal gastrectomy. The rest of the proximal small bowel (biliopancreatic limb) is anastomosed to the distal ileum 50 cm proximal to the ileocaecal junction (Figure 19.8).

The operation causes fat malabsorption and results in malodorous and frequent stools when fat is ingested. Protein absorption is also reduced, and so the patient needs to maintain a high-protein diet, with vitamin and micronutrient supplementation, in order to avoid long-term nutritional complications.

Biliopancreatic diversion with duodenal switch

Biliopancreatic diversion with duodenal switch (BPD/DS) is a modified version of BPD in which the gastric greater curvature is resected to create a gastric sleeve along the lesser curvature (sleeve gastrectomy) and the duodenum is transected 5 cm distal to the pylorus. The distal

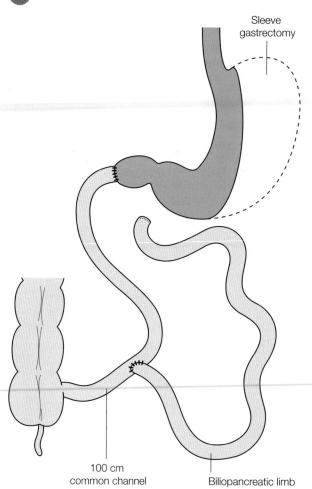

Sleeve gastrectomy

Figure 19.9 ● Duodenal switch/biliopancreatic diversion.

100 cm common channel

Biliopancreatic limb

ileal limb is then joined to the duodenum. Most surgeons use a longer common channel of 100 cm than with a classical BPD, as the sleeve gastrectomy is somewhat more restrictive than the distal gastric resection (Figure 19.9). This reconstruction reduces the incidence of stomal ulcer, reduces dumping and has a lower incidence of protein malnutrition than BPD.

Laparoscopic duodenal switch

Laparoscopic duodenal switch is a long and technically difficult operation. In patients with extreme obesity (BMI > 65), the mortality from the operation may be substantial. The mortality can be reduced markedly by separating the procedure into two stages. The sleeve gastrectomy is performed initially, resulting in weight loss of usually more than 50 kg in the first year. After around 1 year, or at the point that weight stabilises, the duodenal switch/BPD component of the procedure is performed. By this stage, the risks from surgery and anaesthesia are markedly reduced and overall mortality and morbidity are reduced.

Choice of procedure

There is no clear guidance as to which procedure is most appropriate for any particular patient. The decision should be made jointly between the surgeon and the patient after a full explanation of the appropriate procedures, their risks and complications, and lifestyle impact. The patient's expectations of the procedure are often distorted by advertising and media coverage, given the current high profile of obesity surgery.

Factors that may influence the decision include the extent of obesity. Malabsorptive procedures tend to result in greater weight loss and may be more appropriate in super-obese patients. However, the nutritional dangers of such procedures require a thorough understanding and commitment by the patient to adhere to dietary rules. Dietary compliance is also very important for successful weight loss from gastric banding, and patients who are low-volume eaters, snackers and sweet-eaters may not be suitable candidates. Sweet-eaters may find that dumping from sweets after gastric bypass helps to control this aspect of their diet, although dumping is not invariable. The presence of comorbidities such as diabetes and dyslipidaemia are more predictably controlled by gastric bypass or BPD, and patients should be aware of this.

■ KEY POINT

Malabsorptive procedures tend to result in greater weight loss and may be more appropriate in super-obese patients.

The potential morbidity of the procedures differs. Gastric banding is generally perceived to be the least morbid operation. The patient should understand that each operation carries a risk/benefit ratio and that they will need to achieve a good outcome in order to benefit from a low-risk operation. Failure of the patient to control their obesity leaves them at risk, however safe the procedure.

Laparoscopic versus open surgery

In recent years laparoscopic approaches to bariatric surgery have predominated. Although initially patient- and technology-driven, the benefits of laparoscopic surgery have emerged as patients appear to have fewer complications and better early recovery. Several small randomised trials have shown that laparoscopic surgery is associated with shorter hospital stay, a lower incidence of both wound infection and incisional hernia, and a similar incidence of anastomotic leak; however, stomal stricture was higher following laparoscopic surgery, perhaps because of an increased use of staplers. Weight loss does not differ between groups.

All procedures can be completed laparoscopically, but they can be very technically demanding. As such, it is preferable for surgical teams to be specifically trained and to carry out large volumes of cases in order to minimise complications.

● OUTCOMES FROM SURGERY

Weight loss

Weight loss can be presented as actual weight loss, percentage weight loss or percentage of excess weight loss (%EWL). Percentage EWL describes the proportion of weight that is lost of that weight that is over the ideal body weight of the patient; this is the most common term used in surgical literature. Success from weight-loss surgery is generally perceived to be an excess weight loss of 50 per cent or more and ideally should be assessed in the long term – that is, more than 5 years after surgery.

Pure restrictive operations tend to have poorer weight loss than hybrid or malabsorptive operations. A meta-analysis of 22 000 patients in 136 studies showed a mean %EWL of 70.1 per cent for BPD/DS, 61.6 per cent for gastric bypass, 68.2 per cent after gastroplasty, and 47.5 per cent following gastric banding.

Modest weight loss carries quite positive health benefits, but improvement in quality of life as assessed by patients is generally proportional to weight loss.

Mortality

Mortality risk is increased in morbid obese patients compared with the non-obese population, and the risk increases with higher BMI.

The mortality risk from surgery should be less than 1 per cent. Gastric banding is the lowest-risk procedure, and duodenal switch carries the highest mortality. The above meta-analysis gave a mortality of 0.1 per cent for restrictive surgery, 0.5 per cent for gastric bypass and 1.1 per cent for BPD or duodenal switch. Patient factors have a major impact on operative death; males with high BMI (> 65) and hypertension carry the highest operative risk.

> ■ KEY POINT
> Males with high BMI and hypertension carry the highest operative risk.

Surgically induced weight loss significantly reduces mortality in the morbidly obese population and improves numerous obesity-related comorbidities, including diabetes, hypertension and obstructive sleep apnoea. Provided operative mortality is kept at low levels, it is safer for most patients to have surgery than to maintain conservative treatment for morbid obesity. The greatest improvement in mortality risk occurs in the diabetic population.

Comorbidity resolution

Weight loss is usually regarded as the primary outcome for weight-loss surgery. However, the reduction in mortality is related to the reversal of comorbidities, which is brought about by successful weight-loss surgery.

Resolution or improvement of comorbidities is due predominantly to weight loss. However, the foregut reconstruction applied in gastric bypass and biliopancreatic diversion has an immediate effect on diabetic control, which is initially independent of weight loss.

Comorbidities that improve with surgically induced weight loss in addition to diabetes include obstructive sleep apnoea, arterial hypertension, dyslipidaemia, non-alcoholic steatohepatitis, pseudo-tumour cerebri, stress incontinence, venous stasis and gastro-oesophageal reflux disease.

The impact of surgery on type 2 diabetes mellitus is dramatic. The most profound effect occurs with biliopancreatic diversion and gastric bypass, which result in remission of diabetes in around 97 per cent and 85 per cent of patients, respectively. Many patients achieve euglycaemia and are discharged home off medication, within a few days of surgery.

Various theories exist to account for the rapid and prolonged improvement in diabetes. Foregut bypass results in exclusion of the duodenum and alters the gut hormone profile after food. Duodenal exclusion results in improvement in diabetic control through mechanisms that are unclear. The delivery of nutrients into the distal small bowel results in an exaggerated response in the production of gut hormones such as glucagon-like peptide 1 (GLP1). GLP1 is an incretin that increases postprandial insulin production and improves pancreatic beta-cell function.

● COMPLICATIONS OF OBESITY SURGERY

Morbidly obese patients should constitute some of the highest risk patients for surgery, given the surgical, anaesthetic and nursing difficulties in dealing with them, and the range of comorbidities that are prevalent. Reassuringly, in the context of the modern multidisciplinary team approach, complications are quite rare.

Generic complications include bleeding, thromboembolism, chest infection, wound sepsis, dehiscence and wound hernia. All of these risks are increased in the obese population. Thromboembolism is a dangerous complication, and pulmonary embolism is the leading cause of death among bariatric surgical patients, occurring in 0.25 per cent of cases.

> ■ KEY POINT
> Pulmonary embolism is the leading cause of death in bariatric surgical patients.

Wound sepsis and fascial dehiscence are more common with open surgery, and the incidence of ventral hernia can be as high as 20 per cent.

Procedure-specific complications can be technical and usually relate to the stoma or the reconstruction. In addition, the operations can cause nutritional and metabolic disturbances.

Vomiting and solid food intolerance can be due to stomal stenosis and are easily treatable in the context of an adjustable band, which can be partially deflated. If the stenosis is at an anastomosis, balloon dilation is usually effective.

Marginal ulcers occur in up to 10 per cent of gastrojejunal and gastroileal anastomoses. The occurrence of troublesome ulcers is reduced by acid inhibition and is highest within the first year of surgery.

Small bowel obstruction (2%) in the early postoperative phase is of major concern, because of the potential for anastomotic or gastric remnant dehiscence upstream of the obstruction. Following laparoscopic surgery, obstruction may be due to a port site or umbilical hernia. Internal hernia occurs in up to 5 per cent of cases, particularly if internal hernia defects are not closed. Diagnosis of internal hernia can be difficult, with only computed tomography (CT) and re-exploration providing a high degree of diagnostic accuracy. Internal herniae can develop through the mesenteric defect of the jejuno-jejunostomy/ileostomy, the mesocolic defect (retrocolic reconstruction) and the Petersen space (Figure 19.10).

Anastomotic leak is a rare but life-threatening complication. Roux-en-Y reconstruction reduces the impact of a gastric anastomotic leak by diverting duodenal juice downstream.

Figure 19.10 ● Sites of internal hernias. (a) Jejuno-jejunal mesocolic defect. (b) Mesocolic defect in retrocolic reconstruction only. (c) Petersen's defect.

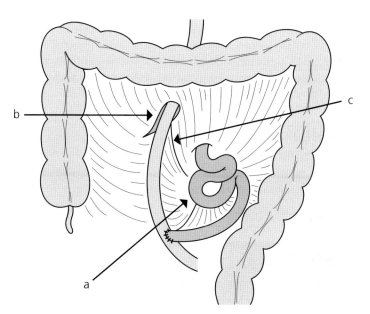

Failure to lose weight is seen in 10–15 per cent of treated patients. Treatment failure varies in different procedures, but it is a complex issue. Weight gain or poor weight loss can be due to technical failure, such as a pouch to remnant fistula, but it is often due to patient compliance. Failure to embrace lifestyle changes and an emphasis on snacking and inappropriate foodstuffs predisposes to weight gain. Good patient support and follow-up and, in some cases, psychological support can minimise the risk of failure.

Micronutrient deficiency occurs because of poor intake, reduced gastric volume and acid production, duodenal and proximal jejunal diversion and, in some cases, fat malabsorption (fat-soluble vitamins):

- Vitamin B12 deficiency is common owing to failure to cleave food-bound vitamin B12. This results from reduced intrinsic factor availability after RYGB and occasionally sleeve gastrectomy.
- Calcium deficiency is common but difficult to detect, because serum calcium is maintained by secondary hyperparathyroidism when intake is poor. Osteoporosis remains a long-term complication of foregut bypass surgery.
- Thiamine deficiency is rare but has serious neurological consequences. It is associated with poor intake and frequent vomiting in the early postoperative phase.
- Trace element deficiencies are common before surgery because of poor diet. Reduced intake and absorption of zinc may contribute to hair loss.
- Fat-soluble vitamin deficiency (vitamins A, D, E, K) can occur in the context of fat malabsorption and is common after biliopancreatic diversion.
- Protein deficiency occurs in 5–10 per cent of patients after malabsorptive surgery. Extreme protein deficiency is a serious concern and can lead to late death and hepatic failure, among others.

Patients should be given dietary support and micro-nutrient supplementation and should undergo long-term follow-up in order to identify and treat these potential deficiencies.

● SUMMARY

Morbid obesity is a complex condition and is associated with comorbidities that affect all of the body's major organ systems. Management of obesity should be multidisciplinary, and surgery for the obese requires a dedicated and well-trained team.

Numerous operations exist, each with its own profile of efficacy and complications. The choice of operation for any individual patient is controversial but should be guided by patient factors as well as the surgeon's expertise. Patients require long-term follow-up after obesity surgery in view of the potential metabolic disturbances. In addition, the results of surgery are improved by postoperative patient support.

● QUESTIONS

1 What are the indications for obesity surgery?
2 Briefly describe the preoperative assessment of a patient waiting to have bariatric surgery.
3 Briefly describe the adjustable gastric banding procedure.
4 Compare the excess weight loss and mortality rates between adjustable gastric banding and gastric bypass.

● REFERENCES

Cleator IG, Gourlay RH (1988). Ileogastrostomy for morbid obesity. *Can J Surg* **31**: 114–16.
Mason EE (1979). Gastric bypass for morbid obesity. *Ann Surg* **11**: 99–126.

● FURTHER READING

Buchwald H, Avidor Y, Braunwald E, *et al*. (2004). Bariatric surgery: a systematic review and meta-analysis. *J Am Med Assoc* **292**: 1724–37.

Fernandez AZ, Jr, Demaria EJ, Tichansky DS, *et al*. (2004). Multivariate analysis of risk factors for death following gastric bypass for treatment of morbid obesity. *Ann Surg* **239**: 698–703.

National Institute for Health and Clinical Excellence (2002). *Guidance on the Use of Surgery to Aid Weight Reduction for People with Morbid Obesity*. Technology Appraisal Guidance no. 46. London: National Institute for Health and Clinical Excellence.

Sjostrom L, Narbro K Sjostrom C, *et al*. (2007). Swedish obese subjects study: effects of bariatric surgery on mortality in Swedish obese subjects. *N Engl J Med* **357**: 741–52.

20 Management of surgery in elderly patients

Qassim F Baker, H Devalia and Tharwat Sulliaman

INTRODUCTION

Surgery in elderly patients, especially in the emergency setting, is associated with a high risk of morbidity and mortality. Due to the increasingly ageing population, especially in Western countries, surgery in elderly patients has become more common. The elderly population is becoming less marginalised and more mainstream, and the number of patients over age 75 years receiving surgery is increasing yearly.

Surgery in elderly patients differs little from surgery in younger populations with regard to the procedures performed and preoperative decision-making. In contrast, special considerations for surgery are required in children and pregnant women. Unfortunately, study of the subject of surgery in elderly patients is incomplete, and therefore current practice aims at compensating for ageing changes in whole-body physiology rather than specific evidence-based practice.

Risk assessment, decision-making and perioperative care are typically more challenging than in younger patients. An understanding of how physiological changes of ageing affect surgical care is essential if the best outcomes are to be achieved.

Elderly patients present with both elective and urgent surgical problems. When possible, it is better to operate in an elective setting than as an emergency – for example, to repair a hernia before it becomes incarcerated. Careful preoperative assessment is needed in order to keep the incidence of complications to a minimum. Any medical requirements must be considered, and a baseline of health status to which the patient is expected to return should be established.

PREOPERATIVE ASSESSMENT

Cardiovascular system

Atherosclerosis affects the entire arterial tree. Progressive narrowing of the coronary arteries leads to ischaemic changes in the heart muscle, including the conductive system, in addition to the atrophy that affects this system with ageing, leading to different types of arrhythmias, such as atrial fibrillation (AF).

Ask the patient about history of hypertension, recent myocardial ischaemia and diabetes mellitus. Cardiac output declines with advancing age. Mobility may be affected by peripheral vascular disease, causing intermittent claudication. Reduced cerebral blood flow can lead to cerebrovascular accidents (CVAs), transient ischaemic attacks (TIAs) and dementia, among other conditions.

Deep vein thrombosis (DVT) is more common in elderly people, especially those undergoing certain operations, such as total hip replacement, internal fixation of fractured neck of femur, and open prostatectomy. Some form of DVT prophylaxis should be considered.

Possible cardiovascular complications in elderly patients include the following:

- *Cardiac:* ischaemic heart disease (IHD), arrhythmias
- *Cerebral:* stroke, TIA, dementia
- *Peripheral:* claudication, trophic changes, gangrene
- *Venous:* DVT, pulmonary embolism
- Abdominal aortic aneurysm (AAA; might be asymptomatic)
- Bowel ischaemia, e.g. ischaemic colitis.

Respiratory system

Chronic obstructive pulmonary disease (COPD) is common in elderly patients and increases the risk of postoperative chest complications, especially after lengthy emergency procedures. In addition to weakness of the muscles of the chest wall and diaphragm, alveolar changes, especially thickening of alveolar walls, lead to a decrease in vital capacity and tissue oxygenation. Elderly patients are also more liable to aspiration pneumonia.

> ■ KEY POINT
> COPD, with chest wall weakness, retention of secretions, and decreased vital capacity and tidal volume, is common in elderly patients.

> ■ KEY POINT
> Elderly patients are more likely to develop aspiration pneumonia and chest infection.

Haematological system

Anaemia is common in elderly patients for a variety of reasons, including bleeding piles, gastrointestinal malignancy such as cancer of the colon or stomach, and malnutrition. Other considerations include iatrogenic blood loss due to aspirin or warfarin. Haematological malignancies are more common in elderly people and are often chronic in nature.

Medications

Elderly patients are often on more than one drug (polypharmacy), in particular diuretics (e.g. to treat hypertension), digoxin and non-steroidal anti-inflammatory drugs (NSAIDs). There is a danger of drug interactions with polypharmacy.

Renal clearance is decreased in elderly patients, and so the dosage of drugs used in surgery (e.g. opiates) should be calculated carefully.

Cardiac arrhythmia can occur in the presence of hypokalaemia, and the action of digoxin is potentiated if the patient is hypokalaemic.

Oral anticoagulants such as warfarin are used for a variety of indications, including atrial fibrillation. Oral anticoagulants pose a real problem (see Chapter 24), especially in emergency situations.

Non-steroidal anti-inflammatory drugs can cause peptic ulcer disease. In this case, the patient may not have abdominal pain but may present with melaena.

Malnutrition

Many elderly patients are malnourished. Patients undergoing elective surgery may need pre-operative nutritional assessment (dietician advice) and some sort of feeding, whether by sips or through a fine-bore nasogastric tube or by parenteral feeding.

Renal system

Renal function decreases with age, due mainly to reduced renal blood flow. The patient should be assessed for clinical features of chronic renal failure (CRF; polyuria, nocturia, frequency, earthy skin colour), urinary tract infection (UTI; dysuria, frequency) and haematuria.

> ■ KEY POINT
> The patient should be assessed for clinical features of CRF, UTI and haematuria.

In all elderly patients, renal function should be checked (estimation of urea, creatinine, serum electrolytes, especially potassium and calcium), and urine output should be monitored. Electrocardiography (ECG) should be used to detect any dysrhythmias.

> ■ KEY POINT
> Urea, creatinine, serum electrolytes (especially potassium and calcium) should be checked and urine output monitored.

Chronic renal failure may be a manifestation of chronic obstructive uropathy due to prostatic pathology in male patients.

Neurological system

With age, there is a decrease in cerebral blood flow and a steady decline in the number of neurons. Communication with elderly patients may be impaired because of deafness and dementia. When taking the patient's history, remember that many elderly patients have short-term memory loss and that some information may need to be checked with the patient's family or general practitioner.

Locomotor system

Joint problems due to osteoarthritis of the hips, knees and hands can affect the elderly patient's mobility and position on the operating table. This also has an impact on mobilisation postoperatively and should prompt the consideration of prophylactic anticoagulation.

Immune system

As the body ages, its ability to fight infection diminishes. The immune system becomes gradually less efficient than that of a younger person. For example, 20 per cent of older adults do not mount a fever to significant bacterial infection, because of the diminished sensitivity of the neurological system to thermoregulation. Although elderly people produce the same quantity of white cells as younger patients, the elderly patient's white cells may have an altered configuration and be less effective. This increases the prevalence of autoimmune disease in the elderly population, another consideration to be taken into account at surgical pre-assessment, particularly with regard to rheumatoid arthritis and atherosclerosis.

Immunity is also reduced by poor nutrition and stress, two factors most prevalent in elderly people.

For details on screening for meticillin-resistant *Staphylococcus aureus* (MRSA) and the risk of *Clostridium difficile*, see Chapter 22.

Social assessment

- Ask about the patient's quality of life before coming to hospital.
- Is the patient independent, mobile, capable of doing their own shopping, etc.?
- Is the patient living alone or with a partner, or living in a nursing home?
- Does the patient have family support? Do members of the family live with or near the patient?

The surgeon and the anaesthetist should speak to the patient's family before the operation, especially if the patient has dementia, to explain all the possible complications, including staying in intensive care or high dependency after the operation, and the potential need for a stoma following bowel resection. Such explanations can keep litigation to a minimum.

Consent in the elderly patient requires special consideration, especially if they do not have the capacity to make an informed decision; for example, if the patient has dementia, their family or carer may be involved in giving consent.

Investigations

Chest X-ray should be done routinely in elderly surgical patients. A full blood count and measurement of urea and electrolytes (U&Es) should be taken, especially in patients on diuretics, steroids and laxatives. Blood sugar levels should be taken. A low serum albumin level can give a rough idea of the severity of patient's malnutrition.

ECG is mandatory in the elderly patient. Further cardiac assessment, such as echocardiography, may be needed, especially for patients undergoing major surgery.

Respiratory assessment, such as pulmonary function testing, may be needed.

Summary of preoperative assessment in elderly patients

Special considerations need to be made in the surgical treatment of the elderly. Perioperative complications can be minimised with careful attention to the unique physiological changes in the aged patient. Recognition and support of these physiological needs is the cornerstone of preoperative management in the elderly population.

Table 20.1 summarises preoperative considerations and their best practice solutions in elderly patients.

● PERIOPERATIVE COMPLICATIONS

Local and general anaesthesia have unwanted effects in elderly patients. Regional anaesthesia, such as spinal block, may be more appropriate for operations such as hernia repair and lower limb amputations, as long as the patient is likely to remain cooperative.

Acute blood loss should be avoided because of the risk of perioperative myocardial infarction. Fluid overload should also be avoided.

● POSTOPERATIVE CARE AND COMPLICATIONS

Most elderly patients tolerate complications of surgery poorly. Try to avoid complications and keep those that do occur to a minimum:

- Oxygen therapy (mask, nasal spectacles) should be continued because of the risk of hypoxia.
- Avoid fluid overload and electrolytes disturbance.
- Confusion can result from hypoxia, retention of carbon dioxide (CO_2), overhydration, urinary retention and overdose of sedative drugs.
- Titrate drug dosages carefully.

Table 20.1 Physiologic limitations of ageing, their clinical consequences and best practices in the elderly surgical patient

Age-related changes	Clinical consequences	Best practice
Body composition		
Significantly decreased muscle mass, accounting for much of decreased lean tissue mass and increased fat mass	Erosion of muscle mass during acute illness may result in strength rapidly falling below important clinical thresholds, e.g. impaired coughing, decreased mobility, increased risk of venous thrombosis	Maintain physical function through effective pain relief; avoid tubes, drains and other restraints; aim for early mobilisation and assistance with mobilisation
	Altered volumes of drug distribution	Minimise fasting; provide early nutritional supplementation or support (protein-calorie and micronutrient)
		Adjust drug dosages for volume of distribution
Respiratory		
Decreased vital capacity	Less effective cough	Provide early mobilisation; assumption of upright rather than supine position
Increased closing volume	Predisposition to aspiration	Ensure effective pain relief to allow mobilisation and deep breathing
Decreased airway sensitivity and clearance	Increased closure of small airways during tidal respiration, especially postoperatively and when supine, leading to increased atelectasis and shunting	Provide routine supplemental oxygen in immediate postoperative period and then as needed
Decreased partial pressure of oxygen	Predisposition to hypoxaemia	Minimise use of nasogastric tubes
Cardiovascular		
Decreased maximal heart rate, cardiac output, ejection fraction	Greater reliance on ventricular filling and increases in stroke volume (rather than ejection fraction) to achieve increases in cardiac output	Use vigorous fluid resuscitation to achieve optimal ventricular filling

Reliance on increased end-diastolic volume to increase cardiac output	Intolerant of hypovolaemia	Non-vasoconstricting inotropes and afterload reduction may be more effective if pharmacological support is required
Slowed ventricular filling, increased reliance on atrial contribution	Intolerant of tachycardia, dysrhythmias, including atrial fibrillation	Decreased baroreceptor sensitivity
Thermoregulation		
Diminished sensitivity to ambient temperature and less efficient mechanisms of heat conservation, production and dissipation	Predisposition to hypothermia, e.g. decline in body temperature during surgery is more marked unless preventive measures are taken	Use active measures to maintain normothermia during surgical procedures and to rewarm after trauma, e.g. warmed intravenous fluids, humidified gases, warm air
Febrile responses to infection may be blunted in frail or malnourished elderly patients, and patients in extreme old age	If there is hypothermia, shivering may result, associated with marked increases in oxygen consumption and cardiopulmonary demands	Maintaining intraoperative normothermia reduces wound infections, adverse cardiac events and length of hospital stay
	Fever may be absent despite serious infections, especially in frail elderly patients	Be aware of hypothermia in trauma resuscitation
Renal function, fluid and electrolyte homeostasis		
Decreased sensitivity to fluid, electrolyte perturbations	Predisposition to hypovolaemia	Predisposition to electrolyte disorders, e.g. hyponatraemia
	Recognise that a 'normal' serum creatinine value reflects decreased creatinine clearance, as muscle mass (i.e. creatinine production) is decreased concurrently	
Decreased renal mass, renal blood flow and glomerular filtration rate	Predisposition to hyperglycaemia	Select drugs carefully: avoid those that may be nephrotoxic, e.g. aminoglycosides, or that may adversely affect renal blood flow, e.g. NSAIDs
Increased renal glucose threshold	Predisposition to hyperosmolar states	Adjust drug dosages as appropriate for altered pharmacokinetics

NSAIDs, non-steroidal anti-inflammatory drugs.

From Watters JM (2002). Surgery in the Elderly. *Can J Surg* **45**(2):104–8.

Reproduced with permission from the Canadian Medical Association.

- Urinary retention from enlarged prostate may necessitate urinary catheterisation. Transurethral resection of the prostate (TURP) may be needed before discharge. Urinary tract infection can result from leaving a catheter in for too long.
- Skin care (proper nursing care, use of special beds) is important in order to prevent pressure sores, which are more common in elderly patients.
- Social circumstances should be evaluated by involving the patient's family and a social worker. Many patients remain on the ward for social reasons and rehabilitation can take a long time.
- Early ambulation is important in order to reduce the incidence of DVT. Respiratory exercises are essential to decrease the incidence of chest complications.

> ■ KEY POINT
> Most elderly patients tolerate surgical complications poorly.

● ACUTE ABDOMEN IN ELDERLY PATIENTS

Abdominal pain in elderly patients can be a greater diagnostic challenge compared with that in younger patients, as elderly patients are more likely to present with vague symptoms due to cognitive impairment. On the other hand, neoplastic and cardiovascular diseases, such as mesenteric ischaemia and aneurysms, are more common in elderly patients. The clinical presentation in the elderly patient may be different from the classical picture, and a high index of suspicion is necessary.

Common surgical disorders

Biliary tract disease

Biliary tract disease includes symptomatic cholelithiasis and ascending cholangitis. Acalculous cholecystitis is rare, but its presentation in the elderly patient may be due to hypovascularity related to atherosclerosis. Asymptomatic gallstones are common, but their incidence varies greatly, depending on sex, age and race. Gallstones affects 25 per cent of women and 10–15 per cent of men over the age of 50 years. The presence of pericholecystic fluid, thickened gallbladder wall, periportal oedema and ultrasound-positive Murphy's sign are characteristic features of acute cholecystitis on ultrasonography. These features are absent in patients with asymptomatic gallstones.

Peptic ulcer disease is a common differential diagnosis in this group.

Complications of biliary tract disease include gallbladder perforation, emphysematous cholecystitis, ascending cholangitis and gallstone ileus.

The management is no different from that in younger patients.

Diverticulitis

Diverticulae are present in 50–80 per cent of patients over 65 years of age. Initial management of acute diverticulitis is conservative and involves resuscitation, admission and antibiotics. Laparotomy may be necessary in patients with peritonitis. Hartmann's procedure is still the procedure of choice in critically ill patients who undergo laparotomy for faecal peritonitis. Bleeding per rectum, colovesical and colovaginal fistulation may complicate chronic diverticular disease. Preoperative stoma marking and postoperative stoma-related rehabilitation are integral parts of the overall management.

Bowel ischaemia

Mesenteric ischaemia can be acute or chronic.

Acute ischaemia may be of arterial or venous origin. Causes of acute arterial ischaemia include cardiac embolus, commonly due to atrial fibrillation, valvular heart disease or recent myocardial infarction. Acute ischaemia may also be due to dislodgement of atherosclerotic plaques. The condition presents with bowel infarction along the superior mesenteric arterial territory. Venous infarction can be segmental.

Causes of venous ischaemia include portal vein thrombosis and low flow state, e.g. hypotension following myocardial infarction. Hypercoagulable venous disorders, such as protein C and S deficiency and factor V Leyden, are present in young patients but are rare in elderly patients.

Chronic mesenteric ischaemia may present as postprandial abdominal pain. Classically, the patient presents with weight loss and is afraid of eating meals, as pain returns few minutes after eating food. On auscultation, an abdominal bruit may be heard in severe stenosis. Chronic ischaemia may manifest as bleeding per rectum, ischaemic colitis and strictures. It is particularly common near the splenic flexure, as this is the watershed area of blood supply between the superior and inferior mesenteric vessels.

Mortality from mesenteric infarction is in the range of 60–90 per cent. Any delay in diagnosis increases the risk of death.

Metabolic acidosis may be the only feature suggestive of bowel ischaemia. Leucocytosis is a typical finding. The patient's consent for the possibility of a stoma should be sought. Although CT scanning may show gas in the bowel wall and portal vein, these may also be entirely normal or may show non-specific changes only. Early laparotomy and resection of gangrenous bowel is indicated, and second-look laparotomy may be required in a few patients.

Bowel obstruction

The most common cause of small bowel obstruction is adhesion, mainly due to previous abdominal surgery. However, femoral, inguinal and incisional hernias must be ruled out before making this diagnosis. Gallstone ileus is another important diagnosis (plain X-ray of abdomen may show pneumobilia).

Common causes of large bowel obstructions are carcinoma, inflammatory stricture, sigmoid volvulus and faecal impaction. Colonic pseudo-obstruction can exactly mimic large bowel obstruction in elderly patients. Meticulous clinical examination, identification and careful correction of electrolyte imbalance help the diagnosis and management.

Water-soluble contrast enema is the first-step investigation in all cases in order to rule out pseudo-obstruction.

Abdominal aortic aneurysm

Abdominal aortic aneurysm can notoriously present as renal colic, particularly left-sided. The classical syndrome of backache, hypotension and pulsatile abdominal mass is present in only 10 per cent of patients. Mortality of ruptured AAA can be as high as 50–80 per cent. Resuscitation with permissive hypotension is an essential step in the management. Abdominal ultrasound is helpful, and CT scanning can be considered the 'doughnut of death' in AAA. The patient must be accompanied by appropriate staff and monitored throughout: these patients benefit from laparotomy and not from investigations.

Appendicitis

Classical symptoms of appendicitis may be absent in elderly patients. Fever and leucocytosis may be not present. The high rate of perforation in elderly patients may be due to delay in diagnosis, depleted immune response and atherosclerosis of the vessels of the meso-appendix.

Pain relief

Non-steroidal anti-inflammatory drugs should be used with caution in elderly patients, as their use can result in increased incidence of renal toxicity and gastric bleeding or perforation. Use of opioids and benzodiazepines should be monitored, and their doses titrated carefully, as elderly patients are more sensitive to sedation and respiratory depression. Surgical review is mandatory if the patient's opioid requirement appears to increase suddenly, in order to rule out postoperative intra-abdominal complications, such as anastomotic leakage, abdominal abscess or abdominal compartment syndrome.

● TREATMENT OF CANCER IN ELDERLY PATIENTS

Common surgical cancers in elderly patients are treated in almost the same way as in younger patients, taking into consideration comorbidities and the high incidence of postoperative complications.

With breast cancer, the patient is given the option of breast-conserving surgery or mastectomy; many elderly patients opt against BCS in order to avoid radiation. Sometimes wide local excision of breast cancer is all that is required for the treatment. Elderly patients with dementia, and patients with very poor quality of life, are probably best treated with hormonal therapy only in order to prevent ulceration.

Although breast reconstruction should be offered to every patient undergoing mastectomy, its morbidity must be taken into account. The procedure should be used sparingly in high-risk elderly patients. The use of chemotherapy, if indicated, can be recommended in a fit patient over the age of 70 years and after discussion in the multidisciplinary team meeting.

● SUMMARY

With the increasingly ageing population, and the increase in people living beyond the age of 80 years, more operations are being performed and there is greater demand for ITU facilities. Physiological changes in all body systems make surgery in elderly patients potentially hazardous. Elderly patients need careful preoperative assessment and intraoperative and postoperative care, including rehabilitation.

● QUESTIONS

1 What cardiovascular changes do you expect in elderly patients?
2 What intraoperative precautions need to be taken in elderly patients?
3 What are the diagnostic problems of acute abdomen in elderly patients?
4 How would you treat a 2-cm oestrogen-receptor-positive breast cancer in a 75-year-old woman?

● FURTHER READING

Parker LJ, Vukov LF, Wollan PC (1997). Emergency department evaluation of geriatric patients with acute cholecystitis. *Acad Emerg Med* **4**: 51–5.

Rusnak RA, Borer JM, Fastow JS (1994). Misdiagnosis of acute appendicitis: common features discovered in cases after litigation. *Am J Emerg Med* **12**: 397–402.

Sanson TG, O'Keefe KP (1996). Evaluation of abdominal pain in the elderly. *Emerg Med Clin North Am* **14**: 615–27.

● ACKNOWLEDGEMENT

We acknowledge Dr Rebecca Ward, senior house office at St Helier Hospital, Epsom, Surrey, for her kind help in writing this chapter.

Day surgery

Karl Mainprize

- Introduction
- Why perform operations as day cases?
- What is necessary for surgery to be carried out as a day case?
- Assessment for day surgery
- What operations can be performed as day cases?
- Anaesthetic management
- Discharge
- Summary
- Questions
- References

● INTRODUCTION

There is some controversy as to the definition of day surgery. Many take day surgery to mean discharged on the same day as admission, but some argue that the term should apply to any patient discharged within 24 h of admission – that is, a 23-h stay.

● WHY PERFORM OPERATIONS AS DAY CASES?

Major morbidity and mortality following ambulatory surgery are exceedingly low. Ambulatory surgery allows earlier return to the preoperative physiological state, is associated with fewer complications and reduced mental and physical disability, and allows earlier resumption of normal activities. In the UK the NHS Plan (DH, 2000) has set a target of 75 per cent of elective surgery to be performed as day cases. The European Charter of Children's Rights states 'Children should be admitted to hospital only if the care they require cannot be equally well provided at home or on a day basis' (Alderson, 1993). There is also evidence of benefit of day surgery in elderly patients, with studies showing a reduction in postoperative cognitive dysfunction.

There are many advantages of day surgery for patients and their families and for hospitals (Table 21.1).

> ■ KEY POINT
> Ambulatory surgery is associated with fewer complications and reduced mental and physical disability.

● WHAT IS NECESSARY FOR SURGERY TO BE CARRIED OUT AS A DAY CASE?

Fundamental principles of day care include the following:

- Good-quality patient information on all aspects
- Preoperative assessment
- Day surgery ward
- Discharge criteria.

Table 21.1 Advantages of day surgery

Advantages to patients and their families	Advantages to hospitals
Reduced risk of cross-infection compared with patients who remain in hospital	Economic savings: day surgery allows treatment of large numbers of patients at less cost than in-patient surgical treatment of the same conditions
Early ambulation reduces risk of thromboembolism	More attractive to nursing staff because less shift work is involved
Avoidance of overnight stay in hospital leads to reduced patient anxiety, especially in children and elderly patients	In-patient beds are freed up as the average length of stay decreases
Quicker return to normal activities, with less time off work	
Savings in time, trouble and accommodation for relatives visiting patient in hospital	

Patients should be selected according to their physiological status and not their age. Fitness for a procedure should relate to the patient's health as found at pre-assessment and should not be limited by arbitrary limits such as American Surgical Association (ASA) status. Obesity is not an absolute contraindication for day care in expert hands and with appropriate resources.

> ■ KEY POINT
> Patients should be selected according to their physiological status and not their age.

As not every patient is fit for day surgery, it is very important that there is a good preoperative assessment service so that patients who require tests are identified and those tests are carried out before the patient is admitted to hospital.

Preoperative assessment

One of the main functions of anaesthetic pre-assessment is to ensure that the patient is able to proceed with the planned procedure on the day of surgery. Cancellations and delays have a negative impact on patients, healthcare personnel and organisations, and they can damage the quality of care provided. Reasons for cancellations include changes in a patient's medical status from the time of pre-assessment to the day of surgery, incomplete medical workup, patients not turning up on the day of surgery, and non-compliance with preoperative orders, such as fasting.

A good service minimises the risk of late cancellations by ensuring that all essential resources and discharge requirements are identified, and that the patient is fully informed and fit to undergo the procedure.

Pre-assessment clinics should be consultant-led and nurse-run, with assessment criteria developed in conjunction with the local department of anaesthesia.

Day surgery team

Day surgery requires a team approach and requires all members of that team to be motivated towards day surgery. This includes both primary care and secondary care practitioners. Healthcare professionals in the community help in assessment, as some factors outlined here are not always easy to assess by secondary care.

Day case surgeons

Surgeons carrying out day surgery need to be skilled in day surgical techniques, both in identifying suitable patients and in applying the surgery. They need to be senior enough to have a low complication rate and skilled enough to provide good-quality surgical care.

Day surgery ward

A DSU, with protected day case beds and with staff motivated to provide day surgery care, yields a much higher day surgery rate than if the patients are admitted to a general ward. Each DSU should have a clinical director who has a specific interest in day case surgery and who will lead the development of local policies, guidelines and clinical governance in this area.

Care should be provided in a facility that is set aside for day surgery, or practised in a dedicated area within the hospital.

Many hospitals provide care for day patients who require anaesthesia in specialised units, such as ophthalmology and dentistry. It may not be appropriate to centralise these services into one DSU, but all such patients must receive the same high standards of selection, preparation, perioperative care, discharge and follow-up.

Simple, rapid and effective exchange of information between hospital and community personnel must be possible.

● ASSESSMENT FOR DAY SURGERY

The assessment of a patient's suitability for day surgery falls into three groups (NHS Modernisation Agency, 2002):

- Social
- Medical
- Surgical.

Social assessment

- A responsible adult should be available to stay with the patient for the first 24 h after surgery.
- The patient and the carer should have access to a telephone.
- General practice/nursing backup should be available.
- The patient's travelling time from the hospital should be 1 h or less.
- The patient should arrive at the ward by 7.30 a.m. for a morning operating list or midday for an afternoon list.
- The patient should agree to surgery on a day case basis.

Medical assessment

- *Age:* the patient should be over 3 years of age (an exception is the paediatric computed tomography (CT) list).
- *General health:* the patient must be assessed as ASA grade 1–3 unless other contraindications are present, and the patient must pass pre-assessment as suitable for day case surgery.
- *Body mass index (BMI):* usually a BMI of up to 40 is suitable for day surgery. Patients with a BMI of 35–40 usually need a full anaesthetic assessment. If the BMI is greater than 40, then day case surgery is contraindicated, although some units are beginning to questioning this. Many units have an absolute weight limit of 150 kg.
- *Specific organ systems and diseases:* generally need to be assessed.

Surgical assessment

Is the operation suitable and does it fulfil the criteria in Box 21.1?

Box 21.1 Requirements for procedures suitable for day surgery

■ Minimal risk of postoperative haemorrhage
■ Minimal risk of postoperative airway compromise
■ Postoperative pain control using outpatient analgesic techniques
■ Postoperative nursing requirements that can be met by community nurse facilities
■ Rapid return to normal fluid and food intake
■ Early commencement of procedures for which a long recovery period is likely
■ Patient should be able to mobilise to some extent.

● WHAT OPERATIONS CAN BE PERFORMED AS DAY CASES?

The fundamental principle is that surgery undertaken as a day case must be based on proven patient safety and quality of care. This requires a degree of common sense and, in some cases, the use of 23-h stay to prove feasible.

In 2000 in the UK, the Audit Commission produced a basket of 25 operations where day surgery should be the standard. The British Association of Day Surgery (2006) has taken this further to give targets for surgeons to achieve and produced the following list of operations that it feels should be done as day cases:

- *General surgery:*
  - Excision of breast lumps, lipomas, sebaceous cysts, etc.
  - Thyroidectomy and parathyroid adenoma, thyroglossal cysts
  - Wide local excision and sentinel node biopsy (e.g. breast, malignant melanoma)
  - Major duct excision
  - Laparoscopic cholecystectomy
  - Varicose vein operations
  - Inguinal hernia repair (including bilateral)
  - Upper and lower endoscopy
- *Urology:*
  - Cystoscopy and endoscopic extraction of calculus from bladder
  - Endoscopic retrograde pyelography
  - Orchidectomy
  - Orchidopexy
  - Circumcision
  - Hydrocele and epididymal cysts
- *Ear, nose and throat (ENT):*
  - Pinnaplasty
  - Myringotomy
  - Submucous resection of nasal septum
  - Septoplasty of nose
  - Tonsillectomy
- *Orthopaedics:*
  - Carpal tunnel release
  - Dupuytren's fasciectomy
  - Diagnostic arthroscopy of knee
  - Bunion operation
  - Autograft anterior cruciate ligament reconstruction.

Box 21.1 outlines the criteria that a procedure should fulfil in order to be suitable as a day case.

● ANAESTHETIC MANAGEMENT

Day surgery anaesthesia should be a consultant-led service. Due to the increasing numbers of procedures carried out as day cases, however, trainees must also be educated in these techniques.

Once a patient has been selected and fully prepared for day surgery, decisions must be made regarding anaesthetic management. High standards of patient monitoring must be met, and assistance provided for the anaesthetist (Association of Anaesthetists of Great Britain and Ireland, 2000).

Each anaesthetist should develop techniques that permit the patient to undergo the surgical procedure with minimum stress and maximum comfort. Analgesia should be long-lasting, but morbidity such as nausea and vomiting must be minimised. For certain procedures (e.g. laparoscopic cholecystectomy), there is evidence that following a standard anaesthesia and analgesia plan minimises morbidity and increases the number of patients who can be discharged.

Policies should exist for the management of postoperative nausea and vomiting (PONV) and discharge analgesia. Routine antiemetics should not be used unless there is a strong history of PONV and in patients undergoing certain procedures, such as laparoscopic sterilisation, laparoscopic cholecystectomy and tonsillectomy. Motion sickness is another strong predictor of potential problems after anaesthesia. If PONV occurs, it should be treated seriously. A standard management protocol can aid the anaesthetist, the nursing staff and the patient.

■ KEY POINT
Routine antiemetics should not be used unless there is a strong history of PONV and in patients undergoing certain procedures.

Prescribing discharge analgesia should be the responsibility of the anaesthetist.

● DISCHARGE

Nurse-led discharge is now widely accepted, as long as the following discharge criteria are met:

- Stable vital signs for at least 1 hour
- Correct orientation in time, place and person
- Adequate pain control
- Minimal nausea, vomiting and dizziness
- Adequate hydration and likelihood of maintenance with oral fluids
- Minimal bleeding and wound drainage
- Patients at significant risk of urinary retention (central neural blockade, pelvic and other surgery) must have passed urine
- Discharge must be authorised by appropriate staff member after discharge criteria have been satisfied
- Written and verbal instructions for all relevant aspects of post-anaesthetic and surgical care must be given to the patient and the accompanying adult; a contact address and telephone number for emergency medical care must be included
- Analgesia should be provided for after discharge, with clear written instructions on how and when it should be used; advice on any other regular medication is also necessary
- Telephone follow-up should be made whenever possible
- A responsible adult must take the patient home; for some patients, it may be important to have an adult escort in addition to the vehicle driver.

It is essential to inform the patient's general practitioner of the nature of the anaesthetic and surgical procedure performed and of the patient's discharge. DSUs must agree with their local primary care teams with regard to how backup is to be provided for patients in the event of problems. Telephone follow-up is highly rated by patients and can be a useful method of auditing any immediate problems.

Factors that affect discharge time in patients undergoing ambulatory surgery are shown in Table 21.2.

Table 21.2 Factors delaying discharge from an ambulatory surgical unit

Preoperative	Intraoperative	Postoperative
Female gender	Long duration of surgery	Postoperative nausea and vomiting, pain, drowsiness
Increasing age	General anaesthesia	No escort
Congestive heart failure	Spinal anaesthesia	

From Junger *et al.* (2001),

● SUMMARY

Day surgery:

- can mean discharged on the same calendar day as admission or a 23-h stay;
- relies on a team approach;
- needs a dedicated day surgery unit (DSU);
- needs a good pre-assessment clinic;
- needs defined discharge protocols.

● QUESTIONS

1 What are the advantages and disadvantages of day surgery?
2 What hospital factors are necessary for day surgery?
3 What patient factors are necessary for an operation to be carried out successfully as a day case?
4 How would you assess a patient as suitable for day surgery?
5 What are the factors that delay discharge of a day surgical patient?

● REFERENCES

Alderson P (1993). European charter of children's rights. *Bull Med Ethics* **93**: 13–15.

Association of Anaesthetists of Great Britain and Ireland (2000). *Recommendations for Standards of Monitoring During Anaesthesia and Recovery*. London: Association of Anaesthetists of Great Britain and Ireland.

British Association of Day Surgery (2006). *BADS Directory of Procedures*. London: British Association of Day Surgery.

Department of Health (DH) (2000). *The NHS Plan*. London: Department of Health. www.dh.gov.uk/en/PublicationsAndStatistics/Publications/PublicationsPolicyAndGuidance/DH_4002960.

Junger A, Klasen J, Benson M, *et al.* (2001). Factors determining length of stay of surgical day-case patients. *Eur J Anaesthesiol* **18**: 314–21.

NHS Modernisation Agency (2002). *National Good Practice Guidance on Preoperative Assessment for Day Surgery*. London: NHS Modernisation Agency.

Antimicrobial prophylaxis, meticillin-resistant Staphylococcus aureus and Clostridium difficile-associated infection

22

Kevin G Kerr

● INTRODUCTION

This chapter outlines the principles of antimicrobial prophylaxis in surgery and considers practical aspects, including a discussion of which procedures require prophylaxis and the selection of antibiotics based on criteria such as the range of bacteria likely to be found at the surgical site and local antimicrobial resistance patterns.

● ANTIMICROBIAL PROPHYLAXIS IN SURGERY

Principles of prophylaxis

In the UK the incidence of surgical site infection is approximately 4 per cent. Patients with such infections remain in hospital for an average of 6.5 days longer than those without.

The complex interplay between a wide array of variables determines the likelihood of infection developing after surgery. These variables include:

- patient-related factors such as obesity and diabetes;
- type of surgery (e.g. contaminated operative site, insertion of prosthetic device);
- other factors relating to surgery (e.g. presence of devitalised tissue, duration of procedure);
- virulence and size of the bacterial inoculum.

Prophylaxis is given for 'clean-contaminated' and some types of clean surgery; therapeutic antimicrobials should be given for dirty and contaminated procedures. Clean surgical procedures that warrant prophylaxis include those in which prosthetic material is inserted, because, although the risk of infection is low, the consequences of an infected prosthesis for the patient in terms of morbidity and mortality are significant. Prophylactic antimicrobials are not, however, recommended for procedures in which the risk of infection is low; studies have failed to show a significant reduction of infection compared with placebo in, for example, clean head and neck surgery and non-mesh herniorrhaphy. It should be acknowledged that prophylaxis in itself can not be relied upon to prevent infection and should not be used to compensate for inadequate preoperative preparation, suboptimal surgical technique or poor postoperative care.

Practical aspects of prophylaxis

What to give

Uncertainties over serum concentrations achievable during surgery coupled with a paucity of evidence for the effectiveness of drugs administered via alternative routes dictate that prophylactic agents should be given intravenously. The doses used for prophylaxis should be the same as those used to treat active infection. The actual choice of agent(s) should reflect:

- the pathogens most commonly isolated from postoperative infection associated with the procedure (Table 22.1);
- local resistance patterns for these pathogens (Scottish Intercollegiate Guideline Network, 2008);
- the need to avoid overly broad-spectrum agents in order to minimise disruption of the regional ('normal') bacterial flora;
- the likelihood of adverse drug reactions, including hypersensitivity;
- cost.

> ■ KEY POINT
> Local antimicrobial resistance patterns should be taken into account.

When to give

Prophylaxis should be started just before or just after the procedure commences, ideally within 30 min of induction of anaesthesia. If a tourniquet is to be used, then antimicrobials should be given before it is applied – 10 min after intravenous administration is recommended. In caesarean section, antimicrobials are given after the cord is clamped.

Note that some agents cannot be given by a bolus injection (e.g. vancomycin must be infused over at least 90 min), and this must be taken into account in the timing of administration.

For how long?

For the majority of procedures, a single dose of each agent is appropriate and additional doses during or after surgery are not required. Exceptions to this recommendation include blood loss in adults of 1500 mL or more in adults and haemodilution to 15 mL/kg or less (Scottish Intercollegiate Guideline Network, 2008).

> ■ KEY POINT
> For the majority of procedures, a single dose of each agent is appropriate.

Penicillin-allergic patients

Many prophylactic regimens rely heavily on cephalosporins, which can create problems when patients give a history of penicillin allergy. Under these circumstances, the following should be considered:

- If possible, document the nature of the 'allergy', as patients sometimes assume, or are told by others, that an adverse event such as nausea, headache or diarrhoea is a manifestation of hypersensitivity.
- Patients with anaphylaxis, urticaria or rash immediately following a dose of a penicillin-class drug should not be given a cephalosporin. The local policy antibiotic policy should be consulted in order to identify an alternative agent.

● METICILLIN-RESISTANT *STAPHYLOCOCCUS AUREUS*

Although meticillin-resistant *Staphylococcus aureus* (MRSA) first emerged over 40 years ago, it remained relatively uncommon until the appearance of epidemic strains (EMRSA). In the UK, EMRSA15 and EMRSA16 are the most common, accounting for more than 90 per cent of all bloodstream infections with the bacterium. These strains appear to be more transmissible than their earlier counterparts, but the exact contribution of other factors to the sharp increase

Table 22.1 Indications for antimicrobial prophylaxis in common surgical procedures

Procedure[a]	Likely pathogens[a]	Typical prophylactic regimens
Gastrointestinal		
Upper gastrointestinal tract	Gram-negative bacilli	Cefradine/cefuroxime[b] or gentamicin
Biliary tract[c]	Gram-negative bacilli, anaerobes	Cefradine/cefuroxime[b] + metronidazole or gentamicin + metronidazole or co-amoxiclav
Colorectal, appendectomy	Gram-negative bacilli, anaerobes	Cefradine/cefuroxime[b] + metronidazole or amoxicillin/ampicillin + gentamicin + metronidazole
Urogenital[d]	Gram-negative bacilli	Gentamicin or cefradine/cefuroxime[b]
Obstetric/gynaecology	Gram-negative bacilli, anaerobes, streptococci	
Caesarean section		Cefradine/cefuroxime[b] or co-amoxiclav[e]
Hysterectomy (abdominal or vaginal)		Cefradine/cefuroxime[b] + metronidazole or gentamicin + metronidazole or co-amoxiclav
Orthopaedic		Cefradine/cefuroxime[b] or flucloxacillin
Prosthetic joint insertion		
Closed fracture fixation		
Hip fracture repair		
Vascular		
Reconstructive arterial surgery	Skin flora, especially *S. aureus* and coagulase-negative staphylococci	Cefradine/cefuroxime[b] or gentamicin[f]
Amputation	*S. aureus*, Gram-negative bacilli, anaerobes	Cefradine/cefuroxime[b] or gentamicin + metronidazole
Cardiothoracic	Skin flora, especially *S. aureus* and coagulase-negative bacilli (if leg veins harvested for bypass procedures)	Cefradine/cefuroxime[b] or vancomycin + gentamicin if prevalence of MRSA is high
ENT		
Clean/clean-contaminated[g]	Streptococci (including pneumococci), *Haemophilus* spp., anaerobes	Cefuroxime + metronidazole or co-amoxiclav
Neurosurgery		
Clean surgery (including craniotomy)	*S. aureus* (less commonly Gram-negative bacilli)	Cefradine/cefuroxime[b]
Clean-contaminated (entering of cranial air sinuses)	Streptococci (including pneumococci), *Haemophilus* spp., anaerobes	Cefuroxime + metronidazole or co-amoxiclav
Insertion of CSF shunt	*S. aureus* (less commonly Gram-negative bacilli)	Cefradine/cefuroxime[b]

[a]All procedures involving a skin incision are associated with a risk of *S. aureus* (less commonly, beta-haemolytic streptococcal) infection.

[b]Narrower-spectrum cephalosporins such as cefradine and cefuroxime are preferable to extended-spectrum (so-called 'third generation') agents, e.g. cefotaxime, as the latter have a greater effect on the normal regional flora and increase the likelihood of *Clostridium difficile*-associated disease and selection for extended-spectrum beta-lactamase-producing bacteria (ESBLs). In addition, narrower-spectrum cephalosporins have better activity than extended-spectrum agents against staphylococci.

[c]Results from some studies suggest that laparoscopic cholecystectomy does not require prophylaxis.

[d]For elective urological procedures, a preoperative urine should be obtained and any urinary tract infection treated before surgery, according to the results of susceptibility tests. The latter can also be used to assist in the choice of prophylactic antimicrobials if preoperative treatment of infection is not possible. Transurethral resection of bladder tumours does not require prophylaxis.

[e]Given after the cord is clamped.

[f]Add metronidazole if high risk of anaerobic infection, e.g. patients with gangrenous changes.

[g]Clean surgery does not require prophylaxis. Nose or sinus surgery and tonsillectomy do not require prophylaxis.

CSF, cerebrospinal fluid; *S. aureus*, *Staphylococcus aureus*.

of nosocomial MRSA infections seen in many countries, such as poor compliance with hand hygiene, a perceived drop in the standards of environmental hygiene in hospitals, and lack of facilities for the isolation of patients known to be MRSA-positive, is difficult to ascertain. Concern over MRSA led to the introduction of national mandatory surveillance for MRSA bloodstream infections in all four countries of the UK and subsequently to the setting of targets for reductions in these infections.

Prevention of MRSA in surgical patients

Much attention has focused on strategies for the prevention of MRSA infection, and many countries have now published national guidelines (Coia *et al.*, 2006). It is worth noting, however, that many guideline recommendations are based on non-controlled trials and descriptive studies. A key element of most guidelines, and central to any debate on preventative strategies, is the issue of screening of patients for carriage of MRSA. Screening aims to identify those patients colonised with MRSA on admission to hospital or upon transfer between or within hospitals (e.g. to an intensive care unit, ICU). Screening can also be performed as part of the preoperative assessment process. Asymptomatic carriers are most frequently colonised in the anterior nares, but some may also have axillary, perineal or throat carriage. Ulcers or pressure sores and the bladder in patients with in-dwelling catheters may also be sites of colonisation. Screening, however, remains contentious and the debate is likely to remain unresolved for some time.

Screening surgical patients for MRSA

Many questions remain unanswered:

- Use universal screening or targeting of high-risk patients (Box 22.1) and procedures (i.e. those where the risk may be low but consequences are severe such as vascular bypass grafting)?
- How many sites to swab – nasal only or include other sites?
- What laboratory methods to use – conventional culture of swabs (cheap but slow – results available in 48 h) or DNA-based methods (expensive but rapid – results available in 2 h).
- Screen once on admission or periodically throughout a patient's stay?
- Dispense with screening to give eradication therapy to all target patients? This counters the problem that screening may produce falsely negative results but increases the risk of resistance to eradication agents.

> ■ KEY POINT
> Screening of surgical patients for carriage of MRSA is becoming increasingly frequent, although optimal screening regimens remain to be defined.

Eradication of MRSA colonisation

Identification of MRSA colonisation in patients serves two principal functions: (i) isolation of the patient to prevent spread of the bacterium to other patients and (ii) to permit eradication of carriage, further reducing the risks of onward transmission to other patients and healthcare staff as well as decreasing the likelihood of endogenous infection. A typical eradication regime for nasal carriers is as follows:

- Mupirocin to the anterior nares three times daily for 5 days.
- 2% triclosan, or similar, body-wash once daily for 5 days. Hair also to be washed twice with this preparation at least twice during this time.

Screening/eradication is not the only element in any comprehensive strategy to prevent MRSA infection. Other measures include the following:

Box 22.1 Risk factors for meticillin-resistant *Staphylococcus aureus* (MRSA) colonisation

- Known previous MRSA colonisation or infection
- Previous hospital admission within past year
- Admitted from another hospital
- Residence in nursing/care home
- Breach in skin such as decubitus ulcer, pressure sore, vascular access devices
- Diabetes or end-stage renal failure
- Repeated courses of antimicrobials
- Healthcare professionals who care for patients likely to have MRSA.

- *Good hand hygiene*: some hospitals have adopted a 'naked below the elbow policy' to enhance the efficiency of hand-cleaning. This became a statutory requirement in England in 2009
- *Well-designed and implemented protocols for the insertion of devices*, e.g. vascular access lines, which can act as a portal of entry for MRSA
- *Cleanliness of the hospital environment*, although the contribution of the environment to the epidemiology of MRSA infection is still unknown
- *Isolation of MRSA-positive patients*: in many UK hospitals, there are insufficient numbers of side rooms for isolation of all positive patients, and some hospitals cohort colonised/infected patients in bays or entire wards; many orthopaedic units have designated MRSA-free wards
- *Prudent use of antimicrobials*
- *Use of perioperative prophylaxis with agents that have anti-MRSA activity in patients known to be MRSA-positive preoperatively*: this can be used for elective surgery in patients in whom preoperative attempts at decolonisation have been unsuccessful and in emergency procedures in MRSA-positive patients
- *Surveillance*: use of resources to reduce MRSA infection will be efficient only if the areas that are most likely to benefit can be identified.

Optimal antimicrobial therapy for MRSA infection

Meticillin resistance indicates resistance to all cephalosporins and penicillins, including flucloxacillin. In addition, EMRSA strains, which are associated with the majority of nosocomial infections, are resistant to other agents, including macrolides (e.g. erythromycin, clarithromycin), clindamycin, ciprofloxacin, and sometimes fusidic acid and gentamicin. Overuse of these agents will select for carriage of MRSA in patients treated with them. Despite this, there are still several antimicrobials that are available to treat MRSA infection (Table 22.2).

■ KEY POINT

As well as resistance to all beta-lactams (penicillins and cephalosporins), hospital-associated strains of MRSA usually manifest resistance to many other classes of antimicrobial.

■ KEY POINT

New agents for the management of MRSA infection include linezolid, quinupristin/dalfopristin and daptomycin.

Table 22.2 Management options for serious meticillin-resistant *Staphylococcus aureus* (MRSA) infection

Agent	Class	Notes
Vancomycin	Glycopeptide	Used widely. Inexpensive, but need for therapeutic drug monitoring increases costs. 'Red man syndrome' (flushing of upper body accompanied by pruritus and, sometimes, hypotension caused by drug-induced release of histamine) precludes bolus dosing
Teicoplanin	Glycopeptide	Used widely. More expensive than vancomycin, but less requirement to monitor levels. Can be given as bolus. Like vancomycin, resistance is very rare in UK
Linezolid	Oxazolidinone	Expensive. Can be given orally, unlike vancomycin and teicoplanin. Requires regular monitoring of full blood count because of possible thrombocytopenia, leucopenia and anaemia
Quinupristin with dalfopristin	Streptogramins	Expensive. Intravenous only, but cannot be given through a peripheral cannula
Daptomycin	Lipopeptide	Expensive. No oral formulation. Once-daily dosing. Monitor creatine kinase levels because of myositis and (rarely) rhabdomyolysis

● *CLOSTRIDIUM DIFFICILE*

The overwhelming majority of cases of *Clostridium difficile*-associated disease (CDAD) follow therapy with antimicrobials. Symptoms typically occur after 5–10 days of therapy, but CDAD can present either earlier or much later (≤ 10 weeks) than this. CDAD represents a continuum of the following syndromes:

- Asymptomatic colonisation with C. *difficile*
- Diarrhoea
- Pseudomembranous colitis
- Toxic megacolon
- Colonic perforation.

> ■ KEY POINT
> *Clostridium difficile* is associated with a spectrum of clinical entities, from asymptomatic colonisation of the gut to colonic perforation. Paradoxically, patients with severe disease may not have diarrhoea.

Damage to the colonic mucosa is caused by the production of two toxins – toxin A (entero-toxin) and toxin B (cytotoxin). Although there is debate about the relative contribution of each in the pathogenesis of the condition, strains that produce only toxin B are known to cause CDAD.

Antimicrobials associated with CDAD

Nearly all classes of antimicrobial agents have been implicated in CDAD, but the following are the most frequently implicated agents:

- Cephalosporins, especially third-generation and extended-spectrum agents such as cefotaxime
- Ampicillin/amoxicillin
- Macrolides, e.g. clarithromycin
- Clindamycin
- Quinolones, e.g. ciprofloxacin.

> ▉ KEY POINT
> Prophylaxis using agents with a broad antibacterial spectrum increases the likelihood of CDAD and the selection of multi-resistant bacteria.

Clostridium difficile-associated disease is particularly likely in elderly patients, especially those with a long duration of hospital stay and who may have had long or repeated courses of antibiotics. The presence of a nasogastric tube and recent gastrointestinal surgery are also risk factors. Receipt of anti-ulcer medication, especially proton-pump inhibitors, is often cited as increasing the likelihood of CDAD, but this remains highly controversial, and conflicting results have been obtained from several studies.

Diagnosis of CDAD

Most laboratories now use commercially available kits for the detection of toxin A and/or toxin B by enzyme-linked immunoassay (EIA) in stools. A cytotoxicity test using tissue culture is often regarded as the gold standard, but this is technically complex, is expensive and takes longer to produce results than EIA. Culture of the stools for *C. difficile* is of limited value as it merely signals the presence of the bacterium and does not given information on whether (i) the strain is capable of toxin production and (ii) the toxin is actually being produced in vivo. It is useful, however, for epidemiological purposes, as strains are available for typing using genetic fingerprinting techniques such as ribotyping (in which DNA fragments produced by digestion of the bacterial chromosome by endonucleases, and that contain all or part of the genes coding for 16S and 23S rRNA, are compared). Endoscopy to identify pathognomic 'pseudo-membranes' is of poor sensitivity and is not without risk to the patient, and its routine use is not recommended.

Management of CDAD

Management includes the following (Bouza *et al.*, 2005):

- Whenever possible, ensure the patient is nursed in isolation.
- Alcohol hand-rub is not effective in vitro against spores of *C. difficile*, and the use of soap and water to physically remove spores is recommended when attending to patients.
- Commence a stool chart: this is helpful for assessing severity of disease and response to therapy. Note that ill patients with toxic megacolon or ileus may not have diarrhoea.
- Commence fluid and electrolyte replacement.
- Stop inciting antimicrobials. (If patient still requires therapy, can narrower-spectrum agents be substituted?)
- Do not use antimotility agents.
- Mild CDAD may respond to cessation of antimicrobials only.
- Treat moderate CDAD with oral metronidazole. A typical regimen is 400 mg three times a day for 10 days. Note that patients may become symptomatically better shortly after commencing metronidazole but should complete a full course of therapy because of the high risk of relapse.
- Treat severe CDAD as described below.

Management of relapsing CDAD

Relapsing or recurring episodes are very common and occur in 20–60 per cent of cases. If the relapses are associated with mild or moderate disease, then a second course of metronidazole can be used. For third episodes, vancomycin is recommended. Management of multiply relapsing patients is problematic; approaches include the use of probiotics, which include bacteria such as *Lactobacillus* spp. (in the form of capsules or dairy products such as live yoghurt) and non-pathogenic yeasts (e.g. *Saccharomyces boulardii*), and prebiotics (substrates for gut microflora). The aim is to correct the ecological imbalance of the normal colonic flora created by broad-spectrum antimicrobials, which have allowed *C. difficile* to flourish and produce toxins. Another, rather more unusual, way of attempting this is through faecal transplants in which faecal material from healthy volunteers is given as an enema. Alternative approaches include neutralisation of *C. difficile* toxins through toxin-binding agents, such as tolevamer, intravenous normal immunoglobulin or monoclonal antibodies directed specifically against *C. difficile* toxins. In addition, the new antimicrobial nitazoxanide is being evaluated for patients with multiply relapsing disease. A *C. difficile* vaccine is also under development. Probiotics appear to be the most promising, thus far, and they have also been advocated for use in the management of first episodes as well as 'prophylaxis' of CDAD. There is still no consensus, however, over their use in routine practice.

> ■ KEY POINT
> Relapsing infection is common. Management of patients with multiple relapses is problematic and the role of probiotics in this setting is still unclear.

Severe CDAD

In recent years, more cases of severe CDAD have been reported (Blossom and McDonald, 2007). Severe CDAD can be defined as two or more of the following:

- Age over 60 years
- Temperature 38.3 °C or higher
- Albumin less than 2.5 mg/dL
- Peripheral leucocyte count greater than 15×10^9/L.

These patients have an increased risk of admission to ICU and requirement for colectomy. There is an attributable mortality rate of 7 per cent. There is much evidence to suggest that this increase in severity may be associated with a new 'hypervirulent' strain of *C. difficile* known as O27 in Europe and NAPI/BI in North America. The strain produces 15–20 times the amount of toxin A and toxin B compared with other strains, as well as another toxin – binary toxin. O27 has been associated with large outbreaks in both UK and North American hospitals. Typically, patients with severe CDAD associated with O27 do not respond to metronidazole, and many authorities now recommend that severe CDAD should be managed with vancomycin 125 mg orally four times a day for 10 days.

> ■ KEY POINT
> A new 'hypervirulent' strain of *C. difficile*, known as O27, has emerged in North America and is becoming increasingly common in the UK and continental Europe.

● SUMMARY

MRSA is emerging as an important cause of infection in the surgical patient, and knowledge of the prevention of infections associated with this bacterium through preoperative screening and the management of MRSA infection is imperative. The incidence of another healthcare-associated infection, CDAD, has also increased in recent years. Nearly all cases of CDAD follow antimicrobial therapy, although the association with some agents is much greater with particular classes of antibiotics. Surgeons may become involved in the management of patients with severe CDAD.

● QUESTIONS

1 Why are narrower-spectrum cephalosporins such as cefradine and cefuroxime preferred over extended-spectrum agents such as cefotaxime and ceftriaxone for surgical prophylaxis?
2 For which surgical procedures are orally administered antimicrobials acceptable alternatives to agents given intravenously?
3 Vancomycin can be used for prophylaxis in procedures where there is a high risk of surgical site infection caused by MRSA as well as in the management of established MRSA infection. Why can this drug not be administered as a bolus dose?
4 Name three sites at which patients may be asymptomatically colonised with MRSA.
5 Why are infections caused by EMRSA strains difficult to manage?
6 What is the most commonly used laboratory method for the diagnosis of CDAD?
7 What clinical or laboratory features suggest that a patient might have severe CDAD?

● REFERENCES

Blossom DB, McDonald LC (2007). The challenges posed by reemerging *Clostridium difficile* infection. *Clin Infect Dis* **45**: 222–7.

Bouza E, Muñoz P, Alonso R (2005). Clinical manifestations, treatment and control of infections caused by *Clostridium difficile*. *Clin Infect Dis* **11** (suppl. 4): 57–64.

Coia JE, Duckworth G, Edwards DI, *et al.* (2006). Guidelines for the control and prevention of meticillin-resistant *Staphylococcus aureus* (MRSA) in healthcare facilities. *J Hosp Infect* **63** (suppl. 1): S1–44.

Scottish Intercollegiate Guideline Network (SIGN) (2008). *Antibiotic Prophylaxis in Surgery*. (Revised 2002.) www.sign.ac.uk/guidelines/fulltext/104/index.html.

Viral hepatitis and HIV infection in surgical practice

23

Walid Al-Wali

● INTRODUCTION

The surgical procedure, because of its invasive nature and the complexities that surround it, may be associated with various complications and risks. An important example of such adverse incidents is the transmission of blood-borne viruses, most importantly the hepatitis viruses and the human immunodeficiency virus (HIV).

There are two facets to this problem: the risk of patients becoming infected as a result of surgery, and the risk of patients who already have such infections transmitting them to the surgical team and other patients.

It is imperative that surgeons and other healthcare workers involved in surgical practice have a thorough understanding, and are cognisant with the mode of transmission of such infective agents. This will help them to prevent these infections by following good infection control practice.

● TYPES OF BLOOD-BORNE VIRUS

The full spectrum of the transmissible blood-borne viruses includes the hepatitis viral agents, the human retroviruses, the herpes viruses and other viruses acquired as a result of animal or human bites (Table 23.1).

However, because surgical patients are frequently given transfusions of blood or blood products, and because hospital staff often incur accidental needlestick injury, it is the viruses that can potentially be transmitted by these routes that are of prime importance to surgeons and their patients.

This chapter focuses on the hepatitis viruses and HIV.

● MODE OF TRANSMISSION OF BLOOD-BORNE VIRUSES

Hepatitis B, hepatitis C and HIV cannot be transmitted through the intact skin and require a route of entry to infect a patient or healthcare worker in the hospital setting. The following are the modes of transmission of hepatitis B virus, hepatitis C virus and HIV:

- Sexual transmission (vaginal, anal)
- Perinatal transmission from mother to child

Table 23.1 Blood-borne viruses potentially transmissible in surgery

Virus	Type
Hepatitis viruses:	
Hepatitis A virus (HAV)	RNA
Hepatitis B virus (HBV)	DNA
Hepatitis C virus (HCV)	RNA
Hepatitis D virus (HDV)	DNA
Hepatitis G virus (HGV)	RNA
Human retroviruses:	
Human immunodeficiency virus (HIV)	RNA
HIV1	
HIV2	
Human T-cell lymphotrophic virus 1 (HTLV1)	RNA
Herpes viruses:	
Cytomegalovirus (CMV)	DNA
Epstein–Barr virus (EBV)	DNA
Herpes simplex virus type 1 (HSV-1)	DNA
Herpes simplex virus type 2 (HSV-2)	DNA
Varicella-zoster virus (VZV)	DNA

- Organ or tissue transplantation and blood product transfusion
- Percutaneous injury from needles, sharp instruments, bone fragments, significant bites that break the skin, etc.
- Intravenous drug injection
- Exposure of broken skin such as abrasions, cuts, eczema, etc.
- Exposure of mucous membranes, including the eye.

NATURAL COURSE AND EPIDEMIOLOGY OF BLOOD-BORNE VIRUSES

Hepatitis viruses

The primary hepatitis viruses are hepatitis A (HAV), hepatitis B (HBV), hepatitis C (HCV), hepatitis E (HEV), hepatitis G (HGV) and hepatitis D (HDV).

Hepatitis A virus

Hepatitis A virus belongs to the picornaviruses family and causes infectious hepatitis. It is transmitted via the faecal–oral route and there is no asymptomatic carrier status.

Hepatitis B virus

Hepatitis B virus (Figure 23.1) is a 42-nm member of the Hepadnaviridae family of DNA viruses. It causes serum hepatitis. The HBV markers can be detected at various times (Table 23.2).

Clinical course

The incubation period ranges from 40 days to 160 days (average 60–90 days). The clinical picture is similar to that of HAV infections, but HBV symptoms tend to be more severe and can

Figure 23.1 ● Electron micrograph of hepatitis B virus.

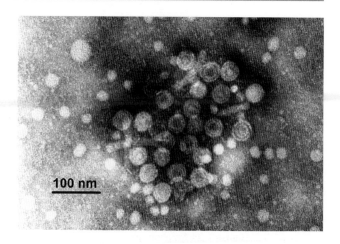

100 nm

Table 23.2 Serological markers of hepatitis B infection

Marker	Comment	Disease stage
HbsAg	Surface antigen not infective	Acute and chronic infections, including antigenaemia
HbeAg	Found in core of virion. Presence in blood indicates infectivity.	Acute and chronic hepatitis
Viral DNA polymerase	As for HbeAg	As for HbeAg
Antibodies:		
Anti-Hbs	Indicates recovery, protects against re-infection	Convalescence
Anti-Hbe	Presence indicates little or no infectivity	Convalescence
Anti-Hbc	In IgM form, indicates recent infection	The first antibody that appears; persists for life as IgG

Hbc, hepatitis B core antibody; Hbe, hepatitis B e antibody; Hbs, antibody to hepatitis B virus surface antigen; HbsAg, hepatitis B virus surface antigen; IgG, immunoglobulin G; IgM, immunoglobulin M.

be life-threatening (Figure 23.2). Chronic hepatitis is defined as persistence of HBsAg (hepatitis B virus surface antigen) in the serum for 6 months or longer. Patients co-infected with both HBV and HIV may have increased hepatic damage if HIV is treated before HBV.

Interferon alfa is clinically useful for the treatment of chronic hepatitis B infections.

Prevention involves either use of a vaccine containing HBsAg produced in yeasts by recombinant DNA technology or the use of hepatitis B immune globulin, which contains high levels of antibodies against HBV prepared from the sera of patients who have recovered from HBV infection. Immunisation against HBV in Taiwan has greatly reduced the incidence of hepatoma in children: this is the first vaccine to prevent human cancer.

Epidemiology

The three main modes of transmission are via blood, from sexual intercourse and perinatally from mother to newborn. The fact that needlestick injuries can transmit the virus indicates

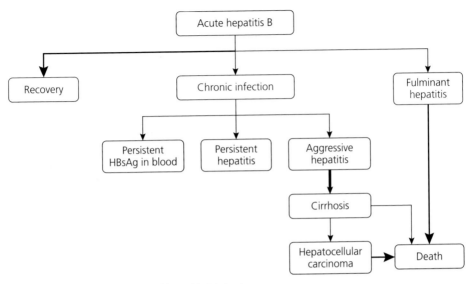

Figure 23.2 ● Clinical outcomes of hepatitis B infection.

Highlighted arrows indicate most likely outcomes. HBsAg, hepatitis B virus surface antigen.

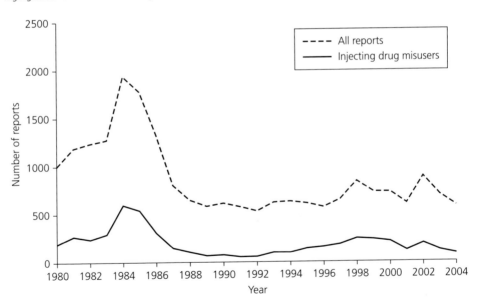

Figure 23.3 ● Laboratory reports of confirmed acute hepatitis B in England and Wales.

that only very small amounts of blood are necessary. Screening of blood for the presence of HBsAg has greatly decreased the number of transfusion-associated cases of HBV infection. The World Health Organization (WHO) has estimated that over 350 million people worldwide are chronically infected with HBV, with a particularly high prevalence in Asia. In high-prevalence areas, infection is acquired primarily in childhood by perinatal transmission or horizontal transmission between young children. In low-prevalence areas, transmission occurs mostly in adulthood via sexual intercourse and via sharing of contaminated needles and equipment among intravenous drug users (Figure 23.3).

Hepatitis C

Hepatitis C is an RNA virus of the Flavivirus family. It is well known to be the major cause of parenteral transmission of non-A, non-B hepatitis. The average incubation period is 7–8 weeks, with a range of 2–15 weeks.

Acute symptomatic disease occurs in less than 10 per cent of individuals. The majority of infections become chronic, leading in 20 per cent of cases to cirrhosis. A small number of patients develop hepatocellular carcinoma.

Transmission by sexual and perinatal exposure is less efficient for this virus than for HBV. Only about 25 per cent of cases of acute infection are icteric, and most patients have no acute illness suggestive of HCV infection. The presence of anti-HCV immunoglobulin G (IgG) does not distinguish acute from chronic hepatitis.

The combination of interferon and ribavirin has been shown to be effective in treatment. Moderate to severe disease can now be treated successfully in up to 55 per cent of cases.

Epidemiology

Hepatitis C virus is transmitted primarily via blood. Transmission by blood transfusion is rare because donated blood is screened, and transmission by needlestick injury is of lower risk than HBV infection. About 0.5 per cent of the general population in England have been infected with HCV (0.4 per cent of the population is chronically infected). Worldwide, about 170 million people are chronically infected with HCV. In the UK, most infected individuals have acquired infection through injecting drug use, mainly by sharing contaminated needles (Table 23.3, Figure 23.4). The majority of infections occur in men aged 25–45 years. Factors associated with more rapid progression of disease are male gender, infection when older and alcohol consumption.

> ■ KEY POINT
>
> In the UK, most infected individuals have acquired HCV infection through injecting drug use.

Hepatitis D

The hepatitis D virus is an incomplete 35- to 37-nm RNA virus that causes infection only in individuals who have active HBV infection. The prevention of HBV infection by immunisation

Table 23.3 Transmission of hepatitis C in England

Risk factor (where reported)	Laboratory reports of hepatitis C infection (n)	%
Injecting drugs use	10 057	91.1
Blood transfusion	279	2.5
Blood product recipient	249	2.3
Sexual exposure	195	1.8
Renal failure	108	0.9
Other known (e.g. organ/tissue transplant, surgical/medical, skin piercing, occupational)	90	0.8
Vertical (mother to baby) or family/household	67	0.6
	11 045	100

Data from Health Protection Agency (2004).

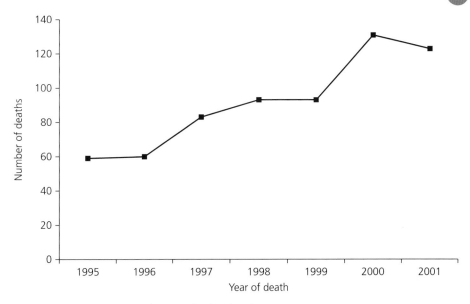

Figure 23.4 ● Hepatitis C mortality in England and Wales.

also prevents HDV infection. Co-infection with HDV is associated with fulminant hepatitis and a mortality of 2–20 per cent. Less than 5 per cent of cases progress to chronic hepatitis D, whereas super-infection with HDV leads to chronic HDV hepatitis, often with cirrhosis in more than 70 per cent of cases. Detection of anti-HDV immunoglobulin M (IgM) is the reliable marker for HDV infection, which can persist in the serum with ongoing infection.

Epidemiology
Hepatitis D virus is found worldwide. It is particularly prevalent in the Amazon Basin, Central Africa, southern Italy and the Middle East. It is less common in the USA and Eastern Europe.

Hepatitis E

Hepatitis E virus has an epidemic potential and is an acute, self-limited disease with a clinical picture similar to the other types of viral hepatitis. It is present in developing countries and is known to spread by the faecal–oral route. It has been implicated in large outbreaks in association with contaminated water.

Hepatitis G

This virus has been described relatively recently. The infection caused by this virus is not fully known; neither is the natural history fully understood.

Human immunodeficiency virus

Human immunodeficiency virus is an RNA virus belonging to the retrovirus family. There are two types: HIV1 and HIV2. HIV1 is the type found most commonly in the UK and Europe. HIV2 is confined mainly to western Africa and is usually less severe than HIV1.

HIV infection can be acquired in the following ways:

● Unprotected sexual intercourse (anal, vaginal or oral)
● Injection or transfusion with infected blood
● Drug users sharing needles and syringes contaminated with HIV-infected blood
● From infected mother and baby during birth or through breastfeeding.

HIV causes progressive destruction of specific immune cells (CD4 cells), leading to the acquired immunodeficiency syndrome (AIDS), which was first reported in 1981.

HIV infection can be divided into three stages: (i) an early, acute stage, (ii) a middle, latent stage and (iii) a late immunodeficiency stage (Table 23.4).

In the acute stage, which begins 2–4 weeks after infection, a mononucleosis-like picture of fever, lethargy, sore throat and generalised lymphadenopathy occurs.

The middle stage is a latent period, which, in untreated patients, usually lasts for 7–11 years. The patient is asymptomatic during this period, while a large amount of the virus is produced by the lymph nodes and remains sequestered there. A syndrome of AIDS-related complex (ARC) can occur, manifested by fevers, fatigue, weight loss and lymphadenopathy.

The late stage of HIV infection is AIDS, manifested by a decline in the number of CD4 cells to below 400/μL and an increase in the frequency and severity of opportunistic infections. The two most characteristic manifestations are *Pneumocystis* pneumonia (Figures 23.5 and 23.6) and Kaposi's sarcoma. Other infections include viral infections such as disseminated herpes simplex, herpes zoster and cytomegalovirus (CMV) infections and progressive multifocal leukoencephalopathy; fungal infections such as thrush (Figure 23.7) and cryptococcal meningitis; protozoal infections such as toxoplasmosis and cryptosporidiosis (Figure 23.8); and disseminated bacterial infections such as with *Mycobacterium avium-intracellulare* and *Mycobacterium tuberculosis* (Health Protection Agency, 2006).

Epidemiology

Sex between men

The majority of infections have occurred through sex between men. In the UK, over 2300 new diagnoses of HIV occur each year. The median age of diagnosis and median CD4 cell count at diagnosis have increased gradually.

> ■ KEY POINT
> The majority of HIV infections have occurred through sex between men, with little change in the incidence.

Sex between men and women

Since 1999 there have been more diagnoses of heterosexually acquired infection than of infections acquired through sex between men. The majority of infections are acquired in Africa, predominantly in eastern Africa, although recently south-eastern Africa has been more

Table 23.4 Clinical stages of human immunodeficiency virus (HIV) infection

CD4+ cells (/mL blood)	Clinical phases		
	A	B	C
	Asymptomatic Acute (primary) HIV or PGL	Symptomatic	AIDS
≥ 500	A1	B1	C1
200–499	A2	B2	C2
< 200	A3	B3	C3

AIDS, acquired immunodeficiency syndrome; PGL, persistent generalised lymphadenopathy.

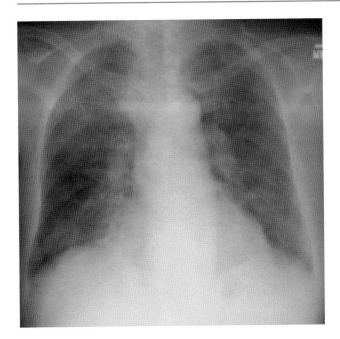

Figure 23.5 ● Chest X-ray of a *Pneumocystis jiroveci* pneumonia in a patient with acquired immunodeficiency syndrome (AIDS).

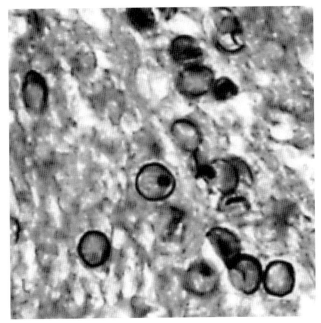

Figure 23.6 ● Lung histological section, showing *Pneumocystis* organisms.

affected. The male : female ratio for all new infections diagnosed in 1985–86 was 14 : 1, whereas in 2004–05 it was about 1.4 : 1. Around 47 per cent of those who are infected via heterosexual sex are being diagnosed with a CD4 count of less than 200 cells/mm^3.

Injecting drug use

In the UK, 5.6 per cent of all new HIV infections by the end of 2005 were due to injecting drug use. Shared needle and syringe use remains an extremely effective means of transmission of

Figure 23.7 ● Oral candidiasis in a patient with acquired immunodeficiency syndrome (AIDS).

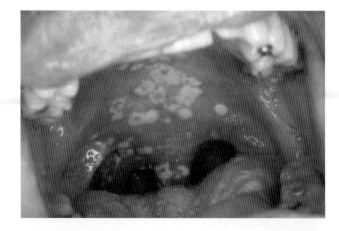

Figure 23.8 ● Cryptosporidium oocysts in a stool sample of an infected patient.

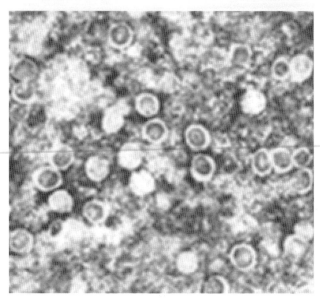

blood-borne viruses. The majority of injecting drug users are male, and HIV-infected injecting drug users are predominantly male.

Mother to child

In England and Scotland during 2005, 1 in every 450 women giving birth was infected with HIV. By the end of 2005, 1781 HIV diagnoses had been reported in children aged under the age of 15 years. Of these, 78 per cent were reported to have acquired their infection from their mother. Forty per cent of the children who acquired their infection from their mother were born abroad.

Intervention to prevent transmission necessitates diagnosis before delivery. Intervention includes antiretroviral therapy, caesarean section and avoidance of breastfeeding, leading to a reduction of transmission to under 3 per cent. In 2005, about 95 per cent of all HIV-infected women giving birth were diagnosed before delivery.

Blood products and blood transfusion

Since the implementation of the viral inactivation process and donor screening in 1985, there have been no documented transmissions via this route. In the UK, a total of 1360 people are reported to have been infected with HIV through this route, of which all but 13 are male. Most diagnoses made more recently have resulted from blood transfusions in areas of the world where it is still difficult to screen for HIV.

HEPATITIS VIRUS AND HIV INFECTION IN SURGICAL PATIENTS AND HEALTHCARE WORKERS

Some patients undergoing surgery may be unknowingly infected with HIV. As a rule, it is always advisable to defer surgery in floridly infected patients with the hepatitis viruses and HIV. Performing surgery on such patients poses a higher infection control risk because of the higher viral load. Universal infection control precautions are always best practice.

Risk of transmission of viral hepatitis and HIV infection to surgical patients

Factors underlying the risk of transmission include the following:

- Type of surgery, e.g. in obstetrics and gynaecology, orthopaedics and cardiothoracic surgery
- Technique of surgery
- Decontamination of medical equipment
- Sterility of tissue and blood products
- Infection status and viral bioload of the surgical team
- Standard of infection control procedures and practice.

The incidence of blood-borne virus infections was found to be similar in trauma and non-trauma surgical patients. Various studies have demonstrated the transmission of the following:

- HBV from healthcare workers to patients
- HCV from healthcare workers to patients
- HIV from healthcare workers to patients.

Risk of transmission to healthcare workers

- Risk of transmission when patient is HBsAg-positive and HBeAg-positive is 1 : 3.
- Risk of transmission of HCV is around 1 : 30.
- Risk of transmission of HIV is 1 : 300.
- Risk of transmission of HIV following mucocutaneous exposure is less than 1 : 2000 (Al-Wali, 2001).
- Most cases of occupationally acquired blood-borne viruses have occurred following percutaneous exposure, of which the majority involved hollow needles.

PROTECTING SURGICAL PATIENTS FROM HEPATITIS VIRUSES AND HIV

General principles

- Biological products such as blood products transfused or transplanted to patients should be screened and hence free from blood-borne viruses.
- Any medical equipment or the environment close to the patient should be sterile/decontaminated from blood-borne viruses.
- Healthcare workers who operate on or are in contact with patients should not be infected with or carriers of blood-borne viruses.

Hepatitis B-infected healthcare workers

- Infected healthcare workers who are also e-antigen-positive must not perform exposure-prone procedures (EPPs) because of their higher degree of infectivity.
- Infected healthcare workers who are e-antigen-negative and who perform EPPs or clinical duties in renal units should be tested for viral load (hepatitis B virus DNA).
- Healthcare workers who have a viral load that exceeds 10^3 genome equivalents per millilitre should be prevented from performing EPPs. Healthcare workers whose viral load does not exceed 10^3 genome equivalents per millilitre need not have their working practices restricted, subject to annual retesting.
- Blood exposure incidents for both healthcare workers and patients should be managed appropriately, including considering the use of HBV passive immunoprophylaxis where indicated (Health Protection Agency, 2004).

Hepatitis C-infected healthcare workers

- Healthcare workers who know that they are carrying HCV or who are found to do so following testing should not perform EPPs.
- Healthcare workers who carry out EPPs and who are known to be infected with HCV or who have antibodies to HCV should be tested for HCV RNA.
- Healthcare workers who are RNA-positive – i.e. carrying the virus – should not be allowed to perform EPPs.
- The same principle should apply to healthcare workers who are intending to undertake professional training for a career that relies upon the performance of EPPs.
- Healthcare workers who perform EPPs and who believe that they may have been exposed to HCV infection should be offered confidential professional advice.
- Healthcare workers who have been treated successfully with antiviral therapy should be allowed to resume EPPs.
- Healthcare workers who remain HCV-RNA-negative for 6 months after cessation of treatment should be allowed to return to performing EPPs at that time. A further check should be done 6 months later.
- Healthcare workers should be provided with information and training about measures to reduce the risk of occupational exposure to HCV.

HIV-infected healthcare workers

HIV-infected surgeons and other healthcare workers should never perform EPPs on patients.

● PROTECTING HEALTHCARE WORKERS FROM VIRAL HEPATITIS AND HIV INFECTION

General principles

- The highest risk of cross-infection to healthcare workers are those associated with a carrier state and persistent viraemia.
- The risk of transmission of blood-borne viruses is greater from patient to healthcare worker than from healthcare worker to patient.

■ KEY POINT

The risk of transmission of blood-borne viruses is greater from patient to healthcare worker than from healthcare worker to patient.

Safe handling and disposal of sharps

- Many percutaneous injuries are preventable.
- Place all disposable sharps in the correct containers immediately after use.
- Provide sharps containers in adequate numbers, and never overfill.
- Avoid resheathing needles manually. Resheathing is permitted only if a device is available to allow this to be done using only one hand.
- Discard disposable syringes and needles whenever possible as a single unit into a sharps container.
- Remove needles from syringes only when essential, e.g. when transferring blood to a container.
- Remove needles and attach blind hubs to syringes containing arterial blood that are to be sent to the laboratory.

Measures to reduce risks during surgical procedures

General principles

- Most percutaneous injuries that occur in the operating theatre or during obstetric/midwifery procedures are caused by sharp suture needles.
- The risk of percutaneous injury to the operator has been found to be associated with the type and duration of the procedure and the use of fingers rather than instruments to hold tissue while suturing.
- The rate of injury varies from 4 per cent for orthopaedic procedures to 10 per cent for gynaecological procedures.
- More than 50 per cent of percutaneous injuries sustained by surgeons have been to the non-dominant index finger, and 20 per cent of injuries are caused by the operator to the assistant.
- Perforations of surgical gloves are common. Double-gloving does not prevent sharps injury but has led to a six-fold decrease in inner-glove puncture.
- The use of blunt-tipped needles can further reduce the incidence of glove puncture and of percutaneous injury.
- Blood–skin contacts pose a risk of blood-borne virus transmission to the healthcare worker if the skin surface is not intact. Non-intact skin on hands is common in surgical healthcare workers because of dermatitis from frequent scrubbing, as are cuts and abrasions incurred during other activities.

Reducing the risk of percutaneous exposure

- Have no more than one person working in an operational/body cavity at any time.
- Use a 'hands-free' technique where the same sharp instrument is not touched by more than one person at the same time.
- Avoid hand-to-hand passing of sharp instruments during an operation.
- Assure safer passage of necessary sharp needles and instruments via a 'neutral zone', and announce when a sharp instrument or needle is placed there. The neutral zone may be a tray, kidney basin or identified area in the operative field.
- Ensure that scalpels and sharp needles are not left exposed in the operative field but are always removed promptly by the scrub nurse.
- Use instruments rather than fingers for retraction and for holding tissues while suturing.
- Use instruments to hand needles and to remove scalpel blocks.
- Direct sharp needles and instruments away from one's own non-dominant hand and the assistant's hands.
- Remove sharp suture needles before tying sutures; tie the suture with instruments rather than fingers.
- Alternative equipment and procedures should be considered where practicable:

- Eliminate any unnecessary use of sharp instruments, needles, etc. by appropriate substitution of electrocautery, blunt-tipped needles and stapling devices.
- Resort to alternative, less invasive surgical procedures where practicable.
- Avoid scalpel injuries associated with assembly/disassembly by using scalpels that are disposable, have retractable blades or incorporate a blade-release device.
- Avoid using sharp clips for surgical drapes; blunt clips are available, as are disposable drapes incorporating self-adhesive operating film.
- Consider double-gloving with a larger pair of gloves innermost for optimum comfort.

Post-exposure prophylaxis

Following significant exposure of the healthcare worker to blood-borne viruses, prophylaxis is recommended in order to reduce the risk of transmission. A baseline blood sample should be obtained and stored for possible future testing.

Hepatitis B

- All healthcare workers should be actively immunised.
- Healthcare workers who have no protective antibodies against HBV and are exposed to significant contamination should be offered immunoglobulin within 7 days of exposure.
- Healthcare workers who are already immunised with the vaccine should be given a booster of the vaccine.
- If the source is unknown, then rapid vaccine acceleration should be offered – i.e. initial dose and at 1 month and 2 months later.

HIV

- Healthcare workers who are significantly exposed to cases of HIV infection should be offered post-exposure prophylaxis.
- The chemotherapy prophylaxis consists of any triple combination of antiretrovirals, ideally within 1 h of exposure.
- HIV testing should be performed at baseline and at 4 weeks, 12 weeks and 24 weeks following exposure.

Hepatitis C

- There are no prophylactic agents available, whether immunoglobulin or antivirals, against significant exposure.
- Exposed healthcare workers should be tested for HCV-RNA alone at 6 weeks, and then both HCV-RNA and anti-HIV antibody testing should be performed at 12 weeks.

● SUMMARY

- The most important blood-borne viruses implicated in cross-infections in surgical practice are HBV, HCV and HIV.
- The modes of transmission of these agents in surgical practice are similar, being mainly through sharps injury and blood contamination.
- HBV is of low prevalence in Western Europe and North America, where transmission is due mostly to intercourse and sharing of contaminated needles and equipment between intravenous drug users.
- In high-prevalence areas, HBV infection is acquired predominantly in childhood by perinatal transmission or by horizontal transmission between young children.
- In the UK, most HCV infections occur via injecting drugs by sharing contaminated needles.

- The majority of HIV infections have occurred through sex between men, with little change in incidence.
- The risk of transmission of blood-borne viruses is higher from patient to healthcare worker than from healthcare worker to patient.
- The risk of transmission is particularly associated with certain types of surgical specialties, including obstetrics and gynaecology, orthopaedics, cardiothoracic surgery and other EPPs.
- The risk of transmission of HBV is the highest, followed by HCV and then HIV.
- The risk of transmission to healthcare workers is the highest in percutaneous injury involving a hollow needle.
- Any blood or tissue product administered or transplanted to patients should be screened for blood-borne viruses.
- All medical equipment in contact with patients should be appropriately decontaminated.
- Healthcare workers who are infected must follow the healthcare recommendations.
- The prevention of transmission of blood-borne viruses to healthcare workers should be based on appropriate risk assessment and categorisation of risks.
- The best infection control practice is to follow universal precautions in addition to specific infection control measures to reduce the risk in surgery.
- Post-exposure prophylaxis to date applies only to HBV and HIV exposure to reduce the risk of transmission.

● QUESTIONS

1   What are the modes of transmission of blood-borne viruses?
2   What are the clinical outcomes and epidemiology of hepatitis viruses?
3   Describe the clinical phases of HIV infection.
4   Following a sharps injury, what is the infectivity risk of HBV, HCV and HIV?
5   List the main infection measures that have to be followed during surgery in order to prevent transmission of blood-borne viruses from healthcare worker to patient and vice versa.
6   Following a needlestick or sharps injury involving blood contamination, what measures should be taken in order to prevent transmission of blood-borne viruses from the patient to the healthcare worker?
7   Is a surgeon who is HBsAg-positive permitted to perform exposure-prone procedures?

● REFERENCES

Al-Wali W (2001). Biological safety. In: Burton J, Rutty G (eds). *The Hospital Autopsy*, 2nd edn. London: Arnold.

Health Protection Agency (2004). *Hepatitis B Infected Healthcare Workers and Oral Antiviral Therapy*. London: Health Protection Agency.

Health Protection Agency (2006). *HIV and Other Sexually Transmitted Infections in the United Kingdom: Annual Report*. London: Health Protection Agency.

● FURTHER READING

Department of Health (2002). *Hepatitis C Infected Healthcare Workers*. Health Service Circular HSC 2002/010. London: Department of Health.

Department of Health (2003). *Health Clearance for Serious Communicable Diseases: New Health Care Workers*. London: Department of Health.

Health Protection Agency (2004). *Surveillance of Significant Occupational Exposure to Blood-borne Viruses in Healthcare Workers, England, Wales and Northern Ireland: Six Year Report*. London: Health Protection Agency.

Health Protection Agency Centre for Infections and Collaborators (2005). *Occupational Transmission of HIV*. London: Health Protection Agency.

Levinson L (2006). *Review of Medical Microbiology and Immunology*. New York: McGraw-Hill.

Lin PH, Bush RL, Yao Q, *et al*. (2004). Abdominal aortic surgery in patients with human immunodeficiency virus infection. *Am J Surg* **188**: 690–97.

Mandell G, Douglas R, Bennett J (2005). *Principles and Practice of Infectious Diseases*. Edinburgh: Churchill Livingstone.

Puro V, De Carli G, Scognamiglio P, *et al*. (2001). Risk of HIV and other blood-borne infections in the cardiac setting: patient-to-provider and provider-to-patient transmission. *Ann N Y Acad Sci* **946**: 291–309.

Puro V, Scognamiglio P, Ippolito G, *et al*. (2003). HIV, HBV or HDV transmission from infected health care workers to patients. *Med Lav* **94**: 556–68.

Souba WW, Mitchell P, Fink MD, *et al*. (2006). Viral infections in surgery. In: *ACS Surgery: Principles and Practice*. New York: WebMD Professional.

Weiss ES, Cornwell EE, 3rd, Wang T, *et al*. (2007). Human immunodeficiency virus and hepatitis testing and prevalence among surgical patients in an urban university hospital. *Am J Surg*. **183**: 55–60.

24 Medical therapy for surgical patients

Samir Abdulla and Suhail Doi

INTRODUCTION

This chapter gives an overview of medications commonly prescribed by surgeons in the peri-operative period and offers advice on how to manage patients with certain medical conditions that are of special importance in surgical practice. Careful medical management of surgical patients reduces the incidence of operative and postoperative complications and reduces the length of hospital stay, length of postoperative recovery, absence from work and total cost of treatment.

DIABETES MELLITUS

Patients are often well informed about their diabetes and its management.

Diabetes mellitus is classified as an intermediate risk factor for increased perioperative cardiovascular risks, so it is wise to screen for the presence of asymptomatic cardiac and renal disease and to be aware of possible silent myocardial infarction.

> ■ KEY POINT
> Diabetes is an intermediate risk factor for increased perioperative cardiovascular risks.

Always try to put the diabetic patient first on the operation list and ensure that the surgeon and anaesthetist are informed early that there is a diabetic patient listed.

> ■ KEY POINT
> Put the patient first on the operation list.

Management of the diabetic patient undergoing surgery depends on the prior treatment of the diabetes, how well it is controlled, and how major the operation is.

Diabetes is classified into type 1 (insulin-dependent diabetes mellitus, IDDM) and type 2 (non-insulin-dependent diabetes mellitus, NIDDM).

Insulin-dependent diabetes mellitus

Patients with type 1 diabetes usually require insulin during surgery. There are a number of described regimens for managing patients with well-controlled IDDM:

1 Patients undergoing minor surgery may be given their usual insulin the night before, fasted overnight and then given one-third of their usual daily requirement of both short-acting and long-acting insulin at 7 a.m. An infusion of 10% dextrose at 100 mL/h should then be started. The patient should be placed first on the list in morning; if the operation is delayed, there is a risk of hypoglycaemia.

2 Alternatively, the morning insulin may be omitted and the blood glucose checked at the time of premedication. If the blood glucose is:
- < 5 mmol/L: start 5% dextrose 1 L every 8 h.
- 5–12 mmol/L: monitor blood glucose hourly.
- 12–20 mmol/L: start insulin infusion of normal saline and potassium 20 mmol/L initially 1–2 units/h of short-acting insulin.
- > 20 mmol/L, or ketotic: treat first and delay the operation.

3 Monitor blood glucose on return from theatre. If it is over 12 mmol/L and the patient is not on insulin infusion, give 8–12 units of short-acting insulin subcutaneously. Repeat blood glucose testing hourly; if blood glucose is not falling, start an intravenous infusion of normal saline with 20 mmol/L potassium and 1–2 units/h of short-acting insulin. The amount of insulin required in the infusion varies widely, depending on initial blood glucose. Patients on steroids will require higher doses.

4 In patients with well-controlled IDDM undergoing major surgery, set up a dextrose-saline infusion on the morning of the operation with 20 mmol/L potassium at an 8-hourly rate and start insulin infusion 1–2 units/h of short-acting insulin. Check blood glucose hourly and maintain it at 5–10 mmol/L. The insulin (50 units short-acting insulin in a total of 50 mL saline) is delivered through a syringe driver piggybacked through a non-return valve on to the dextrose infusion. This is the most flexible regime but requires the most intensive monitoring in order to avoid hypoglycaemia.

Whichever regimen is chosen, the patient should restart subcutaneous insulin when their normal eating pattern is restored.

For patients with poorly controlled IDDM, whether undergoing minor or major surgery, it is important to establish control of diabetes before operating. For non-urgent surgery, diabetic control can be established on an out-patient basis. For urgent surgery, do not operate until the patient is fully rehydrated and blood glucose is less than 13 mmol/L, unless the risk of a few hours' delay is clinically justified.

■ KEY POINT

Whether undergoing major or minor surgery, patients with poorly controlled IDDM must first have their blood glucose controlled.

Non-insulin-dependent diabetes mellitus

Patients on oral hypoglycaemics

Blood glucose levels in patients with NIDDM are usually controlled with oral hypoglycaemics. Do not give long-acting sulphonylureas (e.g. glibenclamide) on the morning of surgery, as they can cause prolonged hypoglycaemia on fasting. Biguanides (e.g. metformin) can cause lactic acidosis, especially if intravenous contrast is administered or the patient has poor renal function.

Patients with well-controlled NIDDM undergoing surgery (minor or major) can fast overnight, omit their hypoglycaemic medication on the morning of operation and have their blood glucose checked preoperatively.

Insulin may be required for patients who are not normally on insulin when they undergo an operation. In patients undergoing minor surgery, check blood glucose on return from theatre and then every 6 h. Use normal saline if fluids are required (avoid dextrose). Give insulin (subcutaneous or intravenous) if the blood glucose level is above 12 mmol/L on two occasions. Restart oral hypoglycaemics when the patient is eating normally again.

> ■ KEY POINT
> Patients with NIDDM should restart oral hypoglycaemics when eating normally after operation.

In a patient undergoing major or urgent surgery, start dextrose-saline 1 L with 20 mmol potassium every 8 h and an intravenous insulin infusion. Check blood glucose hourly.

Patients on oral therapy who are controlled inadequately (i.e. random blood glucose above 15.0 mmol/L or glycosylated haemoglobin (HbAlc) above 9%) should be stabilised on insulin preoperatively and managed in the same way as patients with IDDM.

Diet-controlled diabetes mellitus

Blood glucose usually presents no problem in this group, although some patients may be briefly insulin-dependent postoperatively. Avoid giving dextrose as a fluid replacement, as blood sugar levels will rise.

Insulin treatment

Subcutaneous insulin after surgery

Insulin may be required after surgery when the patient resumes oral intake, even if they were not previously on insulin, because of the stress of the operation. In such patients, soluble insulin is given before meals and isophane insulin (NPH) 8–12 units is given subcutaneously at night, adjusted according to the blood glucose response. Table 24.1 shows an example of a supplemental subcutaneous insulin sliding scale for a patient on 15 units soluble insulin before meals and 15 units NPH before bed.

Table 24.1 Example of a supplemental subcutaneous insulin sliding scale (based on pre-meal measurement of fingerprick glucose) for a patient on 15 units soluble insulin before meals and 15 units NPH before bed.

Fingerprick glucose (mmol/L)	Add subcutaneous soluble insulin (units)*
4–8	+0
8–11	+2
11–14	+4
14–17	+6
17–20	+8
> 20	+10 (check in 1 h and diabetic team review required)

*Regular doses are usually restarted at presurgical doses or a minimum of 6 units before meals (must be on a basal insulin regimen too, e.g. NPH or glargine at about one-third of the total soluble insulin dose). The total daily insulin dose (TDI) for the patient divided by 30 (TDI/30) is then used to calculate the increment needed in the sliding scale.

Table 24.2 Example of an intravenous sliding scale (2-hourly fingerprick glucose check)

Fingerprick glucose (mmol/L)	Intravenous soluble insulin (units/h)
4–8	0.5
8–11	1
11–14	2
14–17	3
17–20	4
> 20	5 (diabetic team review required)

Intravenous insulin

Intravenous insulin is given either on a sliding scale separate from the intravenous fluids or with intravenous dextrose (GKI infusion). This is preferred over subcutaneous insulin intra-operatively when a long and complex surgical procedure such as coronary artery bypass graft is planned or if there is anticipated to be a prolonged postoperative fasting state.

The intravenous sliding scale (Table 24.2) is made up of 49.5 mL of isotonic (normal) saline with 50 units of soluble insulin (e.g. Human Actrapid®) in a 50-mL syringe suitable for a syringe pump.

GKI treatment consists of a combined infusate of 500 mL of 10% dextrose with 16 units of human soluble insulin (e.g. Actrapid®, Novo Nordisk®) and 20 mmol potassium chloride (KCl) administered through a peripheral vein at a fixed rate of 100 mL/h via a metered infusion device. Fingerprick glucose is checked every 2 h: decrease insulin by 5 units if less than 7 mmol/L and increase by 5 units if > 17 mmol/L. Omit potassium if there is renal impairment or the K level is 5 mmol/L or higher.

Management of diabetic ketoacidosis

Hyperglycaemic ketoacidosis occurs in type 1 diabetes. It usually presents as a gradual decline into dehydration and acidosis. If diabetic ketoacidosis is not treated early, the patient goes into a coma. The precipitating factors include infection, surgery, myocardial infarction, non-compliance and wrong insulin dose; all of these possible factors need to be investigated. The patient may require monitoring in an intensive therapy unit (ITU) or high-dependency unit (HDU).

> ■ KEY POINT
> Twenty per cent of myocardial infarctions in diabetic patients may be painless.

> ■ KEY POINT
> In diabetic ketoacidosis, patients require monitoring in HDU or ITU.

Active treatment includes the following:

● Dehydration is a greater threat to life than is hyperglycaemia, so correction of dehydration takes precedence by ensuring good venous access and replacement with normal saline (give 1 L immediately, then 1 L in 1 h, 1 L in 2 h, 1 L in 4 h and then 1 L every 6 h). Use dextrose-containing fluids only when the blood glucose level is less than 15 mmol/L. Monitor and correct electrolytes, particularly potassium (see next point).

- Monitor potassium, glucose, creatinine and bicarbonate (HCO_3^-) hourly initially and then every 4 h once patient is stable.
- Give intravenous soluble insulin 4–8 units immediately and then commence on the intravenous insulin sliding scale as above.
- Monitor vital signs, fluids and urine output on a chart.
- Find and treat infection with the appropriate antibiotics.
- Continue deep vein thrombosis (DVT) prophylaxis until patient is mobile.
- Change insulin to subcutaneous when patient is eating and ketones are 1+ or less (after seeking advice from a diabetologist).

HYPERTENSION

A diastolic pressure over 110 mmHg immediately before surgery is associated with a number of complications, including the following:

- Dysrhythmias
- Myocardial ischaemia and infarction
- Neurological complications
- Renal failure.

Elective surgery in patients with hypertension does not need to be delayed as long as the diastolic blood pressure is less than 110 mmHg and intraoperative and postoperative blood pressure is monitored carefully in order to prevent hypertensive and hypotensive episodes.

An important exception is patients with phaeochromocytoma, in whom operative mortality may be as high as 80 per cent without formal preparation (see below).

Patients on chronic antihypertensive medications can continue with their medication until the time of surgery, by taking the drugs with small sips of water on the morning of surgery.

Management issues before surgery

- The ideal target blood pressure is less than 140/90 mmHg for several months before elective surgery. However, it does not appear to be necessary to postpone elective procedures in patients with blood pressure below 170/110 mmHg.
- Elective surgery should be postponed in patients with blood pressure above 170/110 mmHg.
- Patients with blood pressure above 170/110 mmHg and who require urgent surgery should be treated acutely with a parenteral drug.
- Patients who are taking chronic antihypertensive medications should continue taking their medication until the time of surgery. The drug should be taken with a sip of water on the morning of surgery and then resumed postoperatively.
- It may be reasonable to stop some forms of therapy 48 h before surgery, keeping in mind that alternative therapy needs to be instituted:
  - *Diuretic therapy:* a reasonable alternative to stopping therapy is to be alert to the possibility of volume depletion and hypokalaemia postoperatively.
  - In patients with Conn's syndrome, medical therapy with spironolactone should be given for 4–6 weeks to control blood pressure and replenish potassium stores. The last doses are given on the day of surgery and postoperatively. Blood tests are carried out to check levels of the relevant hormones and potassium levels.
  - Angiotensin-converting enzyme (ACE) inhibitors and calcium channel blockers are associated with some perioperative risk, but they should be continued with monitoring.
  - Beta-blockers and centrally acting agents such as clonidine should not be stopped acutely. If necessary, intravenous beta-blockers or transdermal clonidine can be administered.

Management issues after surgery

- Remedial causes of postoperative hypertension should be excluded or treated. Remedial causes include pain, agitation, hypercarbia, hypoxia, hypervolaemia and bladder distension.
- Therapy should be considered for patients with a persistent diastolic blood pressure above 110 mmHg.
- Patients on chronic antihypertensive therapy should resume their usual medications postoperatively, as needed. Patients who cannot take oral medications should be given a comparable alternative.

Phaeochromocytoma

- Patients require medications that block the excessive amounts of noradrenaline and adrenaline secreted by the tumour.
  - Phenoxybenzamine is started at 10 mg once daily. The dose is increased every few days until the patient's symptoms and blood pressure are controlled. The drug should be started at least 7–10 days preoperatively to normalise blood pressure. Target blood pressure is less than 120/80 mmHg (seated), with systolic blood pressure greater than 90 mmHg (standing). The final target dosage of phenoxybenzamine is typically 20–100 mg daily.
  - Orthostasis and nasal stuffiness occur in almost all patients as the dose is escalated and serve as an indication of therapeutic efficacy. Rarely, miosis, inhibition of ejaculation, diarrhoea and fatigue may occur on the second or third day of alpha-adrenergic blockade.
- There is no consensus on the use of beta-blockade. In some units it is considered unhelpful, as it may cause problems with the management of hypotension once the adrenal vein is ligated. If considered essential for the management of the patient, it is commenced once alpha-blockade has been achieved.
- Once alpha-adrenergic blockade has been achieved, beta-adrenergic blockade is initiated, which typically occurs 2–3 days preoperatively. The beta-adrenergic blocker is never started first because blockade of vasodilatory peripheral beta-adrenergic receptors with unopposed alpha-adrenergic receptor stimulation can lead to a hypertensive crisis.
- Administer the last doses of oral alpha- and beta-blockers on the morning of surgery.
- Hypovolaemia can cause severe perioperative morbidity, and preoperative volume expansion must be given in order to prevent shock after phaeochromocytoma resection:
  - Excess catecholamine causes vasoconstriction, which leads to hypertension and hypovolaemia. The sudden withdrawal of catecholamine when the phaeochromocytoma is resected leads to vasodilation, which in the presence of hypovolaemia can lead to intractable hypotension and shock.
  - The patient should undergo volume expansion with isotonic sodium chloride solution at 60–80 cm^3/h starting 48 h before surgery. Encourage liberal salt intake preoperatively.
- In general, the patient is ready for surgery in 10–14 days.

● CALCIUM HOMEOSTASIS

Calcium metabolism

Ninety-nine per cent of total body calcium resides in bone. Of the remainder, 40 per cent is bound to serum proteins, 13 per cent is complexed with anions, and 47 per cent is free ionised calcium – this is the physiologically active form, regulated by vitamin D and parathyroid hormone (PTH).

Decreased serum calcium stimulates PTH secretion within seconds. The half-life of PTH in serum is 4 min.

The renal effects of PTH include the following:

- Increases calcium reabsorption and increases phosphorus excretion from renal tubules
- Stimulates renal 1-alpha-hydroxylase to activate vitamin D.

The bone effect of PTH is stimulation of osteoclastic bone reabsorption.

Overall, PTH increases serum calcium and decreases serum phosphorus.

The active form of vitamin D (1,25(OH)vitamin D) increases calcium and phosphorus absorption from the gastrointestinal tract. The storage form of vitamin D (25(OH)vitamin D) is the form that is measured and used for clinical decision-making.

Vitamin D deficiency is common in many countries, including the UK.

Hypocalcaemia

Hypocalcaemia is a common problem after parathyroidectomy or thyroidectomy. The fall in serum calcium is due primarily to functional or relative hypoparathyroidism that lasts usually no more than a week. Phosphate rises in this period; if it should drop, then this more likely represents the 'hungry bone syndrome' developing.

Transient hypoparathyroidism leads to reduction in bone reabsorption and intestinal calcium absorption and, in patients with normal renal function, increased calcium excretion.

Hypocalcaemia is transient if the degree of bone disease is mild. Normal parathyroid tissue should recover function within 1 week, even after long-term primary (albeit mild) hyperparathyroidism.

Management issues after surgery

- Vitamin D and calcium supplementation are useful in severe cases to decrease the duration of intravenous therapy or to avoid it altogether. The vitamin D analogue alfacalcidol is given at a starting dose of 0.25 μg/day and titrated up to 4 μg/day. Elemental calcium 2–4 g/day may be introduced with the vitamin D analogue.
- Intravenous calcium is indicated only if the patient develops a rapid and progressive reduction in serum calcium or symptoms related to hypocalcaemia (frank tetany, latent tetany – Chvostek's or Trousseau's sign), or a plasma calcium concentration below 1.9 mmol/L:
  - Administer 0.5 mg/kg/h of elemental calcium as a continuous infusion. This is usually made up as 540 mg elemental calcium (six 10-mL ampoules of 10% calcium gluconate) in 500 cm^3 of 5% dextrose or 0.9% sodium chloride (approximate final concentration is thus about 1 mg/cm^3) and run at an initial rate of 30 cm^3/h continuously in an attempt to get the plasma calcium concentration above 2 mmol/L. An infusion pump is mandatory.
  - There is not much role for intermittent boluses of intravenous calcium, and the continuous infusion is preferred.
  - Serum-corrected calcium must be monitored at least twice daily, or more frequently as indicated, if the patient is on a calcium infusion.

Hungry bone syndrome

Patients who still have low levels of both serum calcium and phosphorus on day 3 postoperatively are said to have the hungry bone syndrome. This phenomenon occurs most often in patients who have developed bone disease preoperatively due to a chronic increase in bone resorption induced by high levels of PTH. The condition requires an abrupt reduction in these high levels of PTH by surgery, leading to a marked net increase in bone uptake of calcium, phosphate and magnesium. The condition is also encountered in some patients with long-standing thyrotoxicosis.

Patients at risk for hungry bone syndrome must be started on an oral vitamin D analogue (alfacalcidol) and calcium immediately postoperatively. If the calcium level drops despite oral therapy, intravenous calcium should also be initiated. Serum magnesium and phosphate concentrations must be monitored. Magnesium supplements are sometimes required.

Hypercalcaemia before surgery

Institution of therapy for hypercalcaemia depends on the degree of hypercalcaemia and the presence or absence of clinical symptoms:

- *Mild hypercalcaemia (< 3 mmol/L):* usually no symptoms, and therefore patient requires no calcium-lowering agents apart from saline therapy (see below) before surgery.
- *Moderate hypercalcaemia (3–3.5 mmol/L) with symptoms:* patient will benefit from calcium-lowering agents before surgery.
- *Severe hypercalcaemia (> 3.5 mmol/L):* patient requires hospitalisation for therapy before surgery.

Calcium-lowering agents

Intravenous normal saline is the initial therapy. Diuretic therapy with furosemide (20 mg with each litre) can be added when euvolaemia is restored. Correction of fluid deficits alone will also produce some decrease in the calcium level. Patients with moderate or severe hypercalcaemia benefit from the starting of an intravenous saline infusion when they become nil by mouth before surgery.

Calcitonin (4–8 IU/kg intramuscularly or subcutaneously every 12 h) is the adjunctive therapy and has the most rapid onset of action. Calcitonin alone rarely normalises serum calcium levels but is useful while waiting for the effects of bisphosphonates to kick in.

Intravenous bisphosphonate is the definitive therapy with pamidronate (single dose of 30–90 mg as an infusion over 4–8 h), usually started after diagnostic tests have been performed. The onset of action for pamidronate is 24–48 h after infusion, with nadir calcium at about 7 days. The treatment effect usually lasts up to 2–4 weeks. It increases the risk of postoperative hypocalcaemia.

● ANTICOAGULANT THERAPY

The main uses of anticoagulant therapy are of heparin and oral anticoagulants such as warfarin for treatment and prophylaxis of DVT and pulmonary embolism and, to a lesser extent, fibrinolytic agents for active thrombolysis.

Heparin

Low-molecular-weight heparin (LMWH)

Certoparin, dalteparin, enoxaparin and tinzaparin have a longer duration of action (two- to four-fold) than unfractionated heparin and are used once or twice daily. This prophylactic regimen does not require monitoring, e.g. dalteparin injections in the prophylaxis of DVT by subcutaneous injection 1–2 h preoperatively to be continued in the dose of 2500–5000 units every 24 h for 5 days. It accumulates in renal failure, so a small dose is given or unfractionated heparin (UFH) is used instead.

> ■ KEY POINT
> The action of LMWH is two to four times longer than that of UFH, so LMWH is given once or twice daily.

Unfractionated heparin

Unfractionated heparin inhibits thrombin, factor Xa and factor IXa and has a rapid onset. The dose is monitored and adjusted by measuring the activated partial thromboplastin time (APTT). Unfractionated heparin can be given by one of the following methods:

- Continuous intravenous infusion pump
- Intermittent intravenous or subcutaneous injections in intervals not exceeding 6 h.

Therapeutic use of heparin is given in a bolus dose of 5000 iu over 30 min (or 10 000 iu in severe pulmonary embolism). Start the infusion at a rate of 1000–2000 iu/h, check APTT at 6 h and aim for APTT ratio of 1.5–2.5.

For longer-term anticoagulation, start warfarin from the first day along with heparin.

Prophylactic use of UFH is by low dose subcutaneously in high-risk patients, e.g. 5000 units twice daily until patient is fully ambulant. For prolonged heparin therapy, the dose can be adjusted according to the estimation of APTT.

Side effects of heparin therapy

- The main side effect is haemorrhage, which usually stops after withdrawing heparin. Protamine sulphate can be given as antidote in a dose of 1 mg/100 units of UFH given in the last dose intravenously
- Skin necrosis and hypersensitivity reaction
- Osteoporosis, thrombocytopenia and, rarely, alopecia after prolonged use.

Oral anticoagulants

Oral anticoagulants (coumarins) antagonise the effects of vitamin K and take at least 48–72 h for the anticoagulant effect to develop fully.

Dicoumarol (warfarin)

Warfarin is used very commonly (1% of the UK population takes warfarin). The international normalised ratio (INR) is used to measure the prothrombin time during warfarin medication; for example, aim for INR of 2.5 for prophylactic therapy of DVT, and INR of 2.5–3 for the treatment of DVT, pulmonary embolism and transient ischaemic attacks (TIA). The INR should be determined on the second and third days of warfarin treatment and then on alternative days until the patient is stable, and then weekly or less often. There is an increased risk of haemorrhage if aspirin or clofibrate has been prescribed in addition to warfarin.

■ KEY POINT

About 1 per cent of the population takes warfarin.

The initial dose post-surgery can be decided based on the following: For patients not previously on warfarin, the drug is initiated at 10 mg on days 1 and 2 (given at 4 p.m.), and the INR at 8 a.m. on day 3 suggests the maintenance dose. If the INR on day 3 is greater than 2 or the patient is over age 50 years, then subsequent doses should be administered cautiously (2–3 mg daily). Subsequent dosing is then adjusted according to the INR. The maintenance dose is to be taken at the same time each day, preferable at 4 p.m. if the INR is monitored in the mornings. Daily INR must be monitored at initiation of warfarin in order to avoid over-anticoagulation. For patients who were previously on warfarin, resume the drug at the previous maintenance dose levels without a loading dose.

Side effects of warfarin include haemorrhage (e.g. bruising, haematuria). Oral anticoagulants are contraindicated during the first trimester of pregnancy.

Warfarin overdose is managed as follows:

- *INR 2–4.5 and minor haemorrhage that needs no other intervention:* reduce warfarin dose only. If haemorrhage is serious or life-threatening give fresh frozen plasma (FFP; 4 units or 1 L for an adult) or factor IX concentrate (50 U/kg). Investigate the local cause of haemorrhage.

- INR > 4.5 with less severe haemorrhage (e.g. haematuria): stop warfarin for 1–2 days and give a single dose of vitamin K 1–2 mg intravenously.
- INR > 4.5 with severe haemorrhage: give FFP or factor IX. Consider giving a single dose of vitamin K 2–5 mg intravenously.
- INR 5–7 without any haemorrhage: stop warfarin and review in 2 days' time.
- INR > 7 without haemorrhage: stop warfarin, give single oral dose of vitamin K 5–10 mg, and review INR daily until stable.

Guidelines on anticoagulant therapy perioperatively

- Once the INR is 2.0 or below, surgery can be performed with relative safety. Following surgery and after warfarin is restarted, it takes about 3–4 days for the INR to rise above 2.0. It is therefore estimated that, if warfarin is withheld for 4 days before surgery and treatment is started as soon as possible afterwards, patients would have a subtherapeutic INR for approximately 2 days before surgery and 2 days after surgery.
- Elective surgery should be avoided in the first month after an acute episode of venous thrombo-embolism or arterial thromboembolism.
- If avoidance of elective surgery is not possible, warfarin should be withheld for 3–4 days and intravenous heparin or LMWH should be given before and after the procedure while the INR is below 2.0:
  - Heparin is not needed before surgery if the patient with venous thromboembolism has been receiving warfarin for more than 1 month but less than 3 months. Intravenous heparin is recommended after surgery in patients who have taken warfarin for more than 1 month but less than 3 months.
  - In arterial thromboembolism, intravenous heparin is administered until 6 h before the procedure, and then restarted as soon as possible after surgery. The dose is adjusted to achieve an APTT that is 2.0 times control. Warfarin is then reinstated before discharge from hospital; the prothrombin time should be in the therapeutic range for at least 48 h before heparin is discontinued.
- The APTT should be monitored during intravenous heparin use and heparin should be continued until 6 h before surgery.
- If acute venous thromboembolism has occurred within 2 weeks or if the risk of bleeding during intravenous heparin is high, a vena caval filter should be considered.
- Heparin or LMWH should not be restarted postoperatively until at least 12 h after major surgery and delayed longer if there is any evidence of bleeding.
- Patients with an artificial prosthetic heart valve and uncontrolled atrial fibrillation may take oral anticoagulant for the rest of their lives.
- Give the lowest dose if the patient is over age 60 years, if the patient has liver disease or cardiac failure, and in rare cases of warfarin sensitivity.
- Vitamin K (oral or parenteral) is the antidote. In emergency cases, FFP or factor IX is used.

Fibrinolytic agents

Streptokinase is used in the treatment of severe acute pulmonary embolism, myocardial infarction and cerebrovascular accident (CVA). It is given either intravenously or via a catheter direct to the site of thrombosis.

STEROID THERAPY

All surgeons require a good knowledge of the use of steroids and their complications, particularly when used in high doses for long periods. Patients on steroids require higher doses after major surgery, severe infection and trauma.

Table 24.3 Steroids of the adrenal cortex

Group	Effect	Example
Glucocorticoids (cortisone)	Metabolism of proteins and carbohydrates	Hydrocortisone, cortisone
Mineralocorticoids (salt-regulating hormones)	Water and electrolyte balance	Aldosterone
Sex hormones (androgenic, oestrogenic)	Secondary sexual characters	Testosterone, oestrogen

The adrenal cortex secretes three groups of hormones (Table 24.3).
Therapeutic uses of steroids include the following:

- Acute adrenal insufficiency, following bilateral adrenalectomy and Addison's disease (hydrocortisone + fludrocortisone)
- Inflammatory bowel disease, e.g. ulcerative colitis (oral, parenteral, retention enema)
- Organ or bone marrow transplantation (postoperatively) as an immunosuppressant to treat rejection
- Topical skin disorders, e.g. pemphigus, eczema
- Connective tissue disorders, e.g. systemic lupus erythematosus (SLE), polyarteritis nodosa
- Cerebral oedema due to intracranial tumours, leading to increased intracranial pressure (ICP) (dexamethasone)
- Septic shock (although use of steroids in this situation is controversial)
- Treatment of rheumatoid arthritis, lymphoma, acute leukaemia, nephrotic syndrome and idiopathic thrombocytic purpura (ITP).

Problems of steroid therapy

To minimise the side effects of steroids, use the lowest possible dose for the shortest period of time. Rapid withdrawal can lead to acute adrenal insufficiency (addisonian crisis) due to suppression of the pituitary–adrenal axis. The dose should be reduced gradually over weeks or months.

> ■ KEY POINT
> Use the lowest possible dose of steroids for the shortest possible period.

> ■ KEY POINT
> Rapid withdrawal of steroids can lead to addisonian crisis.

Side effects include the following:

- Cushing's syndrome, if used for long periods
- Decreased resistance to acute and chronic infections (e.g. opportunistic infections) and increased severity of infections (e.g. chickenpox)
- Gastrointestinal problems such as peptic ulceration, bleeding, perforation pancreatitis and candidiasis
- Diabetogenic effects, with hyperglycaemia and glycosuria
- Tissue atrophy due to increased protein breakdown, resulting in delayed wound bruising, muscle wasting and osteoporosis
- Central nervous system (CNS) changes, such as psychosis, euphoria, depression and aggravation of epilepsy

- Cardiovascular problems, such as hypertension and cardiac failure, due to sodium retention and increased potassium excretion causing hypokalaemic alkalosis
- Fetal growth retardation (when taken in pregnancy) and suppression of growth in children
- Myopathy, osteoporosis and fractures.

Addisonian crisis

An addisonian crisis is precipitated by sudden or rapid withdrawal of long-term steroid therapy, or can be caused by severe infection, trauma or surgery in patients on steroid therapy without increasing steroid dose. The patient may present in shock and may be comatose. An alternative presentation is with hypoglycaemia. If addisonian crisis suspected, the management should be urgent:

- Take blood for cortisol, adrenocorticotrophic hormone (ACTH) and glucose.
- Give intravenous hydrocortisone 100 mg immediately.
- Give intravenous fluid to treat shock: give a plasma expander first and then normal saline.
- Monitor blood sugar in order to avoid the danger of hypoglycaemia.
- Investigate the possible causes, such as infection, and treat accordingly.

Steroid card

All patients taking steroids should carry a card containing details of the steroids he or she is taking, the dosage, the reason for taking the drugs, and any instructions to be followed in the case of stress, such as infection, trauma or surgery.

> ■ KEY POINT
> All patients on long-term steroid therapy should carry a steroid card.

Preparation of a patient on long-term steroids for surgery

Patients who should be assumed to have functional suppression of the hypothalamic–pituitary–adrenal (HPA) function include the following:

- Any patient who has received more than 20 mg/day prednisone or its equivalent (e.g. 16 mg/day methylprednisolone, 2 mg/day dexamethasone, 80 mg/day hydrocortisone) for more than 3 weeks
- Any patient who has clinical Cushing's syndrome
- Any patient who has discontinued glucocorticoids in the year before surgery should have a 1-μg ACTH stimulation test. If the peak cortisol after this is less than 500 nmol/L, then abnormal HPA axis suppression should be suspected and steroid coverage given.

The traditional dosage used for steroid coverage of 100 mg hydrocortisone every 8 h, sometimes with a prolonged taper, is far higher than the physiologic cortisol increase, which peaks at 150 mg/day after major surgery and returns quickly to baseline. There is no evidence to suggest that steroid supplementation needs to be tapered over a prolonged period. A taper over 1–3 days is adequate in uncomplicated situations, and this helps to minimise any adverse effects of high-dose steroids. Caution is advised in patients with hypertension, diabetes mellitus or congestive heart failure, in pregnancy and in children. Stress dosages are given in Table 24.4.

The same preparation is followed after bilateral adrenalectomy, and then oral hydrocortisone is given in two doses, the larger in the morning and the smaller in the evening, mimicking the normal diurnal rhythm of cortisol secretion.

Table 24.4 Perioperative steroid therapy of patients on long-term steroids

Surgery type	Stress dose (mg)	Duration (days)	Order
Minor (outpatient)	25	1	Hydrocortisone 25 mg i.v. before procedure, then resume normal doses
Moderate (e.g. total joint replacement)	50–75	1–2	Hydrocortisone 50 mg i.v. before procedure, then 25 mg every 8 h for 24 h, then resume normal doses
Major (e.g. CABG, adrenal or pituitary surgery)	100–150	2–3	Hydrocortisone 100 mg i.v. before procedure, then 50 mg every 8 h for 24 h, then taper doses to half per day to maintenance level

CABG, coronary artery bypass graft; i.v., intravenous.

Contraindications of steroid therapy

● Systemic infections, such as active pulmonary tuberculosis (TB)
● Active peptic ulcer.

● THYROID CONDITIONS

Thyroid function tests (Table 24.5) should be done whenever there is a suspicion of dysthyroidism on history or examination.

Hypothyroidism

There are no randomised, prospective studies looking at surgical outcomes in hypothyroid versus euthyroid patients. However, evidence suggests that there are no differences between the groups in duration of surgery or anaesthesia and time to hospital discharge. There might, however, be a trend towards more intraoperative hypotension in non-cardiac surgery, more heart failure in cardiac surgery, and more postoperative gastrointestinal and neuropsychiatric complications, and hypothyroid patients are less likely to mount a fever with infection. In view of the fact that surgery can precipitate the development of myxoedema coma in patients with severe hypothyroidism, this also has to be addressed before surgery.

Perioperative management of previously unknown hypothyroidism

Patients with mild to moderate hypothyroidism can undergo urgent or emergency surgery without delay, with the knowledge that minor perioperative complications might develop. On

Table 24.5 Thyroid tests in normal and dysthyroid states

Thyroid function	TSH	Free T4	Free T3
Euthyroid	N (0.3–5 µg/L)	N (11–24 pmol/L)	N (3.5–7.5 pmol/L)
Thyrotoxic	Undetectable	High	High
T3 toxicity	Low	Normal	High
Hypothyroid	High	Low	Low or low normal

N, normal; T3, triiodothyronine; T4, thyroxine; TSH, thyroid-stimulating hormone.

the other hand, surgery should be postponed until the euthyroid state is restored when hypothyroidism is discovered in a patient for elective surgery. If surgery cannot be postponed, begin L-thyroxine treatment in young patients at close to full replacement doses (1.5 µg/kg); elderly patients and patients with cardiopulmonary disease should be started on 25–50 µg with an increase in dose every 2–6 weeks. In patients with angina treated medically, L-thyroxine should be initiated at a lower dose of 25 µg/day, and then increased 25 µg every 2–6 weeks, depending upon response.

Perioperative management of previously known hypothyroidism

Patients receiving chronic thyroxine therapy who undergo surgery and are unable to eat for several days do not need to be given thyroxine if oral intake cannot be resumed for a week. If, after a week, oral intake cannot be started, then thyroxine may be resumed intravenously or intramuscularly at about 80 per cent of the patient's usual oral dose.

Thyrotoxicosis

Thyrotoxicosis often has an autoimmune origin (Graves' disease) and is only very rarely due to overstimulation by thyroid-stimulating hormone (TSH) from the pituitary gland. Other common causes are toxic nodular goitre and toxic adenoma. The advantages of anti-thyroid drugs are that no surgery is required and there is no need for radioactive materials. The disadvantages are that the treatment is prolonged and the failure rate is high (50% or higher) and sometimes goitres become enlarged and very vascular during treatment.

The main anti-thyroid drugs used in the UK are carbimazole and propylthiouracil. These both act primarily by interfering with the synthesis of thyroid hormones. Carbimazole, which is the most commonly used, has an immunosuppressive action on TSH receptor antibody (TSH-RAb) production, which makes it effective in the treatment of Graves' disease.

Uses of anti-thyroid drugs

Medical treatment of thyrotoxicosis

The commonly used anti-thyroids are carbimazole and propylthiouracil. Beta-blockers (atenolol, nadolol) and iodides are also used. Disadvantages of using anti-thyroids as treatment of thyrotoxicosis include the following:

- *Prolonged treatment:* it usually takes 4–8 weeks on carbimazole before the patient becomes euthyroid. Then the patient is kept on a maintenance dose for 18–24 months.
- *High incidence of recurrence of the disease following discontinuation of the drug:* recurrence is about 50 per cent, especially in toxic multinodular goitre.
- *Hypothyroidism:* although sometimes a deliberate 'block and replace' regimen is used.
- *Fetal goitre if used during pregnancy:* however, anti-thyroid drugs can be used from the second trimester and the risk with careful administration is very low.

Side effects of anti-thyroid agents include nausea, rash and, rarely, alopecia and agranulocytosis (suggested by a sore throat).

Preparation of thyrotoxic patients for surgery

Carbimazole, with or without propranolol, is the most commonly used anti-thyroid drug in the UK. It is given at a daily dose of 20–60 mg. It takes 6 weeks to render the thyrotoxic patient euthyroid after initiation of this therapy. Propylthiouracil can be used instead of carbimazole at a dose of 300–600 mg daily in divided doses.

Oral iodides: Lugol's iodine

Three drops in a glass of water three times a day (1 mL/day) may reduce the vascularity of the thyroid gland, but this should only be used as an immediate preoperative preparation in the 10 days before surgery.

Beta-blockers

Propranolol and the long-acting nadolol are used for rapid relief of the symptoms of thyrotoxicosis. These are not anti-thyroid drugs, but they antagonise the adrenergic effects of catecholamines. Propranolol prevents the peripheral conversion of thyroxin (T4) to triiodothyronine (T3) and should be continued for 7 days postoperatively because the hormone levels remain high following thyroidectomy.

Thyrotoxic crisis

Imperfectly controlled thyrotoxic patients may develop an acute form of thyrotoxicosis immediately after or during surgery. This form of acute thyrotoxicosis is associated with hyperpyrexia, tachycardia, respiratory distress and agitation. Treatment is with the following:

- A beta-blocker to control the symptoms induced by increased adrenergic tone
- A thionamide, such as methimazole or carbimazole, to block new hormone synthesis
- An oral iodine solution to block the release of thyroid hormone, e.g. Lugol's solution 10 drops three times daily
- Glucocorticoids may be used in severe cases only, the rationale being to reduce T4 to T3 conversion and possibly treat the autoimmune process in Graves' disease
- Treat hyperthermia if present:
  - Paracetamol is the drug of choice, as aspirin may displace thyroid hormone from binding sites and increase severity of thyroid storm
  - Cooling blankets, ice packs and alcohol sponges encourage dissipation of heat.

It is preferable to monitor the patient in ITU.

Radioactive iodine

Radioactive iodine (^{131}I) is used increasingly for the alternative treatment of thyrotoxicosis, particularly in the following situations:

- When medical therapy or compliance is a problem
- In patients with cardiac disease
- In patients who relapse after thyroidectomy.

Radioactive iodine is contraindicated in pregnancy and in early childhood. The main problem with radioactive iodide is the progressive incidence of thyroid insufficiency, which may reach 75–80 per cent after 10 years, and so indefinite follow-up is essential. The other disadvantage is that a treated parent must be separated from their young children for several days.

● SUMMARY

- Diabetes is one of the more common health problems found in surgical patients. In all but the most urgent cases, diabetic patients must have their diabetes controlled on an outpatient basis before undergoing surgery. In complicated cases, advice from a diabetologist is recommended.
- Hypertension is another common problem that is best treated before surgery.
- Calcium homeostasis can be a significant cause of morbidity, and thus an understanding of basic problems related to perioperative care is required.

- Thromboembolic complications, deep venous thrombosis (DVT) and pulmonary embolism can be minimised with a strict protocol of prophylaxis by medical or mechanical means.
- Steroids are used in the treatment of a wide range of illnesses, particularly chronic inflammatory diseases and as immune suppressants. For the best results and to avoid potential complications in the perioperative period, management of surgical patients taking steroids may be discussed jointly between surgeon and anaesthetist.
- Thyrotoxic patients who choose surgery for long-term control of their condition must be made biochemically and clinically euthyroid before thyroidectomy. Hypothyroid patients should also be rendered euthyroid.
- Surgical site infection is a significant cause of morbidity. Prophylactic antibiotic use is justified in selected patients but is no excuse for shortcuts in maintaining a sterile operative field, improper sterilisation of surgical instruments and bad hygiene on the wards.

● QUESTIONS

1 How would you prepare a diabetic patient for surgery?
2 How would you manage hyperglycaemic (diabetic) ketoacidosis?
3 What are the hypertension-related risks in patients undergoing major surgery?
4 What do you know about the 'hungry bone syndrome'?
5 How would you prepare a patient on anticoagulant therapy for surgery?
6 What precautions would you take when listing a patient on long-term steroid therapy for surgery?
7 What is an addisonian crisis?
8 How would you manage a thyrotoxic crisis?

● FURTHER READING

Ayliffe GAJ, Fraise AP, Geddes AM, Mitchel K (2000). *Control of Hospital Infection*, 4th edn. London: Arnold.

Brooks CGD, Marshall NJ (2001). *Essential Endocrinology*, 4th edn. Oxford: Blackwell Science.

Damani NN (2003). *Manual of Infection Control Procedures*, 2nd edn. London: Greenwich Medical Media.

Kirk RM (2006). *General Surgical Operations*, 5th edn. Edinburgh: Churchill Livingstone.

Kirk RM, Ribbans WJ (2004). *Clinical Surgery in General: RCS Course Manual*, 4th edn. Edinburgh: Churchill Livingstone.

McLatchie GR, Leaper DJ (2007). *Oxford Handbook of Operative Surgery*, 7th edn. Oxford: Oxford University Press.

Russell RCG, Williams NS, Bulstrode CJK (2004). *Bailey and Love's Short Practice of Surgery*, 24th edn. London: Arnold.

Turner HE, Wass JA (2002). *Oxford Handbook of Endocrinology and Diabetes*. Oxford: Oxford University Press.

Williams G, Pickup JC (2004). *Handbook of Diabetes*, 3rd edn. Malden, MA: Blackwell.

25 | Principles of surgical oncology

Qassim F Baker, Steve Allen and Deirdre Pallister

● INTRODUCTION

This chapter gives a general idea about common surgical cancers in terms of aetiology, clinical presentations and current modalities of treatment. The concept of the multidisciplinary team (MDT) may be a new one for clinicians in charge of cancer treatment in developing countries, but it has been a cornerstone in the management of cancer for more than a decade in Western countries.

● DEFINITIONS

The terms 'cancer', 'malignant tumour' and 'neoplasia' are interchangeable. They describe a disease in which there is abnormal and uncontrolled cell growth.

Hyperplasia: an increase in the number of cells within an organ in response to a physiological stimulus (e.g. breast tissue during pregnancy and lactation) or injury. An example is liver hyperplasia and enlargement to compensate for tissue loss, even if massive in magnitude. Hyperplasia can be induced by hormonal stimulation, e.g. endometrial hyperplasia in response to oestrogen.
Hypertrophy: an increase in the size of cells, e.g. skeletal muscle hypertrophy in response to exercise.
Apoptosis: programmed cell death (PCD). The cells are damaged either by intrinsic changes, which inevitably lead to cell death (e.g. endometrial sloughing with menstruation), or by extrinsic factors such as viruses. Apoptosis can be advantageous, e.g. removal of tissues between the fingers and toes during embryonic development prevents syndactyly.
Necrosis: cell death due to acute cellular injury, such as from trauma or virus infection.

● AETIOLOGY OF CANCER

Increasing age is a great risk factor for breast and colorectal cancers (85 per cent of patients are aged over 60 years) and prostate cancer (about 80 per cent of cases and 90 per cent of deaths occur in men over the age of 65 years) (Wilt and Thompson, 2006).

Inheritance of certain genes (family history) that are susceptible to mutation can play a part in the aetiology. Examples include the following:

- BRCA1 and BRCA2 mutations in breast cancer
- Defective tumour suppressor genes in retinoblastoma
- Familial adenomatous polyposis (FAP) and hereditary non-polyposis in colorectal cancer
- Family history of prostate cancer.

Pre-malignant conditions

Pre-malignant conditions include the following:

- Adenoma–carcinoma sequence in colorectal cancer
- Inflammatory bowel disease (ulcerative colitis, Crohn's disease) leading to colonic cancer
- Ductal carcinoma in situ (DCIS) leading to breast cancer
- Liver cirrhosis leading to hepatocellular carcinoma (HCC).

Environmental carcinogens

Table 25.1 lists some of the main environmental carcinogens.

Infectious carcinogens

Table 25.2 lists some of the main infectious carcinogens.

Dietary factors

Table 25.3 lists some of the ways in which diet plays a role in the aetiology of cancer.

● PATHOLOGY OF CANCER

Cancer is typed according to the tissues involved as follows:

- *Epithelial (skin, mucous membrane):* carcinoma
- *Connective tissue, musculoskeletal:* sarcoma
- Nervous *tissue:* e.g. glioma
- *Germ cells:* e.g. ovarian and testicular tumours.

Benign tumours:

- have normal morphology;
- do not metastasise;
- grow slowly;
- may transform into malignant tumours.

Malignant tumours:

- have abnormal morphology;
- demonstrate autonomous proliferation;
- grow rapidly;
- invade local and distal structures, i.e. spread to regional lymph nodes and haematogenously to other organs such as liver and bone.

■ KEY POINT

Prostate cancer is the most commonly diagnosed cancer in men in the UK. Breast cancer is the most common cancer in women worldwide. Colorectal cancer is the second most common cancer in both men and women in the UK.

Table 25.1 Environmental carcinogens

Carcinogen	Neoplastic condition
Aflatoxins	HCC
Asbestos	Respiratory tract neoplasia, pleural/peritoneal mesothelioma
Benzene	Acute myeloid leukaemia
Coal tars	Scrotal (skin) cancer
Tobacco smoke	Cancer of the lung, bladder, pancreatic, oral cavity and oesophageal
Solar radiation	Skin cancers (malignant melanoma, BCC, SCC)
Alcohol	Cancer of the oral cavity, larynx and oesophagus

BCC, basal cell carcinoma; HCC, hepatocellular carcinoma; SCC, squamous cell carcinoma.

Table 25.2 Infectious carcinogens

Carcinogen	Neoplastic condition
Human papilloma virus	Cervical cancer
Helicobacter pylori	Gastric carcinoma
Epstein–Barr virus	Hodgkin's disease, Burkitt's lymphoma
Schistosomiasis	Bladder carcinoma
HIV	Kaposi sarcoma, non-Hodgkin's lymphoma
Hepatitis B and C viruses	HCC
Clonorchis sinensis	Cholangiocarcinoma

HCC, hepatocellular carcinoma; HIV, human immunodeficiency virus.

Table 25.3 Dietary factors in cancer aetiology

Dietary factor	Effect on cancer aetiology
High consumption of vegetables and fruit	Reduced risk of colon cancer
High consumption of meat	Increased risk of colon cancer
Obesity	Increased risk of endometrial, breast, kidney and oesophageal cancers

● CANCER GRADING

Cancer can be graded according to:

- *Depth of invasion*: e.g. Duke's classification for colorectal cancer
- *Tumour thickness*: e.g. Breslow classification for malignant melanoma
- *Mitotic index*: different degrees of proliferation exist, from highly differentiated to poorly differentiated, e.g. Bloom–Richardson classification for breast cancer and Gleason histological scoring for prostate cancer.

Cancer staging

By staging a cancer before therapy, we assess its burden in order to predict the prognosis at presentation and then plan treatment. Staging relies on clinical, pathological and radiological findings.

The TNM (tumour, lymph nodes, metastasis) system is one of the principal methods of staging. It is commonly used in breast cancer:

T: primary tumour:
: T_x: primary tumour cannot be assessed
: T_0: no evidence of primary tumour
: T_{is}: carcinoma in situ
: T_1: size of tumour < 2 cm
: T_2: size of tumour 2–5 cm
: T_3: size of tumour 5–10 cm
: T_4: size of tumour > 10 cm

N: regional lymph nodes:
: N_x: lymph nodes cannot be assessed
: N_0: no lymph node metastasis
: N_1, N_2, N_3: increasing involvement of lymph nodes

M: distant metastasis:
: M_x: metastasis cannot be assessed
: M_0: no distant metastasis
: M_1: distant metastasis is present.

■ KEY POINT

The TNM system is one of the principal methods used to stage cancers.

Investigations

- *Full blood count:* iron-deficiency anaemia due to blood loss (see above)
- *Renal, liver, bone profiles, deranged LFT:* hypercalcaemia due to secondary bone metastasis
- *Immunoglobulins:* monoclonal gammopathy in multiple myeloma.

Tumour markers

Tumour markers are substances in the blood or tissues related to the presence of cancer in the body. Tumour markers can be measured by immunoassay, immunohistochemistry and fluorescent in situ hybridisation (FISH), e.g. for *HER2* receptors in breast cancer. They can be used for:

- screening, e.g. prostate-specific antigen (PSA);
- follow-up after surgical or other modality treatment, e.g. carcinoembryonic antigen (CEA) to monitor the response of treatment or recurrence of colorectal cancer;
- diagnostic purposes and monitoring of therapy, e.g. alpha-fetoprotein (AFP) for hepatocellular and germ-cell testicular tumours.

Carcinoembryonic antigen

The normal CEA value is less than 2.5 ng/mL in adult non-smokers and less than 5 ng/mL in adult smokers. The presence of CEA is non-specific: it can be positive in several cancers, including gastric, lung and pancreatic cancers, and in benign conditions such as liver cirrhosis and inflammatory bowel disease.

Alpha-fetoprotein

Alpha-fetoprotein is produced by the fetal liver and yolk sac. The normal AFP value is less than 10 µg/L. The AFP level can be elevated in various malignant conditions, including gastrointestinal and lung cancers and hepatitis.

Prostate-specific antigen

This is produced specifically by the prostate gland. It is not cancer-specific, as it can be elevated in prostatitis and benign prostatic hyperplasia. The normal value varies between races but is around 0–4 ng/mL. The PSA level is predictive of recurrence and the response to treatment of prostatic cancer.

Human chorionic gonadotrophin

Human chorionic gonadotrophin (HCG) may indicate gestational trophoblastic disease and certain germ-cell tumours. The HCG level correlates with the tumour mass and thus has prognostic value.

Other tumour markers of surgical importance

- Calcitonin in medullary thyroid cancer
- Catecholamines in phaeochromocytoma (rarely malignant)
- CA15-3 in breast carcinoma
- CA125 in non-mucinous ovarian carcinoma: the level correlates with patient response and is non-specific (can be elevated in other cancers, such as endometrial and breast cancer)
- CA19-9 for pancreatic cancer.

Radiological imaging

Radiological imaging has the following applications in cancer:

- Screening
- Staging
- Determination of response to treatment
- Planning for radiotherapy
- Identification of disease recurrence
- Assessment of tumour complications

Mammography

The standard four-view technique includes bilateral craniocaudal (CC) and mediolateral oblique (MLO) views. It is sensitive in diagnosing invasive and in situ breast cancer. Lesions can appear as well- or ill-defined densities, micro-calcifications (in situ disease; Figure 25.1), distortions or asymmetric soft tissue. Mammography is less efficacious in dense breasts (often found in younger women), as it is difficult to distinguish disease from normal breast tissue.

Chest radiography

With chest radiography, look for the following:

- *Pulmonary lesions:* areas that may be overlooked include lesions overlapped by ribs or clavicles, anterior or posterior to the pulmonary hila, behind the heart and behind the diaphragm (bronchogenic or metastatic cancers) (Figures 25.2 and 25.3)
- *Lung collapse*

Figure 25.1 ● Mammogram, showing calcifications.

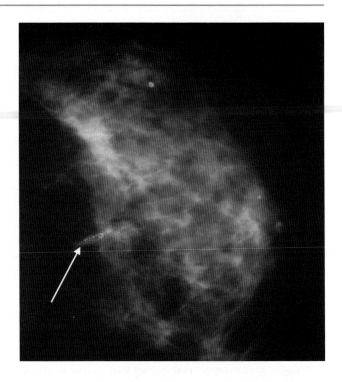

- *Pleural effusions*
- *Mediastinal lesions:* look for lymphadenopathy, especially at the hilae and paratracheal areas
- *Bone lesions:* osteolytic or osteoblastic lesions in the ribs (typical osteolytic bony lesions: lung, breast, renal cancers; typical osteoblastic bony lesions: prostate, lymphoma, some breast cancers), clavicles, pathological fractures in the thoracic spine
- *Lesions within the soft tissues.*

Fluoroscopy

Barium and other gastrointestinal contrast techniques are increasingly being superseded by advanced computed tomography (CT) and magnetic resonance imaging (MRI) techniques. Filling defects are often diagnostic of cancer.

- Barium swallow is useful for diagnosing pharyngeal and oesophageal cancer.
- Barium follow-through is useful for assessing the small bowel.
- Barium enema is performed in assessment of the large bowel.

Fluoroscopy is used to guide a range of interventional oncological procedures, including biopsies, drainages, diagnostic angiography and, increasingly, tumour embolisation techniques such as radiofrequency ablation.

Ultrasound

Ultrasound is a simple, quick and safe investigation that can be used in many body areas. It is an excellent modality at guiding many percutaneous procedures, such as biopsies and drainages. Uses of ultrasound in cancer include the following:

- Thyroid gland and lymph nodes
- Breast and axilla (within the breast, ultrasound distinguishes cystic from solid lesions)

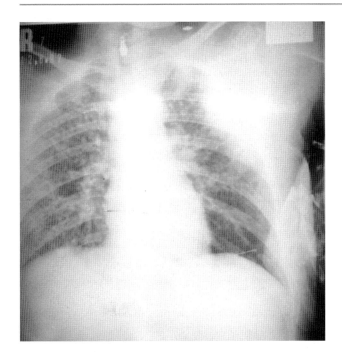

Figure 25.2 ● Lymphangitis carcinomatosa in a 45-year-old patient with breast cancer.

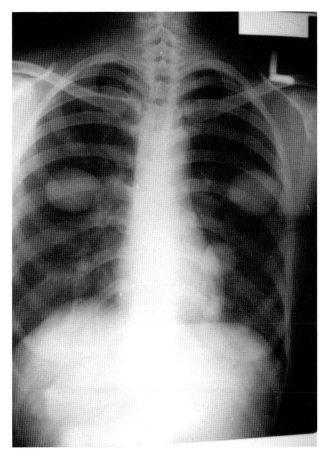

Figure 25.3 ● Cannon-ball metastasis due to choriocarcinoma.

- Scrotal lesions (fine-needle aspiration (FNA) is contraindicated because of the risk of malignant dissemination)
- Endocavity scanning, including transrectal (prostatic cancer to guide biopsy) and transvaginal scanning (for diagnosis and screening of ovarian tumours)
- Guiding interventional procedures such as biopsy and drainage
- Doppler ultrasound to assess deep venous thrombosis, and renal and hepatic vessel flow
- To detect and characterise solid abdominal organ lesions, such as liver metastases; this is complementary to cross-sectional imaging techniques such as CT and MRI.

Computed tomography

This is the radiological examination of choice in the detection and staging of many solid organ malignancies. For staging of colonic cancer, CT chest, abdomen and pelvis is performed. For rectal cancer, MRI of the pelvis is added.

Oral contrast or water is used in abdominal and pelvic scanning in order to differentiate bowel loops from lymph nodes and other normal anatomy.

Intravenous contrast is useful for differentiating blood vessels from lymph nodes and allows the correct timing of the scan in order to improve the accuracy of lesion detection and characterisation.

High-resolution CT (HRCT) of the chest can be used to distinguish lymphangitis carcinomatosa from infection, pulmonary oedema and infection, and is used to diagnose fungal chest infection in patients undergoing immunosuppressive treatments such as chemotherapy.

Computed tomography colonography is an emerging technique that can accurately assess the large bowel with regard to mucosal lesions. It is particularly suitable in patients otherwise unfit for conventional colonoscopy.

Magnetic resonance imaging

This technique is superior to CT in the CNS, head, neck and pelvis and in assessing musculoskeletal neoplasms. It is complementary to CT in many other indications.

Although MRI protocols are continually developing with advances in imaging software and hardware, T1-weighted images are still used to identify normal anatomy, and T2-weighted images are still often used to distinguish normal from pathological tissue.

Intravenous gadolinium contrast is often used in a similar way to the CT iodine-based agents to look for lesional enhancement. However, intrinsic body water provides MRI with significantly more 'natural' contrast, and so gadolinium is generally utilised less than iodine-based contrast agents for CT. Gadolinium does, however, have a common use in distinguishing scar from recurrent disease in many body areas.

Nuclear medicine

Nuclear medicine provides functional information and, to a variable extent, anatomical information from the organ or system imaged. The patient is injected with a radioactive isotope, and the radiation emitted is detected, usually using a gamma-camera.

Uses of nuclear medicine in cancer include the following:

- *Isotope bone scan:* to detect bone metastasis
- *Mecaptoacetyltriglycine (MAG3) renogram:* to assess renal function before chemotherapy
- *Ventilation/perfusion ($\dot{V}/\dot{Q}$) scan:* to evaluate the presence of pulmonary embolism
- *Radioiodine thyroid scan:* to investigate and treat thyroid cancer
- *Lymphoscintigraphy in sentinel node imaging:* to stage melanoma, breast, penile and vulval cancers.

Positron-emission tomography

Positron-emission tomography (PET) is an emerging technology in the detection of occult primary and recurrent disease. In the UK, PET is available in only a few centres, but it is increasingly being approved for the diagnosis and staging of various cancers. It is increasingly combined with CT imaging (PET-CT), which allows the functional information to be perfectly fused with the anatomical information, with improved accuracy.

PET has shown particular promise in staging lung and oesophageal cancers, as it can detect occult nodal deposits in the mediastinum, where the nodes themselves are normal in size and shape and, hence, normal by traditional CT criteria. In this situation, unnecessary complex major surgery can be avoided if a curative result is shown to be impossible.

PET has also shown promise in staging many lymphomas, as treated fibrosed inactive tissue following treatment is often residual on standard CT imaging if there was a significant original bulk of disease. With PET-CT, the activity of such scans be assessed and 'burnt-out' fibrosed tissue can be distinguished from low-activity disease.

Planning management following diagnosis of cancer

Management following diagnosis is a multifactorial decision that depends on life expectancy, comorbidities, the natural course of the cancer, the available resources and the patient's priorities. The patient's family should also be involved in the management.

An increasingly used concept in the management of malignant disease is a weekly meeting of the multidisciplinary team comprising all the specialties involved in the treatment of patients with cancer, including surgeons, clinical and medical oncologists, pathologists and radiologists. There is usually a separate meeting for each specialty, such as upper gastrointestinal, colorectal, breast, lymphoma and hepato-pancreatico-biliary (HPB) surgery. The specialist nurses are the link between the multidisciplinary team and the patients. Each patient is discussed; a plan for management is then agreed on and may need to be discussed further in future meetings with feedback from the treating surgeon or oncologist.

> ■ KEY POINT
> An increasingly used concept in the management of malignant disease is a weekly meeting of the multidisciplinary team.

Surgery

Surgery is the most important and most successful treatment modality for most tumours. It has a role in diagnosis and staging and in treatment.

Diagnosis and staging

The main surgical techniques used in the diagnosis and staging of cancers are as follows:

- *Biopsy*:
  - FNA
  - Core-needle biopsy
  - Incisional biopsy
  - Excisional biopsy, e.g. lymph node, suspicious skin lesion
  - Punch biopsy for skin recurrence, Paget's disease of nipple
- *Endoscopy (fibre-optic, rigid)*: according to the most suspected diagnosis – oesophagogastroduodenoscopy (OGD), colonoscopy, endoscopic retrograde cholangiopancreatography (ERCP), bronchoscopy, endoscopic ultrasound – for direct visualisation and biopsy

- *Diagnostic laparoscopy:* for peroperative assessment of spread, e.g. pancreatic and gastric cancer
- *Sentinel node biopsy (SNB):* the principle is to identify the first lymph node within the drainage area from the lesion, based on the assumption that, if the sentinel lymph node is free of metastasis, then the remaining nodes should also be free of tumour spread. SNB was initially used for penile cancer, and then in malignant melanoma and breast cancer. The biopsy can be performed with intradermal injection of blue dye with or without injection of radioactive material before surgery. Intraoperatively the sentinel node can be identified by colour (blue node) or increased radioactivity (hot node) via a handheld gamma-probe at the site of draining lymph nodes.

Treatment

The principle of radical surgery is to remove all cancerous growth with adjacent tissues, if feasible, to leave a cancer-free margin in addition to the draining lymph nodes, thus leading to cure. Common examples include the following:

- Wide local excision (WLE) or mastectomy, with axillary surgery (clearance, sampling, SNB), complete excision of malignant skin lesion with clear microscopical margin
- Colectomy (right, left, total)
- Radical prostatectomy
- Lobectomy or pneumonectomy for lung cancer.

> ■ KEY POINT
>
> The principle of radical surgery is to remove all cancerous growth with adjacent tissues and to leave a cancer-free margin.

Cytoreductive surgery (debulking) is used to remove the bulk of the tumour and may increase the probability of disease control with other modalities. Examples include debulking of ovarian and brain tumours.

Surgical emergencies in patients with cancer include bowel perforation and obstruction, spinal cord compression and raised intracranial pressure.

Palliation is used to relieve symptoms and to improve the patient's quality of life. Examples of palliative surgery include the following:

- Relief of obstruction, e.g. bypass surgery or stoma formation for gastrointestinal malignancies
- Surgery for masses causing pain
- Stenting for oesophageal and biliary obstruction
- Surgery to fix a pathological fracture
- Surgical pleurodesis for recurrent pleural effusion
- Shunt procedures for recurrent ascites.

A good example of reconstructive surgery is a latissimus dorsi myocutaneous flap following mastectomy. Other flaps, such as transverse rectus abdominus myocutaneous (TRAM) and deep inferior epigastric perforator (DIEP) flaps, are performed less commonly.

Surgical procedures may be used to treat metastases, such as liver resection for metastatic colorectal cancer.

Chemotherapy

Chemotherapy is the use of drugs to kill or inhibit the growth of cancer cells (Bhosie and Hall, 2006). The main principles of cancer chemotherapy are as follows:

- Cancer chemotherapy is most commonly used in the adjuvant and palliative settings, but it may be used as a neoadjuvant to reduce the size of cancer, thus enabling conservative surgery in breast cancer.
- Some tumours, such as germ-cell tumours and lymphomas, are potentially curable with chemotherapy.
- Most chemotherapy agents have a narrow therapeutic index and therefore a high incidence of toxicity.
- Chemotherapy is given in cycles in order to allow recovery of normal tissue.
- Chemotherapy is given in combinations in order to reduce the chance of resistance.

Classification of chemotherapy treatment

Cancer chemotherapy drugs are classified as follows:

- *Alkylating agents:* damage cellular DNA by alkylation; examples include the platinums, nitrogen mustard, melphalan and chlorambucil
- *Antimetabolites:* act by causing enzyme inhibition and DNA malfunction; examples include methotrexate, 5-fluorouracil (5-FU) and capecitabine
- *Antibiotics:* inhibit normal DNA replication, resulting in DNA catabolism; examples include anthracyclines such as doxorubicin and epirubicin, and non-anthracyclines such as bleomycin and mitoxantrone
- *Mitotic spindle inhibitors:* inhibit cell division; examples include vincristine and the taxanes
- *Topoisomerase inhibitors:* inhibit DNA synthesis; an example is etoposide.

Chemotherapy can be used as adjuvant treatment following surgical treatment (e.g. lymph node positive or grade 3 breast cancer, especially in younger patients) or as neoadjuvant treatment (e.g. to down-stage breast cancer and enable breast-conserving surgery (BCS)).

Fluorouracil, epirubicin and cyclophosphamide (FEC) is one of the most common combination chemotherapy regimes for breast cancer.

5-FU and folinic acid are used as adjuvant treatment for stage III colorectal cancer.

Side effects of chemotherapy

Side effects of cancer chemotherapy include the following:

- *Blood:* myelosuppression, with neutropenia, thrombocytopenia and anaemia
- *Pyrexia:* with or without sepsis
- *Gastrointestinal effects:* vomiting, mucositis (with sore mouth), diarrhoea
- *CNS toxicity:* peripheral neuropathy (e.g. with taxanes), cerebellar signs, encephalopathy
- *Infertility*
- *Alopecia:* usually reversible
- *Genitourinary tract effects:* e.g. haemorrhagic cystitis with cyclophosphamide
- *Cardiac effects:* 5-FU can cause cardiac ischaemia, and anthracyclines can affect left ventricular function (multiple uptake gated acquisition (MUGA) scanning measures the left ventricle ejection fraction).

Hormonal therapy

Hormonal therapy in breast cancer

The aim of hormonal therapy in breast cancer is to reduce oestrogenic growth stimulation of cancer cells. About 70 per cent of oestrogen receptors and progesterone receptors respond positively to hormone manipulation (Stokes and Chan, 2006). Hormonal therapy in breast cancer is mainly used as an adjuvant following surgical removal of breast cancer, but it can be used in neoadjuvant setting, e.g. the use of letrozole to down-size the tumour and enable BCS.

Examples of hormonal therapy in breast cancer include the following:

- *Ovarian ablation (the ovaries are the main source of oestrogen in premenopausal women)*: oophorectomy (open or laparoscopic), ovarian radiation and luteinising hormone-releasing agonists (medical oophorectomy), e.g. goserelin 3.6 mg subcutaneously every 28 days
- *Tamoxifen*: non-steroidal oestrogen receptor blocker that also has some oestrogen agonist activity. It is given as a 20-mg tablet once daily for 5 years. It improves bone mineral density in postmenopausal women. The main side effects are hot flushes, increased risk of thromboembolic disease and endometrial cancer
- *Raloxifene*: oestrogen receptor modulator that is not associated with endometrial cancer but is associated with a high risk of thromboembolic disease
- *Aromatase inhibitors*: used in postmenopausal women to inhibit the peripheral conversion of steroidal androgens into oestrogens by acting on the peripheral aromatase system. The non-steroidal aromatase inhibitor anastrozole (1 mg daily) is the most commonly used aromatase inhibitor in the UK. It has a reduced risk of endometrial cancer but an increased risk of osteoporosis compared with tamoxifen. Dual-energy X-ray absorption (DEXA) bone density scanning is done before starting and after 2–3 years of aromatase inhibitor therapy. Other aromatase inhibitors include letrozole (non-steroidal) and exemastane (steroidal).

Hormonal therapy in prostate cancer

Examples of hormonal therapy in prostate cancer include the following:

- *Surgical castration*: subcapsular orchidectomy
- *Medical castration*: gonadotrophin-releasing hormone analogues such as goserelin inhibit the secretion of the gonadotrophins follicle-stimulating hormone (FSH) and luteinising hormone (LH) from the pituitary gland. Before goserelin therapy, the patient is started on an anti-androgen such as cyproterone to counteract the testosterone flare. Side effects include impotence, gynaecomastia and depression
- *Oestrogen*: very effective but has limited use due to increased incidence risk of cardiovascular disease.

Radiotherapy

Radiation causes DNA damage and hence tumour cell death. Its use is limited by the small therapeutic window between tumour cure and normal tissue damage. In cancer, radiotherapy is used for radical and adjuvant treatment and palliatively.

Radical treatment

Cure may be achieved as monotherapy (e.g. in early prostate cancer) or in combination with surgery and chemotherapy (e.g. in lymphomas). The total dose is divided into fractions and given once daily over 4–6 weeks.

Adjuvant treatment

Adjuvant treatment is used to eradicate residual microscopic disease following surgery. Examples include:

- in breast cancer, routinely following WLE and in some patients following mastectomy for T3 cancers or when the cancer reaches deep surface;
- in head and neck tumours.

Neoadjuvant treatment is used before surgery to increase the operability and treat microscopic disease. Examples include rectal, breast and oesophageal cancers.

Palliative radiotherapy

Radiotherapy is commonly used for control of symptoms. Examples include pain from:

- bone metastases;
- spinal cord compression;
- superior vena cava obstruction;
- cerebral metastases.

The total dose of radiotherapy given in the palliative setting is lower than that used in treatment, but in the palliative setting it is given in a larger fraction over a shorter period of time.

Interstitial radiation therapy is used mainly for head, neck and anal cancers. Brachytherapy is used mainly for cervical and prostate cancers.

Side effects

Early side effects of radiotherapy include the following:

- *Eye:* conjunctivitis
- *Skin:* pain, redness, ulceration
- *Gastrointestinal tract:* mucositis, proctitis
- *Lung:* pneumonitis
- *Bladder:* cystitis.

Late effects of radiotherapy include the following:

- Skin telangiectasia
- Delayed wound healing
- Fibrosis, fistula and stricture (small bowel)
- Secondary solid malignancy and leukaemia

Immunotherapy

The basic premise of immunotherapy is that cancer cells express mutated proteins or over-express differentiation antigens that can then be recognised by antibodies or T-cells (Durrant and Scholefield, 2006). The following forms of immunotherapy are used in the treatment of cancer:

- *Interferons:* have antiproliferative and immunomodulatory functions; used in lymphoma, chronic myelogenous leukaemia (CML), myeloma and renal tumours
- *Interleukin 2:* stimulates the production of natural killer cells; has been used in malignant melanoma and renal cell carcinoma
- *Monoclonal antibodies:* target specific cell markers of the tumour antigens; examples include:
  - Anti-CD20 antibody (rituximab) for non-Hodgkin's lymphomas
  - Anti-HER2 receptor antibody (trastuzumab – Herceptin®) for breast cancer
  - Gemtuzumab for treatment of advanced acute myeloid leukaemia (AML)
  - Bevacizumab for treatment of advanced colorectal cancer.

Angiogenesis inhibitors

Angiogenesis inhibitors block blood vessels formation, which results in inhibition of tumour growth. Examples are thalidomide in multiple myeloma and bevacizumab in colorectal cancer.

● CANCER SCREENING

The World Health Organization (WHO) lists the following principles for screening for a certain cancer:

- The condition should pose an important health problem.
- The natural history should be understood well.
- There should be a recognisable early stage, and treatment at that stage should be of more benefit than treatment started at a later stage.
- There should be a suitable test that is acceptable to the population.
- There must be adequate facilities for diagnosis and treatment of any abnormalities detected.
- The chance of harm to those screened should be less than the chance of benefit.
- The cost of a screening programme should be balanced against the benefit.

English experience of screening for breast cancer

The English National Health Service Breast Screening Programme (NHSBSP) started in 1988 in response to the report of an expert committee (Forrest, 1986) that had conducted a review of the evidence at the time and concluded that 'screening by mammography can lead to prolongation of life for women 50 and over'. The report recognised that there would be a need to develop services alongside the screening programme to assess and treat the breast problems detected. Initially it was decided to invite women aged 50–64 years every 3 years for two-view mammography at the first round and oblique-view mammograms only thereafter. Since then, the programme has evolved, responding to emerging evidence and changing technology, and new guidelines and targets have been set. The age range was extended up to 70 years, and a move was made to two-view screening throughout the programme, as this was shown to increase the small-cancer detection rate. In recent years, an overall uptake rate of 75 per cent has been achieved, and about 1.3 million women have been screened in England, Wales and Northern Ireland between 1998 and 1999; approximately 10 000 cancers have been detected annually. The screening interval is still every 3 years.

Since the onset of the screening programme, however, there have been changes in the incidence of breast cancer in the population as well as more effective treatment methods, and the contribution of screening in terms of mortality reduction has been questioned.

It has been recognised that there are negative as well as positive aspects to screening. In particular, there are concerns regarding anxiety caused by false-positive recalls, risks associated with radiation exposure and possible over-diagnosis of very early-stage disease.

In 2002, a review of breast screening by the International Agency for Research on Cancer (IARC) concluded that routine mammographic screening was effective in reducing mortality from breast cancer in women aged 50–69 years. The IARC stated that the mortality benefit was likely to be in the region of 25 per cent in those invited for screening but that the effect would not be seen until an interval of 5–12 years from the start of any programme.

This overview of the English experience of screening is based largely on a report issued in 2006 by the Advisory Committee on Breast Cancer Screening, which summarised progress to date and looked forward to future developments.

Since 1988, the number of cases of breast cancer recorded in women aged 50–64 years in England has increased by about 50 per cent. It is thought that half of this increase is due to screening and half is due to a real change in the incidence of the disease. The latter is probably associated with a large increase in the use of hormone replacement therapy (HRT) over this time. Data have shown clearly that, although women participating in screening are more likely to be diagnosed with breast cancer, their cancers are significantly smaller and less likely to be treated with mastectomy than in women presenting symptomatically. Statistics show that death rates from breast cancer have fallen since 1990 in all age groups, partly as a result of earlier diagnosis but also due to improvements in the management of the disease, particularly hormonal therapy (e.g. tamoxifen). Attempts to measure the exact contribution of screening have included looking at surrogate measures of mortality based on the size, nodal status and grade of the cancers detected. One striking feature has been the large increase in the number of cases of DCIS since screening was introduced, representing about 20 per cent of all cancer cases currently detected by screening. About 70 per cent is high-grade disease and thus more likely to develop into invasive cancer. There have been concerns about over-diagnosis of DCIS, and some low-grade invasive cancers may never develop into clinically significant disease, thus leading to over-treatment. It is not possible currently to predict how individual lesions will behave and, until this is the case, treatment continues to be offered appropriate to each woman's circumstances. Interval cancer rates have also been used as a measure of the success of the screening programme. The number of cancers detected between screens depends on several factors, including the geographical variation of underlying risk factors in the population and HRT use, as well as the quality of mammograms produced and their interpretation. Quality-assurance monitoring and the setting of increasingly rigorous targets have played important parts in ensuring that all aspects of the service have continued to develop and maintain high standards. Statistics concerning uptake, screening intervals, recall rates, numbers and sizes of cancers diagnosed, preoperative diagnosis and benign biopsy rates are collected regularly and fed back to screening units, and action is recommended if targets are not reached in any of these areas.

■ KEY POINT

Since 1988, the number of cases of breast cancer recorded in women aged 50–64 years in England has increased by about 50 per cent. However, death rates from breast cancer have fallen since 1990 in all age groups.

It has been estimated that about one in eight women screened regularly in the NHSBSP will experience a recall for assessment at least once in 10 years; recall is more likely for premenopausal women, women who have had previous breast surgery and women who are taking HRT. False-positive recalls can create high levels of anxiety in the short term, but studies have shown that few women suffer serious long-term consequences. The aim is always to reduce recall rates to as low a level as possible, while maximising the detection of small cancers. The overall recall rate is highest for the prevalent screen at 7.6 per cent, which compares favourably to that in the USA (12.5–14.6 per cent), but this varies between units due to local circumstances, film-reading protocols and experience.

The introduction of double reading of mammograms has been shown to improve cancer detection rates by about 10 per cent. Film-reading performance figures are audited regularly, and it is encouraging that improvement in the detection of small cancers, alongside a fall in recall rates, has occurred consistently since the start of the programme. The assessment process has generated improvements in biopsy techniques, including core biopsy largely replacing fine-needle aspiration, digital stereotaxis and, more recently, sophisticated wide-bore needle biopsy systems.

High-quality film-screen mammography is still the only screening method of proven value through randomised controlled trials. Clinical and ultrasound examinations are extremely important tools at assessment. Ultrasound has shown benefits, particularly in younger women and in women with dense breasts; however, ultrasound has low sensitivity for DCIS, is time-consuming, and is dependent on the quality of the equipment and the experience of the operator.

It is in the introduction of full-field digital mammography that future improvements are anticipated. Studies have indicated that this has a similar sensitivity and better specificity when compared with film screening, and it enables a lower radiation dose to be used. Multiple other advantages are apparent, such as the ability to manipulate images avoiding additional exposures, better visualisation of dense breast tissue, and opportunities for improved image storage and transmission. The application of computer-aided detection (CAD) to digital systems continues to be evaluated and may have a future role, although current systems generate too many false-positive prompts to be helpful.

Magnetic resonance imaging has been shown to be highly sensitive for the detection of invasive breast cancer. Its use as a screening method is limited, however, by expense, lower specificity, and difficulty of throughput of large numbers. It has not been recommended for screening in the general population, but it is advised for women under age 50 years who have a high risk of developing breast cancer for genetic reasons, such as women who are carriers of the BRCA1, BRCA2 and TP53 gene mutations.

> ■ KEY POINT
> MRI is advised for women under age 50 years who have a high risk of developing breast cancer for genetic reasons.

In summary, in England the NHSBSP has undergone many improvements and changes since its introduction and is now considered successful and well established. Screening has been estimated to save 1400 lives each year, at a cost of approximately £3000 for each life-year saved. Screening has aided research that has led to improvements in the early diagnosis of breast cancer, and it continues to stimulate and support studies relating to the prevention, diagnosis and management of the disease. The benefit has also been seen outside the screened population of women in a general increase in awareness and thus earlier presentation of symptomatic disease and the development of improved services for the diagnosis and treatment of all women with breast problems.

Challenges for the near future include extending the service to include women between the ages of 47 years and 73 years, including the screening of younger women with a significant family history of breast cancer in the programme, and embracing digital technology.

Screening for other cancers

- *Cervical cancer:* in the NHS cervical screening programme (NHSCSP), women aged 20–64 years are screened every 3–5 years. The Papanicolaou (Pap) smear test is used for cytological screening. Approximately 3.9 million women are tested in England each year.
- *Colorectal cancer:* the main tests are faecal occult blood test and sigmoidoscopy. Colonoscopy is used to screen high-risk cases with previous colon tumour, polyps, ulcerative colitis and family history of colorectal cancer.
- *Prostate cancer:* screened for by estimation of plasma PSA levels.
- *Ovarian cancer:* screened for by measuring CA125 levels and transvaginal ultrasound.

Cancer prognostic index

The Nottingham prognostic index (NPI) is used to determine the prognosis of breast cancer:

$$NPI = (0.2 \times \text{tumour size}) + \text{grade} + \text{LN stage}$$

where LN is lymph node stage:

LN1 = no node
LN2 = one to three nodes
LN3 = more than four nodes.

Grade is numbered 1 for grade 1, 2 for grade 2, and 3 for grade 3.

SUMMARY

Management of patients with cancer is an ever developing issue. This chapter summarises the latest updates in cancer diagnosis, especially imaging. It briefly describes surgical therapy, radiotherapy, chemotherapy and hormonal therapy. It also emphasises the importance of cancer screening, in particular for breast cancer.

QUESTIONS

1. What types of biopsy are used in the diagnosis of solid cancers?
2. Which early complications can follow the use of chemotherapy?
3. What are the late complications of radiotherapy?
4. What tumour markers can be of benefit in the diagnosis of suspected testicular cancer?
5. Outline the imaging techniques used in diagnosing breast cancer.
6. What types of surgical management are in common use in treating colorectal cancer?
7. How does screening affect the management of breast cancer?
8. Is there any relation between immunotherapy and treatment of breast cancer?
9. Describe the use of lymph node biopsy in the diagnosis of malignant disease.
10. Describe the role of hormonal therapy in breast and prostate cancer.

REFERENCES

Bhosie J, Hall G (2006). Principles of cancer treatment by chemotherapy. *Surgery* **24**: 66–9.

Dixon JM (2005). *ABC of Breast Diseases*, 3rd edn. London: BMJ Books.

Durrant LG, Scholefield JH (2006). Principles of cancer treatment by immunotherapy. *Surgery* **24**: 55–8.

Forrest P (1986). Report to the health ministers of England, Wales, Scotland and Northern Ireland. London: Department of Health and Social Security.

Stokes Z, Chan S (2006). Principles of cancer by hormone therapy. *Surgery* 59–62.

Wilt TJ, Thompson IM (2006). Clinically localised prostate cancer. *Br Med J* **333**: 1102–6.

FURTHER READING

DeVita VT, Hellman S, Rosenberg SA (2005). *Cancer Principles and Practice of Oncology*, 7th edn. Philadelphia, PA: Lippincott Williams & Wilkins.

National Institute for Health and Clinical Excellence (NICE) (2006). *Familial Breast Cancer*. NICE clinical guideline. London: National Institute for Health and Clinical Excellence.

Peedell C (2005). *Concise Clinical Oncology*. Edinburgh: Elsevier.

26 Sutures, surgical incisions and surgical anastomoses

E Philip Perry and Naif El-Barghouti

● INTRODUCTION

This chapter deals with aspects of basic operative principles that are useful for basic surgical trainees.

● SURGICAL INCISIONS

All surgical incisions should be planned carefully in order to give a good view of the deeper structures and to avoid underlying large vessels and nerves. Incisions should be made parallel to and not across their long axis.

Table 26.1 summarises the common incisions and closures used.

Table 26.1 Summary of common incisions and closures

Location	Type	Use	Closure
Face	Transverse	Removal of skin lesions	Vicryl or glue Interrupted prolene or subcuticular vicryl if longer wound (remove in 3–5 days)
Neck	Collar Oblique	Thyroidectomy	Continuous PDS to fascia Subcuticular vicryl to skin
Chest	Median sternotomy	Cardiac artery bypass graft	Wire to sternum Vicryl to fascia Subcuticular vicryl to skin
Abdomen	Laparotomy	Large bowel resection	Mass closure with PDS Clips to skin
	Laparoscopic	Laparoscopic cholecystectomy	Glue or Steristrips® or vicryl to skin
Limbs	Vein harvesting	Veins for CABG graft	Vicryl to fascia Clips or subcuticular vicryl to skin

PDS, polydioxanone.

Skin incisions

For best results, place skin incisions along skin tension lines. Skin tension lines run parallel to the dermal collagen bundles but at right-angles to the direction of contraction of the muscles underneath. To find skin tension lines:

- *Face:* look for wrinkles
- *Limbs and trunk:* handle the skin to find the maximum wrinkling direction.

Skin tension lines do not always correspond to Langer's lines. Langer's lines are lines of cleavage and were first described by Langer in 1861. Their existence is due to the fact that collagen fibres in the dermis lie mostly in parallel bundles. Surgical incisions made along Langer's lines heal with a minimum of scar tissue. Elsewhere in the body, cleavage lines tend to be longitudinal in the limbs and circumferential in the neck and trunk.

> ■ KEY POINT
> Skin tension lines do not always correspond to Langer's lines.

All incisions are described as vertical, horizontal (transverse), oblique or continuous (S-shaped).

Common abdominal incisions

Figure 26.1 shows the common abdominal incisions, and Table 26.2 gives their main uses.

Figure 26.1 ● Common abdominal incisions.

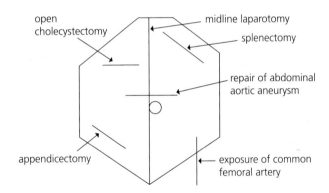

open cholecystectomy — midline laparotomy — splenectomy — repair of abdominal aortic aneurysm — appendicectomy — exposure of common femoral artery

Table 26.2 Common abdominal incisions and their uses

Incision	Main use
Left subcostal	Splenectomy
Right transverse	Cholecystectomy
Midline	Colectomy
Left flank	Nephrectomy
Right transverse	Appendicectomy
Subumbilical	Laparoscopic camera
Left groin (vertical)	Femoral artery

Compared with longitudinal incisions, transverse incisions in the abdomen:

- heal with minimum scarring (along skin tension lines) and are more cosmetically pleasing;
- have a decreased incidence of subsequent incisional hernia;
- are associated with less postoperative pain and fewer chest problems.

> ■ KEY POINT
> Transverse abdominal incisions are associated with less postoperative pain and fewer chest problems compared with longitudinal incisions.

Chest incisions

Table 26.3 lists the common chest incisions and their main uses.

Table 26.3 Common chest incisions and their uses

Incision	Main use
Median sternotomy	Heart
Anterior thoracotomy	Main vessels, including subclavian
Posterior lateral thoracotomy	Fifth space
Posterior lateral thoracotomy	Seventh space

Laparoscopic incisions

Port sites include the following:

- *Umbilical port*: the laparoscopic camera port should be inserted by cut-down and insertion into the peritoneal cavity under direct vision
- *Other abdominal ports*: depend on the procedure, but should be inserted under direct vision using an intra-abdominal camera.

● SUTURES

Sutures are used to:

- close the edge of a wound or incision;
- repair damaged tissue;
- secure foreign bodies, e.g. drains.

The following five main characteristics should be considered when selecting an appropriate suture material:

- Strength
- Physical structure
- Absorbability
- Tensile behaviour
- Biological behaviour.

Types of suture

All sutures can be described in the following categories or types:

- *Absorbable/non-absorbable:*
  - Non-absorbable sutures persist and are used when persistent strength is needed, e.g. polypropylene to close the abdominal sheath.
  - Absorbable sutures have a finite life, e.g. vicryl is used in the biliary tree and urothelium as persistent sutures could be a nidus for stone formation.
  - Different absorbable sutures last for different lengths of time, measured by half-life – the time taken for the suture to lose 50 per cent of its tensile strength.
- *Braided/monofilament:*
  - Monofilament sutures cause less tissue damage when passing through structures, e.g. 6/0 polypropylene sutures for vascular anastomoses.
  - Braided sutures have a capillary action and should be avoided if there is a risk of infection, e.g. do not use silk sutures to close skin.
- *Coated/non-coated:*
  - Sutures may be coated with silicone, polytetrafluoroethylene (PTFE) or polybutyrate for easier tissue passage.
  - Coatings reduce the problem of premature locking and facilitate the tightening problem of the suture.
- *Dyed/non-dyed:*
  - Absorbable sutures may be dyed to make them more visible, e.g. vicryl (which is usually white) may be dyed purple.
  - Dyed sutures should be avoided in the skin, as they may cause tattooing.
- *Natural/synthetic:*
  - Natural sutures such as silk and catgut may elicit a marked tissue reaction and may cause foreign body (protein) reactions. Catgut is not used any more because of the risk of contamination with Creutzfeldt–Jakob disease (CJD).
  - Synthetic sutures such as polydioxanone (PDS) and polypropylene have largely replaced natural sutures.

> ■ KEY POINT
> Catgut is no longer used because of the risk of contamination with CJD.

Needles

Suture needles are made of stainless-steel or carbon steel and are packaged in water-resistant foil. Most sutures are inserted in the base of a drilled needle.

Table 26.4 shows the various suture needle points used.

The needle body may interact with a needle-holder or be handheld. The following bodies are used:

- Straight
- Half-curved
- Curved (1/4, 3/8, 1/2, 5/8)
- Compound curved
- J-shaped

Needle-holders

The needle-holder must be selected carefully to match the size and strength of the needle. Larger needle-holders may damage smaller needles. Old or worn needle-holders may result in needle rotation.

Table 26.4 Types of suture needle point

Type	Use	Shape
Cutting	Tough tissue, e.g. tendon	△
Reverse cutting	Tough tissue, e.g. tendon	▲
Taper cutting	Tough tissue, e.g. calcified vessel	△
Round body, taper point	Small holes in soft tissue, e.g. bowel anastomoses	○
Blunt point	Friable tissue, e.g. liver, kidney	○

Table 26.5 Summary of suture sizes

Standard gauge	11/0	9/0	7/0	6/0	5/0	4/0	3/0	2/0
Metric gauge	0.1	0.3	0.5	0.7	1.0	1.5	2.0	3.0
Diameter limits (mm)	0.010–0.019 0.100–0.149		0.030–0.039 0.150–0.195		0.050–0.069 0.700–0.249		0.070–0.099 0.300–0.399	

Standard gauge	0	1	2
Metric gauge	3.5	4	5
Diameter limits (mm)	0.350–0.399	0.400–0.499	0.500–0.599

■ KEY POINT

The needle-holder must be selected carefully to match the size and strength of the needle.

Suture size

Table 26.5 summarises the suture sizes used.

● TYPES OF SKIN CLOSURE

Skin closures can be categorised as follows:

- *Subcuticular:*
  - Most popular sutured skin closure
  - Continuous stitch through the dermis
  - May be non-absorbable (suture may be removed) or absorbable
  - Very neat scar.
- *Interrupted over and over or mattress:*
  - May be over and over
  - Mattress sutures may be vertical or horizontal
  - Used when the wound may be under tension.
- *Continuous:*
  - Identical to interrupted sutures, except that, after tying the first knot, the rest of the sutures are inserted in a continuous manner until the far end of the wound is reached, when the suture is then knotted
  - Used for closure of the abdominal wall.

- *Purse-string sutures:*
  - Continuous sutures placed around a lumen and tightened like a drawstring to invert the opening
  - Example: burying the appendix stump after appendicectomy.
- *Buried sutures:*
  - Sutures placed so that the knot protrudes on the inside, under the layers to be closed
  - Example: prolene sutures closing the linea alba.

OTHER METHODS OF TISSUE CLOSURE

Staples and clips

- Quick
- More expensive than sutures
- Reduce infection, as they rest on the skin
- Produce a neat scar
- Taken out using a special staple remover.

Glue and tissue adhesive

Glues are composed of fibrinogen and thrombin and tend to be based upon a solution of *n*-butyl-2-cyanocrylate.

- May need subcutaneous sutures to give strength to closure
- Sprayed on cut surfaces, e.g. liver during resection.

Self-adhesive tape and Steristrips

- Quick
- No need for local anaesthetic
- For tension-free wound, e.g. face or digit lacerations.

Stainless-steel and wire

- Non-absorbable and inert
- Approximate bones
- Example of use: sternum.

Tables 26.6 and 26.7 summarise the various skin and tissue closures available.

LIGATURES

Principles of knot-tying

- Approximate, do not strangulate.
- The knot must be firm and unable to slip.
- The knot must be as small as possible in order to minimise foreign material.
- Do not 'saw' the suture during tying, as this will weaken the thread.
- Except when knot-tying, do not grasp the suture with instruments such as artery forceps, as this will damage the thread.
- Avoid tearing the tissue being ligated when 'bedding down' the knot – control the tension carefully using the index finger.

Base knots

- Reef knot
- Surgeon's knot.

Table 26.6 Summary of skin closures

Closure	Advantages	Disadvantages
Sutures	Inexpensive	Longer time to insert
		May need to be removed
Clips/staples	Minimal tissue reaction	More expensive
	Quick and east to insert	May be uncomfortable in situ
		Requires special device for removal
Glue	Quick	Not to be used under tension
	No local anaesthetic required	Expensive
Steristrips®/adhesive tape	Inexpensive	No local anaesthetic required
	Quick	May come off if wound becomes wet
		Not to be used if wound under tension

Table 26.7 Summary of tissue closures

Closure type	Closure used
Skin	Clips, subcuticular vicryl
Fascia	PDS or polypropylene
Muscle	Vicryl
Intestine	Polypropylene
Tendon	Polypropylene
Blood vessel	Prolene

PDS, polydioxanone.

Knot behaviour

Fashion all knots with care:

- Use the first 'throw' for position.
- Use the second throw for tension.
- Use the third and subsequent throws for security. For example, use four throws for PDS and six throws for polypropylene.

More throws may only increase the bulk of the knot.

● ANASTOMOSES

Bowel anastomoses

The principles of bowel anastomosis are as follows:

- No tension
- Good blood supply

- Accurate opposition
- Serosa to serosa without mucosal protrusion
- Avoid rotation of the bowel.
- Hand sewn: one layer – preferable, as less reduction in lumen size, and less loss of blood supply.

For interrupted single-layer serosubmucosal or extramucosal anastomosis, individual sutures are placed 5 mm apart and deep. Recommended sutures are 3/0 PDS using an atraumatic, round-bodied needle.

For end-to-end extramucosal anastomosis:

1 Resect lesion.
2 Use soft bowel clamps to prevent spillage and orient ends of bowel. Ensure no tension.
3 Suture from the serosal surface, including the muscle layer and submucosa, and emerging between the mucosa and submucosa.
4 It is essential to include the submucosa for strength but to invert the mucosa.
5 Insert stay sutures at the mesenteric and antimesenteric borders (do not ligate them but place in haemostats).
6 Starting from the mesenteric border, place interrupted sutures along the anterior border (5 mm deep and apart).
7 On completing the anterior border stay sutures, place in haemostats and pass the antimesenteric stay sutures under the bowel to emerge at the mesenteric defect. (This will reverse the bowel and the posterior border will now be anterior.)
8 The 'new' front wall is now closed in a similar manner with interrupted extramucosal sutures.
9 On completion, return the stay sutures to their original position.
10 Close the mesenteric defect with interrupted vicryl sutures without damaging the mesenteric vessels. (Suture to the peritoneum or previous knots and tissue.)
11 The blood supply of the bowel ends should be adequate. Avoid rotation and tension.

For the continuous extramucosal single-layer anastomosis, a similar technique is used:

1 Place a full-length stay suture at the mesenteric border and ligate.
2 Place a stay suture at the antimesenteric border and place in haemostat.
3 Suture the anterior border with the continuous suture.
4 Care must be taken not to purse-string or narrow the anastomosis.

Complications of bowel anastomosis include:

- leakage due to poor technique, poor blood supply or tension on the anastomosis;
- stenosis, which could lead to obstruction.

Vascular anastomoses

Intima to intima with everting sutures:

- Require more delicate handling compared with bowel, in order to prevent injury to the delicate wall.
- The artery wall should never be grasped between forceps, as this may cause intimal loss or a full-thickness tear.
- The suture material is passed from inside to out on the arterial wall (from intima to adventitia) to fix atherosclerotic plaques and to prevent the formation of intimal flaps.

- Non-absorbable monofilament sutures such as polypropylene, which move smoothly through the wall, should be used.
- A smooth suture and suture line, preserving as much endothelium as possible, is essential in order to prevent platelet aggregation, which may narrow or occlude the anastomosis.
- Do not grasp the suture material with forceps or a needle-holder, except when tying the knot, as this can fracture or break the suture.
- Accurate, fine, water-tight sutures need to be inserted at even tension.
- Insert the needle at right-angles to the wall and use the curve of the needle to allow the needle to travel through the wall.
- The finer the vessel, the finer the sutures required and the smaller the bites taken.

■ KEY POINT

Do not grasp the suture material with forceps or a needle-holder, except when tying the knot, as this can fracture or break the suture.

Stapled anastomoses

- Circular stapling devices are used for end-to-end anastomoses.
- Linear stapling devices along or combined with circular stapling devices may be used for side-to-side anastomoses.
- The bowel must be cleaned of mesentery and fat in order to reduce bulk before stapling.

The types of anastomosis used include the following:

- Vascular: end to end
- Single layer: continuous
- Renal: ureter to ureter, ureter to bladder
- Fistulae: bowel to skin, loop or end colostomy or ileostomy.
  Table 26.8 summarises the various anastomoses used.

Table 26.8 Summary of anastomoses used

Type	Anastomosis	What to use	
		Hand-sewn	Stapled
Intestinal	Small bowel to small bowel →	Single-layer PDS	Ease of use
	Small bowel to large bowel		May be quicker
	Large bowel to large bowel		Where placement of sutures is difficult
			Discrepancies in size
	Stomach to skin (gastrostomy) →	Interrupted undyed vicryl	Not applicable
	Small bowel to skin		
	Large bowel to skin		
Vascular		6/0 polypropylene	Not applicable
Urological		3/0 PDS or 3/0 vicryl	Not applicable

INCISIONAL HERNIAE

An incisional hernia is an acquired hernia at the site of previous laparotomy. Precipitating factors relate to poor wound healing, including the following:

- General factors, e.g. diabetes, malnutrition, malignancy, jaundice, obesity, pulmonary disease, abdominal distension
- Infection
- Technical factors, e.g. type of suture material, length of suture material, technical errors, emergency surgery, re-do surgery.

Principles and types of repair

Open repair

1 Excise the old scar and redundant skin.
2 Dissect out the hernial sac.
3 May invaginate the sac; or, open the sac, free any adhesions and then excise the sac.
4 Mobilise the fascia.
5 Oppose the fascia with 1-polypropylene.
6 If hernia greater than 4 cm, apply either polypropylene darn or mesh.

Laparoscopic repair

1 Reduce contents of hernia.
2 Dissect any adhesions from peritoneum.
3 Identify area of defect and measure.
4 Secure a large mesh or meshes over the defect with polypropylene sutures (sutures secured through small skin incisions and ligated).

Complications of incisional herniae

- Infection
- Seroma
- Enterocutaneous fistula
- Recurrence of incisional hernia.

SUMMARY

This chapter deals with the principles and mechanics of operative surgical techniques for all surgeons, including surgical incisions, skin closure, sutures, anastomoses and repair of incisional herniae.

QUESTIONS

1 What are Langer's lines?
2 What is the incision used for an exploratory laparotomy?
3 Why are transverse incisions better than longitudinal incisions?
4 How do you place the umbilical port for a laparoscopy?
5 What is the difference between absorbable and non-absorbable sutures? Give examples.
6 How do you perform a bowel anastomosis?
7 What type of suture is used for vascular anastomosis?
8 What are the causes of incisional hernias?

● FURTHER READING

Lewis MH, Galland RB (2002). *A Handbook of Basic Vascular Technique*. London: Bard Impra.

Thomas WEG (2002). Sutures, ligature materials and staples. *Surgery* **20**: 97–107.

Thomas WEG, Darzi A, Cheshire N, Royal College of Surgeons of England (1999). *Specialist Registrar Skills Course in General Surgery*. London: Royal College of Surgeons of England.

Principles of anaesthesia

27

Ramanathan Kandasamy

- Introduction
- Preoperative assessment
- Premedication
- General anaesthesia
- Intravenous sedation
- Regional anaesthesia
- Anatomy of the spinal cord
- Summary
- Questions
- Further reading

● INTRODUCTION

The word 'anaesthesia' comes from the Greek roots *an–* (not, without) and *aesthe_tos* (perceptible, able to feel). The word was coined by Oliver Wendell Holmes, Senior, in 1846. The first anaesthetic was administered by WTG Morton of Boston, MA, USA. Anaesthesia is very safe these days due to the use of modern technology in designing the machines and monitoring devices. The death rate for modern anaesthesia is one in 1 million general anaesthetics administered for a fit patient. The purpose of this chapter is to provide surgical trainees with a brief knowledge of the importance of preoperative assessment and the types of anaesthetic used – general, regional and local anaesthesia.

● PREOPERATIVE ASSESSMENT

The purposes of preoperative assessment are to:

- establish rapport with the patient;
- evaluate the patient's physical condition and any coexisting medical problems;
- optimise any coexisting medical conditions, e.g. arrhythmia;
- obtain an informed consent and to discuss the risk of anaesthesia;
- prescribe premedication and to advise the patient on stopping or continuing pre-existing medication during the perioperative period.

Inadequate preoperative preparation of the patient may increase the morbidity and mortality in the perioperative period. Ideally, all patients coming for an operation should be seen in a preoperative assessment clinic and the anaesthetic plan discussed well in advance, thus allowing the patient to make an informed decision regarding the whole procedure – remember that failure of communication is one of the most important causes of medicolegal problems. This also gives ample time for the anaesthetist to prepare the patient for the surgery and anaesthesia and to optimise any coexisting medical conditions. Many operations are now performed as day surgery procedures, and the patient may see the anaesthetist for the first time just before surgery.

> ■ KEY POINT
> Failure of communication is one of the most important causes of medicolegal problems.

Table 27.1 American Society of Anesthesiologists (ASA) grading for evaluating the physical status of a patient

ASA grade	Physical status
1	Normal healthy individual
2	Mild systemic disease
3	Severe systemic disease that is not incapacitating
4	Incapacitating systemic disease that is a constant threat to life
5	Moribund patient who is not expected to survive 24 h with or without the operation
E	Added as a suffix for emergency operation

Anaesthetists use the American Society of Anesthesiologists (ASA) grading to evaluate the physical status of the patient (Table 27.1).

The physical status determined by the ASA grade is not synonymous with risk. The disadvantage is that the ASA system does not include all aspects of anaesthetic risk, such as smoking, age and difficult intubation.

● PREMEDICATION

Premedication is the administration of drugs 1–2 h before anaesthesia. These drugs include sedatives and also the patient's regular medication for any pre-existing medical problems. The purpose of premedication is to:

- allay the patient's anxiety and fear;
- decrease the secretions of the respiratory tract;
- enhance the potency of the general anaesthetic agents used;
- decrease the incidence of postoperative nausea and vomiting (PONV);
- produce amnesia;
- reduce the volume and increase the pH of gastric secretions;
- attenuate vagal and sympathoadrenal responses;
- provide postoperative analgesia.

Not all premedication principles are applicable in all patients. For example, some premedication drugs are used in specific situations, such as the administration of H_2 receptor antagonists and sodium citrate antacid in obstetric anaesthesia. In modern anaesthesia, the use of atropine or glycopyrrolate to reduce secretions is not a routine practice except in difficult intubations, e.g. where fibre-optic laryngoscopy is used to intubate the trachea. A benzodiazepine such as temazepam 20 mg 2 h before surgery is commonly given.

● GENERAL ANAESTHESIA

Intravenous and inhalational anaesthetics can be used to induce general anaesthesia. Commonly, intravenous agents are used to induce anaesthesia and inhalational agents are used to maintain anaesthesia. In certain clinical situations, such as difficult airway, an inhalational agent is used to both induce and maintain anaesthesia. In this section we discuss the pharmacology of the commonly used intravenous and inhalational anaesthetic agents and opioid analgesics.

Intravenous anaesthetic agents

Thiopental sodium:

- is a barbiturate derivative;
- is one of the most commonly used intravenous anaesthetic agents;
- depresses the central nervous system (CNS), cardiovascular system and respiratory system;
- does not have a significant effect on skeletal muscle and uterine smooth muscle;
- decreases intraocular pressure;
- induces the hepatic microsomal enzyme system, which may increase the metabolism and elimination of other drugs.

Propofol

- is a phenol derivative;
- is extremely lipid-soluble;
- is formulated in a white emulsion containing soya bean oil and egg phosphatide;
- depresses the CNS, cardiovascular system and respiratory system.

There are several differences between thiopental and propofol:

- Propofol causes greater hypotension.
- Propofol causes hypotension mainly by vasodilation, whereas thiopental causes hypotension by myocardial depression.
- Propofol causes apnoea more commonly and of longer duration.
- Propofol is eliminated more quickly than thiopental by extrahepatic metabolism. Therefore, propofol is associated with a quicker recovery and less drowsiness postoperatively.

Propofol has revolutionised day surgery, as it is eliminated rapidly and causes less drowsiness postoperatively. The use of thiopental is slowly reducing in the UK, although it is still a common induction agent in most parts of the world.

> ■ KEY POINT
> Propofol has revolutionised day surgery.

Inhalational anaesthetic agents

Inhalational anaesthesia is the most popular method of maintenance of anaesthesia. There are similarities between all inhalational agents, with only minor differences between the individual agents. Total intravenous anaesthesia (TIVA) is increasingly being used these days. The incidence of PONV is significantly less with TIVA compared with that seen with inhalational agents.

The advantages of inhalational anaesthesia are that it:

- can be used for both induction and maintenance;
- produces immobility and amnesia;
- can produce muscle relaxation and potentiate the effects of neuromuscular blocking agents;
- decreases oxygen consumption;
- assists in the protection of the heart and brain from hypoxic injury;
- suppresses the stress response to surgery;
- offers easy control of depth of anaesthesia with the use of agent monitors, which allow breath-by-breath assessment of the concentration of the drug.

All inhalational anaesthetics have an enviable safety record and have been administered tens of millions of times.

The disadvantages of inhalational anaesthesia are that it:

- causes PONV, particularly with nitrous oxide (N_2O);
- decreases blood pressure in a dose-dependent manner;
- depresses respiration;
- depresses vital organ (brain, kidney, heart, liver) function in a dose-dependent manner;
- can precipitate malignant hyperthermia (see below);
- can cause postoperative drowsiness, depending on the lipid solubility of the drug used.

Halothane specifically predisposes to ventricular arrhythmias.

Malignant hyperthermia is a rapid increase in body temperature of at least 2 °C/h. This is a potentially fatal condition. In susceptible individuals, contact with specific inhalational anaesthetics or muscle relaxant suxamethonium can abnormally release calcium from the sarcoplasmic reticulum into the cytoplasm of the cells. Malignant hyperthermia is treated with intravenous dantrolene 1–2 mg/kg body weight and supportive measures as required;

The commonly used inhalational agents are isoflurane, sevoflurane, desflurane and nitrous oxide. Sevoflurane is the least irritant to the airway; desflurane and isoflurane can cause laryngospasm and airway obstruction during induction. Isoflurane, sevoflurane and desflurane are not arrhythmogenic and protect against myocardial ischaemia.

Opioid analgesics

Analgesia is an important part of anaesthesia in the perioperative period. Opioids are used in anaesthetic practice to provide pain relief supplementation of general anaesthesia, regional anaesthesia and local anaesthetic procedures. Opioids can also be used as part of the intravenous sedation along with a benzodiazepine such as midazolam. The management of postoperative pain is covered in Chapter 3; however, in this chapter we look briefly at the commonly used intraoperative analgesics fentanyl, alfentanil and morphine. Non-steroidal anti-inflammatory drugs (NSAIDs) such as parecoxib are also used to supplement opioid analgesia.

Opioid analgesics act by binding to the opioid receptors in the CNS. Opioid receptors are located in the brainstem, thalamus, hypothalamus and spinal cord. Three receptors, designated mu (μ), kappa (κ) and delta (δ), have been described (the sigma (σ) receptor is no longer considered to be an opioid receptor):

- *Mu receptor:* stimulation causes supraspinal analgesia, a feeling of wellbeing, euphoria, respiratory depression and physical dependence.
- *Kappa receptor:* stimulation causes spinal analgesia, sedation and anaesthesia.
- *Delta receptor:* function is unclear – may be responsible for modulation of the activity of the mu receptor.

Fentanyl:

- is a synthetic opioid that acts on the mu receptor;
- is 50–100 times more potent than morphine;
- has a duration of action of approximately 30 min;
- is highly lipid-soluble, so the affinity for the receptor is very high;
- produces marked analgesia, respiratory depression and, at high doses, sedation and unconsciousness;
- is associated with good cardiovascular stability, provided that ventilation is maintained;
- can cause bradycardia and muscular rigidity in high doses;
- can cause delayed respiratory depression – the postulated mechanism is the release of fentanyl in gastric secretions and absorption from the alkaline small bowel, causing a secondary elevation of the plasma fentanyl concentration.

Alfentanil:

- is a synthetic opioid related to fentanyl;
- acts on the mu receptor;
- is five to ten times less potent than fentanyl;
- has a duration of action of approximately 15–20 min;
- can be used for continuous intravenous infusion because of its shorter duration of action;
- causes muscular rigidity, particularly of the chest wall.

Morphine

- is the standard opioid against which all the others are compared;
- is obtained from opium;
- acts on the mu receptor, causing analgesia, respiratory depression, suppression of the cough reflex and a reduced level of consciousness (dose-dependent);
- lowers the blood pressure due to a decrease in systemic vascular resistance;
- releases histamine.

Adverse effects of opiates

All opiates:

- cause nausea, vomiting, itching, sedation and constipation;
- delay gastric emptying;
- cause respiratory depression and urinary retention;
- can cause visual hallucinations.

Practical conduct of anaesthesia

The anaesthetic machine and all related equipment must be checked before the operation. Depending on the type of operation, the patient may need endotracheal (ET) intubation and controlled ventilation, or laryngeal-mask airway (LMA) and spontaneous ventilation. The introduction of the LMA revolutionised the general anaesthetic administration. The LMA is inserted like an oral airway without the aid of a laryngoscope. The LMA is a supraglottic device and does not protect against aspiration.

Some of the most commonly used equipment in anaesthesia includes the following:

- Laryngoscope with light source
- Various sizes of ET tube
- Gum elastic bougie
- Various sizes of LMA
- Oropharyngeal airway
- Magill's forceps
- Anaesthetic breathing circuits with different sizes of facemask
- Bandage or tape to secure the ET tube.

General anaesthesia is induced with an intravenous agent (propofol, fentanyl, alfentanil) and may be followed by a muscle relaxant to facilitate ET intubation. If the patient does not require intubation, the LMA is inserted in order to maintain the airway, and spontaneous breathing is maintained. The use of an ET tube is influenced by various factors, such as the body cavity involved, whether laparotomy or thoracotomy is being performed, and the positioning of the patient. If the patient is in the prone or lateral position, ET intubation may be the best option to secure the airway intraoperatively.

Anaesthesia is maintained with an inhalational agent. The effects of non-depolarising muscle relaxants are reversed with neostigmine and glycopyrrolate or atropine at the end of the procedure.

Rapid sequence induction (RSI) is practised in emergency anaesthesia where there is a risk of aspiration of the gastric content into the lungs. After pre-oxygenation for at least 3 min, the intravenous anaesthetic agent is given, followed quickly by a short-acting depolarising muscle relaxant such as suxamethonium. Cricoid pressure is applied to occlude the oesophagus against the vertebral column as the patient goes to sleep – the patient should be warned about the use of cricoid pressure, as it may cause a chocking sensation as pressure is applied. The cricoid bone is used because it forms a complete ring and the tracheal lumen is not distorted.

The following are indications for RSI:

- Full stomach or delayed gastric emptying, e.g. due to trauma or opiate administration
- Obstetric anaesthesia with risk of acid aspiration
- History of regurgitation or hiatus hernia
- Patient starved for less than 6 h and requiring emergency surgery
- Clinical bowel obstruction or peritonitis.

Problems of RSI include:

- haemodynamic instability due to excessive or inadequate intravenous anaesthetic agent, leading to hypotension or hypertension and awareness;
- difficulty in intubating the trachea.

● INTRAVENOUS SEDATION

Intravenous sedation is a technique in which the use of a drug or drugs produces a state of depression of the CNS enabling treatment to be carried out, but during which verbal contact with the patient is maintained throughout. The level of sedation must be such that the patient remains conscious, retains protective reflexes, and is able to respond to verbal commands.

Midazolam is a commonly used intravenous sedative for upper and lower gastrointestinal endoscopy. Midazolam:

- is a member of the benzodiazepine group of drugs;
- causes dose-dependent transition from sedation to hypnosis;
- can produce loss of consciousness and anaesthesia at higher doses;
- is a smooth muscle relaxant.

The dosage of midazolam is 0.1–0.35 mg/kg body weight, depending on the age and the physical status of the patient. The drug should be administered in small incremental doses.

Flumazenil antagonises the effects of midazolam. The half-life of flumazenil is less than 1 h.

Intravenous sedation generally creates smooth conditions for carrying out minor procedures. Occasionally it produces loss of inhibition and agitation from the pain. Intravenous sedation works very well in combination with opiates such as fentanyl. Used together, midazolam and fentanyl have a potentially respiratory-depressant effect, especially in elderly patients, and it is important to have to hand all the necessary equipment for resuscitation and facilities to administer oxygen.

● REGIONAL ANAESTHESIA

The practice of regional anaesthesia as a whole anaesthetic or in combination with general anaesthesia has increased significantly. In this chapter we look specifically at spinal and epidural blocks and the pharmacology of the local anaesthetic agents.

Advantages of regional anaesthesia include the following:

- The patient can be awake, which may be an advantage in obstetric patients undergoing a caesarean section – the mother experiences the birth and can quickly establish a bond with her baby. Lower abdominal and lower limb operations can be done easily with spinal anaesthesia.
- Patients with significant respiratory disease such as chronic obstructive pulmonary disease (COPD) benefit from regional block, and opiates can be avoided completely.
- Regional anaesthesia provides intra- and postoperative analgesia.
- Regional anaesthesia attenuates the stress response to surgery.
  Disdvantages of regional anaesthesia include the following:

- The patient may be anxious of being awake during the operation
- The patient's fear of neurological complications
- Failure of the regional block, depending on the experience of the operator.

Mechanism of action of local anaesthetics

Stimulation of a nerve fibre results in an action potential, leading to the movement of sodium ions (Na^+) into the cell and potassium ions (K^+) out of the cell. This depolarises the nerve fibre and conducts the impulse. Local anaesthetics prevent the conduction of impulses along nerves by blocking the sodium channels. A second mechanism involves the disruption of ion channel function by the incorporation of local anaesthetic molecules into the cell membrane (Figure 27.1).

Ester and amide groups of local anaesthetics are used. Lidocaine (lignocaine), bupivacaine, L-bupivacaine and ropivacaine are the commonly used amide agents in the UK. Cocaine is the only ester agent used.

Lidocaine:

- has a rapid onset of action;
- has a duration of action of approximately 1 h when used without adrenaline (epinephrine) and of 2–2.5 h when given with adrenaline;

Figure 27.1 ● Mechanism of action of local anaesthetics.

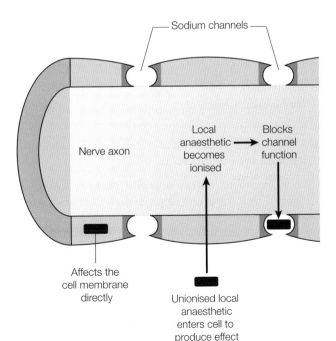

- is used to produce various blocks, from local skin infiltration to subarachnoid block;
- is given as a dose of 3–4 mg/kg body weight without adrenaline or 7 mg/kg body weight with adrenaline;
- is commonly used in dental procedures in a preparation of 2% lidocaine with 1 : 80 000 adrenaline.

Bupivacaine:

- has a slower onset of action compared with lidocaine;
- is four times more potent than lidocaine;
- has a duration of action of approximately 3–4 h, depending on the block;
- action is not prolonged by the addition of adrenaline, but adrenaline can reduce the absorption from the local injection site and may avoid local anaesthetic toxicity;
- is given as a dose of 2 mg/kg body weight with or without adrenaline.

L-Bupivacaine is the levo-isomer of bupivacaine.

The safe dosage suggested above is only a clinical guide and is for regional (epidural and nerve blocks) and local infiltration, not for subarachnoid block.

Local anaesthetic toxicity

The most common cause of local anaesthetic toxicity is inadvertent intravascular injection of the drug. This is avoided by aspirating before injecting the drug. Negative aspiration does not guarantee that the needle is not in the vessel. The drug should be injected slowly. Talking to the patient (if he or she is awake) can alert the drug administrator to the possibility of intravascular injection.

> ■ KEY POINT
> Negative aspiration does not guarantee that the needle is not in the vessel.

CNS effects of local anaesthetic toxicity include the following:

- The earliest feature of toxicity is circumoral numbness or a tingling sensation of the tongue.
- Light-headedness, anxiety and tinnitus may follow.
- This is followed by loss of consciousness and convulsions.
- The patient may become apnoeic and cardiovascular collapse may follow.

Cardiovascular effects of local anaesthetic toxicity include:

- hypotension due to vasodilation;
- arrhythmias due to slow intracardiac conduction, leading to first-degree heart block, atrioventricular block and widened QRS complex.

Local anaesthetic toxicity is usually treated by supportive measures ('ABC'). Convulsions are treated with thiopental or midazolam. Cardiovascular support is mainly with ionotropic drugs to maintain the perfusion pressure to the vital organs. Cardiac arrest is treated with 20% Intralipid® 100-mL bolus, repeated and continued as an intravenous infusion until a stable cardiac rhythm is achieved. It is a requirement that Intralipid is immediately available in all areas where potentially toxic doses of local anaesthetic are injected.

● ANATOMY OF THE SPINAL CORD

The spinal cord lies within the vertebral canal. The nerve roots emerge between the vertebrae through the intervertebral foramen. The vertebral bodies are attached together posteriorly by the supraspinous, interspinous and ligamentum flavum (Figure 27.2). Anterior and posterior longitudinal ligaments attach the bodies of the vertebrae and the intervertebral discs. The spinal cord extends from the base of the medulla oblongata and terminates as conus medullaris at the level of the lower border of the L1 or the upper border of the L2 vertebrae. In neonates, the apex of the conus medullaris lies between the third and fourth lumbar vertebrae. Below the level of the conus medullaris, the nerve roots form the cauda equina ('horse tail').

It is important to perform subarachnoid block below the L2 level without damaging the spinal cord. Three membranous layers cover the spinal cord:

- *Dura mater*: a fibrous layer attached above to the foramen magnum and below to the second sacral vertebra. The spinal dura mater represents the extension of the cerebral dura mater. The epidural space lies between the dura mater and the vertebral column.
- *Arachnoid mater*: a thin membrane closely applied to the dura mater. It covers the spinal nerves to the intervertebral foramen.
- *Pia mater*: closely applied to the spinal cord. The space between the pia mater and arachnoid mater represents the subarachnoid space, within which cerebrospinal fluid (CSF) circulates.

> ■ KEY POINT
> It is important to perform subarachnoid block below the L2 level without damaging the spinal cord.

Spinal anaesthesia

- Local anaesthetic is injected into the CSF in the subarachnoid space in small amounts (Figure 27.3).
- Injection is usually made below the second lumbar vertebra in order to avoid damage to the spinal cord.
- Spinal anaesthesia provides good anaesthesia and analgesia for operations below the umbilicus.
- Spinal anaesthesia blocks autonomic, sensory and motor nerve fibres:
  - Autonomic blockade produces vasodilation below the level of the block.
  - Sensory and motor blockade produces loss of pain, temperature and touch sensation and loss of movement.
- Spinal blockade produces denser motor blockade than epidural blockade because the drug is deposited directly into the CSF.
- 0.5% bupivacaine hyperbaric solution (mixed with 5–10% dextrose) is commonly used for spinal anaesthesia. The hyperbaric solution makes the bupivacaine settle in a gravity-dependent fashion, which allows the anaesthetist to control the level of the block by positioning the patient after injecting the local anaesthetic into the subarachnoid space.
- The onset of the block is usually within 5 min and lasts for 2–3 h.
- Opiates such as diamorphine may be added in order to provide postoperative analgesia.

Epidural anaesthesia (analgesia)

- The local anaesthetic is injected into the epidural space between the dura mater and the vertebral column (Figure 27.3).
- The total amount and volume of the drug required to produce a block is higher than that required for spinal anaesthesia.
- Epidural anaesthesia can be performed at any level of the spinal column.
- Epidural block produces autonomic and sensory blockade, but it has a slower onset of action than spinal anaesthesia, as the drug has to penetrate the dura mater to act on the spinal cord and nerves.

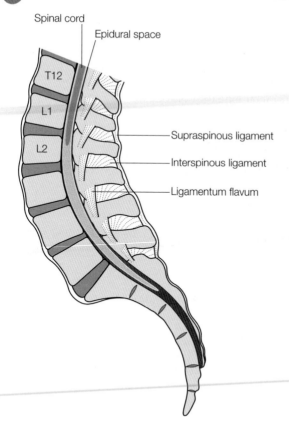

Spinal cord

Epidural space

T12

L1

L2

Supraspinous ligament

Interspinous ligament

Ligamentum flavum

Figure 27.2 ● Anatomy of the spinal column.

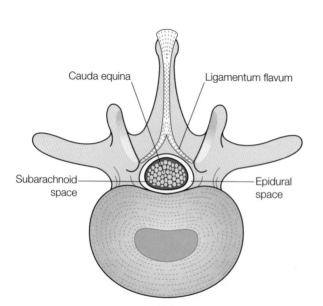

Cauda equina

Ligamentum flavum

Subarachnoid space

Epidural space

Figure 27.3 ● Cross-section of the spinal cord, showing subarachnoid and epidural spaces.

- Epidural block does not produce complete blockade. It may be difficult to operate on the patient with epidural block alone.
- 0.125% bupivacaine plain solution or with fentanyl 2 μg or 4 μg per 1-mL concentration is commonly used. The drug is infused continuously at a rate of 0–10 mL/hour to provide postoperative analgesia.
- The main advantage of epidural analgesia is that it can be used both intra- and postoperatively and it provides continuous analgesia.

Contraindications to spinal and epidural blockade

Absolute contraindications include the following:

- Bleeding diasthesis
- Patient on anticoagulation, e.g. warfarin
- Patient refusal
- Acute neurological disease, e.g. raised intracranial pressure.

Relative contraindications include the following:

- Severe stenotic valvular heart disease
- Hypovolaemia
- Sepsis – local or systemic.

Table 27.2 Complications of subarachnoid and epidural block

Subarachnoid block (spinal)	Epidural block
Hypotension due to sympathetic blockade	Hypotension due to high levels of block causing sympathetic block
Postdural puncture headache: can be avoided by using smaller-gauge pencil-point needle. This is more of a problem in younger individuals, e.g. obstetric patients	Dural tap: accidental dural tap with a 16 or 18G epidural needle can cause severe headache. This is usually treated with rehydration and simple analgesics. If the patient is not responding, epidural blood patch may be required
Urinary retention may be associated with administration of large volume of intravenous fluid	Total spinal anaesthesia may occur because of the large volume of the epidural solution injected into the subarachnoid space accidentally
Labyrinthine disturbances	Massive epidural block and subdural block
Cranial nerve palsy (sixth nerve palsy): usually temporary. The longer intracranial course of the sixth nerve causes stretching of the nerve due to intracranial hypotension	Intravenous toxicity
Meningitis and meningism: strict aseptic precaution is mandatory	Urinary retention
Nausea, vomiting and itching due to the addition of opiates to the local anaesthetic agent	Shivering
Spinal cord damage due to inappropriate level of needle insertion, leading to permanent neurological damage or paraplegia: extremely rare	Epidural haematoma and abscess. Spinal cord damage: damage to single nerve root or paraplegia is rare

Monitoring

Epidural analgesia requires monitoring the level of the local anaesthetic block on the ward at regular intervals. High levels of sympathetic blockade due to continuous infusion of local anaesthetic can precipitate hypotension. Patients usually respond to bolus fluid administration or decreased rate of infusion, or both. It may not be advisable to stop the epidural infusion completely, because of the recurrence of pain, unless the patient has severe hypotension – call for anaesthetic review. Remember that hypotension may occur because of postoperative bleeding.

Complications of subarachnoid and epidural block

Table 27.2 shows the main complications of subarachnoid and epidural block.

Local infiltration

Local anaesthetic infiltration may be used as the sole anaesthetic to carry out procedures such as excision biopsy of a lymph node. It is routine practice to infiltrate the wound at the end of surgery in order to keep the patient pain-free and to reduce the use of other analgesics such as morphine. Cutaneous nerves require less concentration of local anaesthetic agent to produce the block; this gives the flexibility of using more volume of local anaesthetic solution to produce a reliable block. The addition of a vasoconstrictor agent such as adrenaline may be useful to prolong the effect and to improve the surgical field; however, it may be detrimental in places where there are end arteries, such as the digits, toes, tip of the nose, ears and penis.

● SUMMARY

This chapter provides an idea of practice in general and regional anaesthesia with particular reference to the pharmacology of intravenous, inhalational anaesthetics, opiate analgesics and local anaesthetics. An understanding of opioid analgesics and local anaesthetics is important for surgeons because they provide pain relief and manage epidurals on the ward before the arrival of the anaesthetist. The text also outlines the principles of the intravenous sedation and local anaesthetic toxicity management because many of the procedures are done under local anaesthesia and sedation by the surgeons themselves.

● QUESTIONS

1 What is the purpose of preoperative assessment?
2 What is the ASA classification?
3 What are the disadvantages of ASA classification?
4 How is general anaesthesia performed?
5 What are the common intravenous anaesthetic agents?
6 What are the problems of intravenous induction?
7 What are the common inhalational anaesthetic agents?
8 What are the indications for inhalational induction?
9 What is intravenous sedation? What are the common drugs used?
10 What are the common opiates? How do they act?
11 What are the side effects of opiates?
12 What is regional anaesthesia?
13 Describe spinal and epidural anaesthesia.
14 What are the complications of spinal anaesthesia?

15 What are the complications of epidural anaesthesia?
16 What are the commonly used dosages of local anaesthetic?
17 What are the features of local anaesthetic toxicity?
18 How would you prevent and treat local anaesthetic toxicity?
19 What are the contraindications for the use of adrenaline along with local anaesthetic?

● FURTHER READING

Aitkenhead AR, Rowbotham DJ, Smith G (2001). *Textbook of Anaesthesia*, 4th edn. Edinburgh: Churchill Livingstone.

Anaesthesia UK. www.frca.co.uk.

Wood M, Wood AJJ (1990). *Drugs and Anaesthesia: Pharmacology for Anaesthesiologists*, 2nd edn. London: Lippincott Williams & Wilkins.

28 | *Surgical considerations in hydatid disease*

Vikram J Anand, Qassim F Baker and Samie Safar

● INTRODUCTION

Hydatid disease has been a well-known entity since the era of Hippocrates. Three species of tapeworm are of importance in human hydatid disease worldwide: *Echinococcus granulosus*, *Echinococcus multilocularis* and *Echinococcus vogeli*. The most common causative organism for hydatid disease is the helminth *E. granulosus*. The classification of helminths is shown in Tables 28.1, 28.2 and 28.3 (Chatterjee, 1973).

Echinococcus granulosus is distributed throughout the world. The infestation is common in sheep-farming areas of Greece, Turkey, the Middle East, Australasia, South Africa, parts of America, and India. The disease is endemic in central India. Due to its varied morphological presentations and involvement of various body sites, it gives rise to varying clinical symptomatology. The dog is the primary host, and the sheep is an intermediate host. Humans are usually accidental hosts. Hydatid disease can be found in any age group and in any part of the body, except the hair and nails. Common sites of involvement in humans, and their respective incidences, are: liver (75%), lung (15%), muscle (4%), kidney (2%), spleen (2%), bone (1%), and other sites (e.g. brain, breast, heart, orbit, 1%) (Taori *et al.*, 2004).

Table 28.1 Nomenclature and classification of helminths

Platyhelminthes	Nemathelminthes
Cestodes, Trematodes	Nematodes
Flattened, leaf-like, segmented	Elongated, cylindrical, unsegmented
Mostly hermaphrodite	Sexes separate
Alimentary canal incomplete or entirely lacking	Alimentary canal complete
Body cavity absent	Body cavity present

Table 28.2 Nomenclature and classification of Platyhelminthes – the Cestodes and Trematodes (flattened, leaf-like, segmented)

Cestodes	Trematodes
Fish tapeworm (*Dyphyllobothrium latum*)	Classically Schistosomiases
Beef tapeworm (*Taenia saginata*)	*Schistosoma haematobium* causing haematuria
Pork tapeworm (*Taenia solium*)	*Schistosoma mansoni* causing dysentery
Larval stage of pork tapeworm (cysticercus cellulose of *T. solium*)	*Schistosoma japonicum* causing dysentery and cirrhosis
Dwarf tapeworm (*Hymenolepis nana*)	
Dog tapeworm (*Echinococcus granulosus*)	

Table 28.3 Nemathelminthes – the nematodes (elongated, cylindrical, unsegmented)

Whip worm (*Trichuris trichiura*)

Hook worm (*Anchylostoma duodenale*)

Thread worm or pin worm (*Enterobius vermicularis*)

Round worm (*Ascaris lumbricoides*)

Filariasis (*Wuchereria bancrofti*)

African eye worm (*Loa loa*)

Guinea worm (*Dracunculus medinensis*)

In the UK, the important intermediate hosts for *E. granulosus* are sheep. Current evidence suggests that the main areas for hydatid disease in Wales are Powys, Monmouthshire, and farms on the southern slopes of the Brecon Beacons and the Black Mountains. A pocket of disease is also present in the part of southern Herefordshire adjacent to southern Powys (Health Protection Agency, 2007).

● LIFECYCLE OF *ECHINOCOCCUS GRANULOSUS*

Figure 28.1 shows the lifecycle of *E. granulosus*.

The adult worm (Figure 28.2) is a small tapeworm, measuring 3–6 mm in length. It comprises a scolex (head), neck and strobilia consisting of three segments. The terminal segment is by far the biggest, measuring 2–3 mm in length and 0.6 mm in breadth. The scolex bears four suckers and a protrusible rostellum with two circular rows of hooks. The neck is short and thick.

● SYMPTOMS OF HYDATID DISEASE

Patients present with a wide range of symptoms, depending on the following factors:

● *Involved organ*: with liver involvement there are often no symptoms and the problem comes to light only on investigation of unrelated complaints; hepatomegaly may be a presentation. In

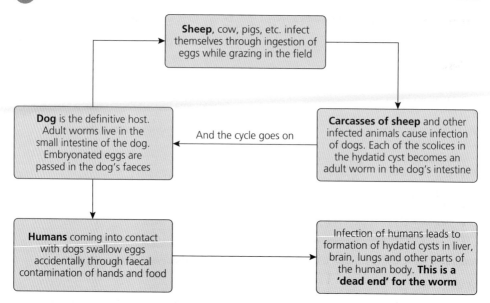

Figure 28.1 ● Lifecycle of *Echinococcus granulosus*.

Figure 28.2 ● The adult *Echinococcus granulosus* worm. Total length 3–6 mm. Head has four suckers. Neck is short and thick. Strobila has three segments, terminal segment is largest, measuring 2–3 mm.

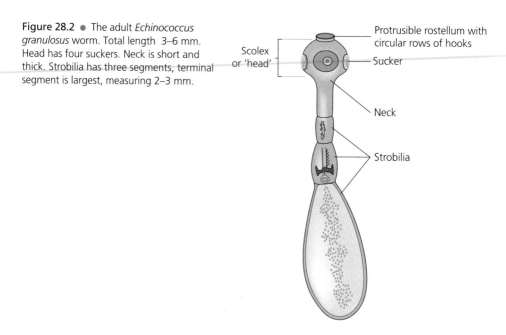

pulmonary hydatid disease, there may be no pulmonary symptoms and the disease may come to light while doing a routine chest X-ray.

- *Size of cyst:* small cysts may cause no symptoms, unless they are located in the brain, where they may cause neurological symptoms, depending on the specific location of the cyst.
- *Complications caused by untreated hydatid disease:* may produce a variety of symptoms (see below).

Immunological reactions such as asthma and anaphylaxis may be due to the release of hydatid fluid into the body.

Complications of untreated hydatid disease

Complications in untreated hydatid disease can arise due to the following reasons:

- *Pressure effects on adjacent organs:* this may cause obstructive jaundice, dysphagia, dyspepsia or dyspnoea, depending on the location of the cyst. Pressure effects in the brain may produce a variety of neurological symptoms.
- *Infection and abscess formation:* the patient may present with intercostal pain, sepsis or septicaemia.
- *Calcification of cyst wall:* this is a late presentation and implies a dead or living parasite.
- *Rupture of the hydatid cyst into:*
  - *Biliary tree:* may cause cholangitis and obstructive jaundice
  - *Peritoneal cavity:* may cause anaphylaxis and widespread dissemination, causing acute abdomen; carries a poor prognosis
  - *Pleural cavity or the lung:* causes pleural effusion or bronchopleural fistula
  - *Pericardium:* produces cardiac tamponade
  - *Blood vessels:* causes anaphylactic reaction or severely allergic manifestations.

● DIAGNOSIS OF HYDATID DISEASE

Eosinophil count is raised in about 25 per cent of patients with hydatid disease (Orloff, 1978). Diagnosis of hydatid disease can be made based on the following tests:

- Radiological tests
- Ultrasound examination
- Computed tomography (CT) scan
- Magnetic resonance imaging (MRI)
- Immunological tests, which include:
  - Intradermal test (Casoni test)
  - Complement fixation test
  - Indirect haemagglutination test
- Fine-needle aspiration (FNA) of the cyst.

Radiological tests

An abdominal X-ray may show the calcified wall of the cyst, suggesting a diagnosis of hydatid cyst. Chest X-ray may show an elevated right dome of the diaphragm in a patient with hydatid disease involving the right lobe of the liver. All radiological tests are indirect tests and may only suggest the presence of hydatid disease; they are not diagnostic of the disease.

> ■ KEY POINT
> All radiological tests are indirect tests and may only suggest the presence of hydatid disease; they are not diagnostic of the disease.

Ultrasound examination

This is a reliable screening test. However, if only a single cyst is present, then the reliability of the test is not good. Simple cysts with well-defined borders and uniform anechoic contents are not pathognomonic for echinococcal cysts because non-parasitic cysts have the same appearance. Cysts with a visible split wall inside (floating membrane or water lily sign) are pathognomonic of hydatid cysts (Brunetti and Filice, 2008).

In several studies, a correct diagnosis was made using ultrasound examination of the cyst complemented by immunological tests (Babcock *et al.*, 1978).

Figure 28.3 ● Contrast Enhanced CT Scan of upper abdomen showing typical findings of hydatid disease in liver.

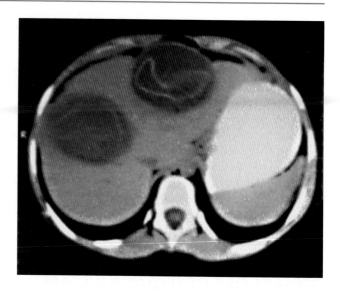

Computed tomography

Computed tomography is more descriptive and has a better reliability for hydatid cyst than ultrasound examination. In developing countries, the cost of CT may be prohibitive (Figure 28.3).

Immunological tests

The Casoni test is associated with a large number of false-positive results and therefore has been replaced in Western countries by indirect haemagglutination and serum immunoelectrophoresis, which have a diagnostic accuracy of 85–90 per cent (Amir-Jahed et al., 1975). However, Casoni's test is still used in many developing countries the world to diagnose hydatid disease.

In Casoni's test, 0.2 mL of sterile hydatid fluid is injected intradermally. A weal occurring in 20 min is a positive test. The weal is generally large (5 cm in diameter (Chatterjee, 1973). The test is positive in 90 per cent of cases of hydatid disease. However, the test remains positive for many years after the hydatid cyst has been removed (Evans, 2003).

Serological tests that indicate hydatid infection, such as the indirect haemagglutination test, the complement fixation test and immunoelectrophoretic assay, are easily available (Orloff, 1978). The indirect haemagglutination test and enzyme-linked immunosorbent assay (ELISA) are the most widely used methods for detection of anti-Echinococcus antibodies (immunoglobulin G, IgG) (Brunetti and Filice, 2008). It is generally accepted that the indirect haemagglutination test is more specific than the other tests (Garabedian et al., 1959).

Fine-needle aspiration of the cyst

Ultrasound-guided FNA can be used to obtain a sample of the cyst fluid for histological examination in order to confirm the presence of hydatid disease. Microscopic examination after centrifugation of the specimen reveals numerous hooklets, and parts of the laminated membrane and scolices, which confirm the diagnosis of the disease (Handa et al., 2005).

During FNA, contrast medium can be injected into the cyst to exclude communication between the cyst and the biliary tree. The communication, if present, can be obliterated during surgery.

A word of caution: Even though recent publications bear out that chances of anaphylactic reaction are not as high as was previously thought, it still needs to be emphasised that each time puncture of the hydatid cyst is considered we should be fully prepared for management of an anaphylactic reaction, should it occur.

● MEDICAL TREATMENT OF HYDATID DISEASE

The drugs commonly used for medical treatment of hydatid disease are:

- Albendazole
- Mebendazole
- Praziquantel.

Albendazole and mebendazole are the only antihelminthic drugs that are effective against cystic echinococcosis. Albendazole is the drug of choice against this disease because its degree of systemic absorption and penetration into hydatid cysts is superior to that of mebendazole. Albendazole in combination with percutaneous aspiration (see below, Surgical treatment of hydatid disease) can lead to a reduction in cyst size. Presurgical use of albendazole in echinococcal infestations reduces the risk of recurrence and facilitates surgery by reducing intracystic pressure (Brunetti and Filice, 2008).

Albendazole

Albendazole causes death of the worm by energy depletion and immobilisation of the worm. Treatment with albendazole results in a cure in as many as 70–80 per cent of patients. Patients who do not show obvious initial evidence of response may be found to be cured when observed over several years. The standard dose of albendazole is 400 mg twice daily or 15 mg/kg/day for 1–6 months.

There are two regimens for treatment with albendazole:

- *Daily uninterrupted therapy:* albendazole 400 mg twice daily for 3 months.
- *Cyclical therapy:* Albendazole 400 mg twice daily for 4 weeks separated by 1–2 weeks without drugs. Patients receive three such cycles.

Perisurgical use of albendazole consists of 400 mg of albendazole twice daily 1 week before and 4 weeks after surgery. This reduces the risk of recurrence and facilitates surgery by reducing intracystic pressure.

Albendazole is absorbed poorly from the gut. Absorption increases five-fold when the drug is taken with a fatty meal (40 g).

> ■ KEY POINT
> Albendazole is absorbed poorly from the gut. Absorption increases five-fold when taken with a fatty meal (40 g).

The side effects of albendazole include hypersensitivity and hepatic toxicity. The toxicity of the drug increases when co-administered with dexamethasone, cimetidine, ritonavir or praziquantel (Brunetti and Filice, 2008). The safety of albendazole during pregnancy is not established.

Mebendazole

Mebendazole causes worm death by selectively and irreversibly blocking the uptake of glucose and other nutrients by the worm. The dose of mebendazole is 50 mg/kg/day orally for 3 months (Brunetti and Filice, 2008).

The side effects of mebendazole include hypersensitivity. Carbamazepine and phenytoin decrease the effects of mebendazole, whereas cimetidine may increase mebendazole levels. The safety of mebendazole during pregnancy is not established.

Praziquantel

Praziquantel is used for the treatment of schistosomiasis. However, it has been suggested that praziquantel offers greater efficacy of treatment for hydatid disease. The drug is administered once a week in a dose of 20–40 mg/kg during treatment with albendazole. Praziquantel is available in 600-mg film-coated tablets. The use of praziquantel with rifampicin is not recommended because rifampicin may make praziquantel less effective (Karawi et al., 1995; MayoClinic.com, 2008). Praziquantel has toxic side effects; it is hepatotoxic and causes alopecia. The role of praziquantel in the treatment of hydatid disease is evolving and is not firmly established.

● MEDICAL TREATMENT IN INOPERABLE AND RECURRENT HYDATID DISEASE

Inoperable hydatid disease

Surgery is contraindicated in patients at the extremes of age, in pregnant women, in patients with comorbid diseases, in patients with extensive or recurrent disease and in patients with cysts that are difficult to access. Operative mortality varies from 0.5 per cent to 4 per cent in centres with adequate medical and surgical facilities. Cyst fluid spillage can occur during surgery, resulting in anaphylactic reaction (Khuroo, 2002).

No satisfactory therapy for inoperable multiple hydatid disease was available until Heath et al. (1975) demonstrated the effect of mebendazole in experimental hydatid disease. Subsequently, benzimidazoles have been used clinically for multiple, inoperable hydatidosis with encouraging results (Bekhti et al., 1977; Morris et al., 1983). In one study, a child with inoperable hydatid cysts in the liver was treated successfully with albendazole; the cysts regressed and disappeared after treatment (Singh et al., 1995). The child, who had 15 cysts in the liver, was given albendazole 600 mg/day for 3 weeks. The course was repeated for 9 months with a week's break between each course.

Recurrence of hydatid disease

Recurrence of hydatid disease can be treated satisfactorily with medical treatment. Surgery is often technically more demanding in recurrent cases and carries higher morbidity.

● ANATOMY OF THE HYDATID CYST AND SURGICAL TREATMENT

Anatomy of the hydatid cyst

In order to plan surgical management of a case of hydatid disease, it is important to understand the anatomy of the hydatid cyst (Figure 28.4):

- The *pericyst* is the condensed host tissue. For instance, in the case of hydatid cyst of the liver, the pericyst consists of condensed liver tissue. Normal liver tissue lies peripheral to the pericyst.
- The *cyst wall* has two layers:
  - The *ectocyst* is the laminated hyaline membrane. To the naked eye, the ectocyst has the appearance of the white portion of hard-boiled egg. The ectocyst is elastic and, when incised or ruptured, curls in on itself, thereby exposing the inner layer containing the brood capsule and daughter cysts.

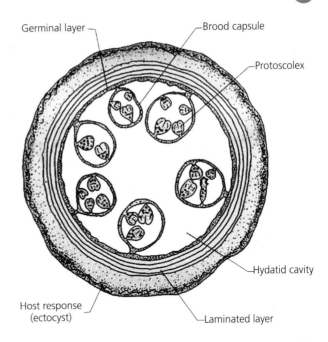

Figure 28.4 ● Diagrammatic scheme showing the anatomy of the hydatid cyst.

- The *endocyst* is the very thin, highly cellular, inner germinal layer. This is the living part of the parasite. It is the vital layer, giving rise to the brood capsules with scolices. This layer also secretes the specific hydatid fluid.
- *Hydatid fluid* is a clear, colourless fluid with a specific gravity of 1005–1010. The fluid has a pH of 6.7. The fluid is antigenic and is used for immunological tests. The fluid contains sodium chloride, sodium sulphate, sodium phosphate, and sodium and calcium salts of succinic acid. The fluid is highly toxic and, when absorbed, gives rise to anaphylactic symptoms.
- *Hydatid sand* is a granular deposit that settles to the bottom. It consists of liberated brood capsules, free scolices and loose hooklets (Chatterjee, 1973).

Surgical treatment of hydatid cyst

Based on the understanding of the anatomy of the hydatid cyst, the following surgical options for management of hydatid disease are available:

Cystopericystectomy

The complete cyst is excised, with the dissection starting between the pericyst and the normal tissue (plane C in Figure 28.5). The dissection causes significant blood loss.

Peripheral and unilobar echinococcal cysts can also be treated with laparoscopic surgery using partial cystopericystectomy and drainage. Laparoscopic surgery is indicated only for superficial and anteriorly located lesions.

Ectocystectomy

The cyst is removed by dissecting between the ectocyst and the pericyst (plane B in Figure 28.5). It is technically difficult to get into this plane.

Endocystectomy

The plane for dissection is created between the endocyst and the ectocyst (plane A in Figure 28.5). Blood loss is considerably less and the procedure is effective in treating the echinococ-

Fig 28.5 ● Hydatid cyst. Planes A, B and C are the three key planes which form the basis of surgical intervention. (Figure modified substantially and redrawn from http://www.pathobio.sdu.edu.cn /sdjsc/webteaching/Course/webt each/Cestoda/Echinococcus-20granulosus/broodcapsule.jpg)

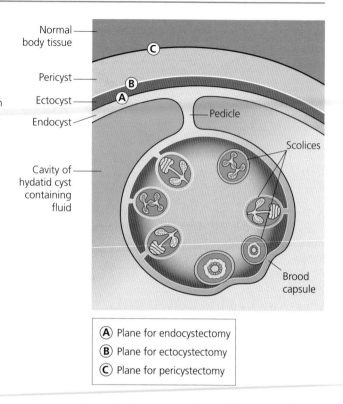

Normal body tissue

Pericyst

Ectocyst

Endocyst

Pedicle

Scolices

Cavity of hydatid cyst containing fluid

Brood capsule

(A) Plane for endocystectomy
(B) Plane for ectocystectomy
(C) Plane for pericystectomy

Fig 28.6 ● Specimen of surgically removed hydatid cyst by endocystectomy.

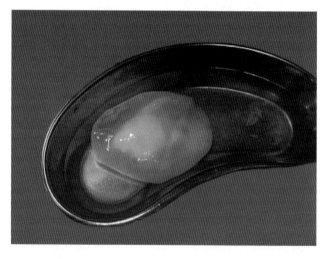

cus cyst. Figure 28.6 shows a specimen after endocystectomy. This is the most commonly performed procedure. Before injecting the scolicidal agent, it is important to make sure that no bile-stained fluid is aspirated (this indicates communication with the biliary system).

■ KEY POINT

Before injecting the scolicidal agent, it is important to make sure that no bile-stained fluid is aspirated.

Liver resection

This procedure is adopted for cysts located on the borders of the liver and for lesions involving the left lobe of the liver. Part of the liver bearing the hydatid cyst is removed.

Liver transplantation

This procedure is required in extreme cases where the hydatid cyst involves the entire liver.

Securing the area around the cyst

It is imperative to secure the area around the cyst during cystopericystectomy, ectocystectomy and endocystectomy. This is to ensure that there is no spillage into the peritoneal cavity if the cyst ruptures during removal. The area can be secured using one of the following methods:

- Packing the area around the cyst with packs soaked in scolicidal agents such as silver nitrate, hypertonic saline, povidone–iodine or any of the scolicidal agents listed in the section Scolicidal agents (see below).
- Use of a plastic drape sutured around the margins of the cyst (Aarons, 2003). This ensures that, in the event of a spillage, the hydatid fluid containing daughter cysts does not come into contact with the peritoneal cavity.
- Saidi and Nazarian (1971) describe the use of a cryogenic cone, which was made to adhere to the cyst surface by freezing. This was an effective means for the purpose but had some drawbacks: (i) the risk of damage to other structures, such as bowel, coming into contact with the freezing ring; (ii) the need to excise the part of the cyst damaged by freezing; and (iii) if the cyst fluid at body temperature flowed into the cone, the frozen seal thawed and the protection was frequently lost (Kune, 1985).
- Aarons and Kune (1983) developed a suction cone that adhered to the cyst wall. The cones are supplied in sets of two. An area of the cyst wall slightly larger than the base of the cone is exposed, the cone is placed in position, and suction is applied. Once the cone is firmly adherent to the cyst wall, the operation of removal of the hydatid cysts can proceed (Kune, 1985).

Incisions for surgical approach

The choice of incision depends on the following factors:

- Organ involved
- Location of the cysts within the involved organ
- Presence of any additional complicating factors.

Hepatic hydatid disease

Since the liver is the site of involvement in over 75 per cent cases, we will consider hepatic hydatid disease here:

- *Right paramedian incision:* used to deal with a cyst involving the right anterior lobe of the liver.
- *Right thoracoabdominal approach:* required for a posteriorly or posterolaterally located cyst in the liver.
- *Upper midline or left paramedian incision:* required for cysts located within the left lobe of the liver. However, midline incision with full mobilisation of the liver ligaments can approach most hydatid cysts, even in difficult locations. Intraoperative ultrasound scanning, if available, is a useful tool to ensure that no further cyst has been missed (which is a common cause for recurrent hydatid cyst).

After removal of hydatid cyst from the liver, management of the residual cavity involves the following:

- Closure of the cavity if the cyst is small
- Drainage of the cavity until the drainage stops, which may take a few days or longer
- Marsupialisation of the cavity
- Omentoplasty by filling the hydatid cavity with omental plug. This is the most frequently done procedure.

Abdominal hydatid disease

This requires suitably placed incisions, depending on the location of the disease within the abdomen.

Pulmonary hydatid disease

Cysts located within the lung require a thoracotomy. The intercostal space used for approach depends on the location of the cyst within the lung. Frequently, surgeons go through the bed of a rib after doing a rib resection. This is a matter of personal preference for the surgeon. While going through an intercostals space, it is safe to remain close to the upper border of the rib, since the intercostal vessels are located close to the lower border of the rib. Having dealt with the cyst, the thoracotomy incision is closed with an intercostal drain.

Splenic hydatid disease

The spleen is involved in approximately 2 per cent of cases of hydatid disease (Taori *et al.*, 2004). Diagnosis of the disease is made by tests (see above). Medical treatment is the treatment of choice when the spleen is involved. Splenectomy is resorted to only in cases where the spleen is massively enlarged and there is a danger of rupture of the spleen due to trauma. Splenectomy is avoided as far as possible, because of the risk of causing overwhelming postsplenectomy infection (OPSI; Box 28.1), a life-threatening infection caused after the spleen has been removed (Brigden and Pattullo, 1999; Working Party of the British Committee for Standards in Haematology Clinical haematology Task Force, 1996).

The incision used is the same as that used for splenectomy for any other indication. Upper left paramedian is frequently found to be suitable. However, for a very large spleen due to multiple cysts, a left thoracoabdominal approach is required. Polar hydatid cysts can be managed in the same way as endocystectomy of the liver, unless the spleen is involved with multiple hydatids or is massively enlarged.

● SCOLICIDAL AGENTS

The instillation of scolicidal agents into the cyst has been considered part of the classic surgical approach to minimise the possibility of recurrent disease attributable to peritoneal spillage. The following scolicidal agents can be used:

- Hypertonic saline (20% saline) (normal saline – 0.9% – is not effective as a scolicidal agent)
- Chlorhexidine gluconate 0.04%
- Hydrogen peroxide 3%
- Silver nitrate 0.5%
- Povidone–iodine (polyvinylpyrrolidone–iodine) 1%, 5% or 10%
- Cetrimide 0.5%
- Ethanol 95%.

Formalin 2% or 5% is contraindicated as a scolicidal agent because of the danger of causing irreversible sclerosing cholangitis.

Box 28.1 Overwhelming post-splenectomy infection (OPSI) and its prevention

■ Infection occurs after splenectomy in 4 per cent of patients who have not received prophylaxis.

■ Encapsulated bacteria cause the infection. Over 50 per cent of the infections are caused by *Streptococcus pneumoniae, Haemophilus influenzae* and *Neisseria meningitides*. Other pathogens include *Escherichia coli, Pseudomonas aeruginosa, Capnocytophagia canimorsus*, group B streptococci, and protozoa such as plasmodium, leading to malaria (Lipman, 2005).

■ The greatest risk of OPSI occurs in the first 2 years after splenectomy.

■ Mortality from OPSI is high, reaching as much as 50 per cent.

Prevention of OPSI can be done by two methods:

■ *Antibiotic prophylaxis with penicillin or amoxicillin:* the chief medical officer in the UK recommends lifelong prophylaxis with oral phenoxymethylpenicillin (or erythromycin for people allergic to penicillin). Patients who develop infection despite vaccination and antibacterial prophylaxis should go into hospital for treatment with broad-spectrum systemic antibiotics (Lipman, 2005). Amoxicillin has been recommended for antibiotic prophylaxis. This drug is less well tolerated in young children and is more expensive. The advantages of amoxicillin over penicillin in adults include better absorption, broader spectrum and longer shelf-life. Prophylaxis is required in children up to the age of 16 years.

■ *Immunization:* pneumococcal, meningococcal and *Haemophilus* vaccinations are recommended 2 weeks before the planned operation. Vaccination should be done immediately postoperatively for emergency cases and then repeated every 5–10 years.

● MINIMALLY INVASIVE TREATMENT – PUNCTURING THE CYST

Puncture of echinococcal cysts traditionally has been discouraged because of the risks of anaphylactic shock and spillage of the fluid. Now an increasing number of articles have reported its effectiveness and safety in treating liver echinococcal cysts (Filice *et al.*, 1990).

In a compilation of series, 4209 cysts had been punctured for diagnostic or therapeutic purposes (Brunetti and Filice, 2008). There were 16 cases of anaphylactic shock; two of these (0.047%) were lethal. Peritoneal seeding has never been reported.

From a diagnostic point of view, cyst puncture is the only method that provides a direct histological diagnosis of the parasitic cysts in hydatid disease. The procedure shortens the time of treatment and recovery and, therefore, is a valuable alternative to surgery in terms of reduction in costs and hospital stay.

Puncture–aspirate–inject–re-aspirate (PAIR)

With albendazole cover, cysts are punctured using ultrasound or CT guidance. An anaesthetist should be present during the procedure in case of allergic manifestations or anaphylactic shock. Usually, a small quantity of fluid is aspirated first and examined by light microscope to look for the presence of scolices. If they are present, the cyst is aspirated completely. A scolicidal agent, usually hypertonic saline solution or ethanol, is injected and left for a variable period of time (usually 5–30 min) and then re-aspirated. The destruction of proto-scolices can be observed in the fluid sample aspirated after the injection of a scolicidal agent.

Contrast medium can be injected into the cyst at this point to exclude the possible connection of the cyst with the biliary tree.

MANAGEMENT OF INTRABILIARY RUPTURE OF HYDATID CYST

According to Kune (1985), intrabiliary rupture of hydatid cyst can often be predicted before surgery because of the clinical presentation of symptoms of cholestasis, such as jaundice, dark urine and pale stools, sometimes accompanied by fever and rigors. The cause of jaundice in association with hepatic hydatid cysts is almost always rupture into the biliary tree. It is therefore relevant to do a cholangiogram in order to exclude the presence of hydatid material in the common bile duct (CBD).

If the presence of hydatid tissue in the CBD is ascertained before surgery, then endoscopic sphincterotomy of the sphincter of Oddi should be performed before undertaking surgical intervention. This ensures the automatic expulsion of the small bits of hydatid tissue from the biliary tree after exploration of the CBD.

The hepatic cyst is dealt with in the usual manner. Care must be taken to identify and suture the communication that caused the hydatid elements to enter the biliary tree. At an appropriate juncture during surgical management, an operative cholangiogram should be performed to identify the communication.

Exploration of the CBD is done in the usual manner and the hydatid material is removed. A Fogarty catheter can be passed proximally into the duct system to ensure the removal of the hydatid tissue from the proximal reaches of the biliary tree. After exploration, the CBD is closed with a T-tube. A T-tube cholangiogram is done after 10–14 days before the T-tube is removed. The gallbladder is not removed during the exploration of CBD as this is not the seat of any disease. After surgery, the cavity of the hydatid cyst is obliterated with omentoplasty; a drain is always left in, or very close to, the cavity.

A persistent biliary fistula after surgery is diagnosed by the persistence of bile drainage from the tube left in or near the cyst. This situation can be resolved by adding an endoscopic sphincterotomy if one has not already been done. If this fails to stop the bile drainage, internal drainage by cystoenterostomy can be done, which ensures the drainage of bile into the small intestine.

MANAGEMENT OF INFECTED HYDATID CYSTS

Infection in a hydatid cyst usually does not occur primarily. Infection is a sequel to a complication such as rupture of the cyst into the biliary tree. Often the infection develops following surgical intervention when the communication with the biliary tree is not recognised or not dealt with effectively. If the infection is recognised preoperatively due to rupture of the cyst, then appropriate steps can be taken to obliterate the communication during surgery. The patient should be started on appropriate antibiotics before surgery. The cavity of the cyst should be treated with omentoplasty after the contents of the cyst have been removed.

Omentoplasty consists of using the omentum to fill the cavity of the cyst. Once the omentum is packed into the cyst cavity, the omentum is stitched to the margins of the cavity by a few interrupted stitches using absorbable suture material. This ensures the retention of the omentum in the cyst cavity. A drain is left near the cavity for a suitable period of time.

INFECTION WITH *ECHINOCOCCUS MULTILOCULARIS*

This hydatid disease is totally different from that caused by *E. granulosus* and is a rarer form of hydatid disease. The larval worm causes alveolar or multilocular hydatid disease in humans.

The definitive hosts are dogs, foxes and wolves. Intermediate (larval) hosts are field mice and rats and, occasionally, humans. The disease is frequently seen in Russia, Canada, Alaska, Switzerland and China.

The size of the adult worm is 1.2–3.7 mm – much smaller than *E. granulosus*. The infection is acquired in humans following the consumption of vegetables contaminated by faeces of dogs or foxes. The liver is the most frequently involved organ. There are numerous cysts, usually small in size and containing gelatinous material. Central necrosis with infection is sometimes seen.

Patients present with an enlarged liver with a localised swelling, which may resemble primary carcinoma of the liver. Jaundice may also be a presenting feature if the biliary tree is involved. Contrast CT or MRI helps to differentiate the condition from hepatoma.

Diagnosis can be made by immunological tests such as complement fixation, indirect haemagglutination and enzyme immunoassay (Kune, 1985). Untreated cases have a high chance of death due to jaundice, cholangitis and, sometimes, metastatic spread of the worm (Wilson and Rausch, 1980).

Surgical resection is the most effective treatment. In advanced cases with jaundice, drainage of the biliary tree is required in addition to surgical treatment of the cyst.

● SUMMARY

The chapter begins with prevalence of hydatid disease across the world including specified areas in the UK. Liver is involved in nearly 75 per cent of the cases followed by lung involvement in about 15 per cent of cases. A perspective is given to *Echinococcus granulosus* by including a classification of the helminths. The life cycle of *E. granulosus* shows dog as the definitive host. The worm comes to a dead end when it enters the human being. It is highlighted that the symptoms depend on the organ involved, size of the cyst and any complications present. Diagnosis is made by a variety of tests.

Medical, surgical and minimally invasive treatments are discussed. Albendazole and mebendazole are the two main stay drugs for medical treatment. Methods of securing the area around the cyst are highlighted when attempting surgery to ensure that there is no spillage of the contents of the cyst into the peritoneal cavity in the event of a rupture of the cyst during removal. Splenic involvement is discussed and details of OPSI (overwhelming post-splenectomy infection) and its prevention are provided following splenectomy for hydatid disease of the spleen.

Details of minimally invasive treatment are provided along with a list of various scolicidal agents. The technique of PAIR (puncture aspirate inject re-aspirate) is discussed. Details are provided for management of intrabiliary rupture of hydatid cyst and management of infected hydatid cyst. The chapter ends with a discussion on infection with *Echinococcus multilocularis*.

● QUESTIONS

1 What are the complications of liver hydatid disease?
2 How would you diagnose and treat intrabiliary rupture?
3 What is the role of medical therapy in hydatid disease?
4 What is the surgical approach for a hydatid cyst on the superior surface of the liver?
5 What scolicidal agents are available?
6 What is meant by PAIR?

● REFERENCES

Aarons B (2003). Hydatid disease of the liver in pregnancy. *ANZ J Surg* **73**: 78.

Aarons BJ, Kune GA (1983). A suction cone to prevent spillage during hydatid surgery. *ANZ J Surg* **53**: 471.

Amir-Jahed AK, Fardin R, Farzad A, *et al.* (1975). Clinical echinococcosis. *Ann Surg* **182**: 341–6.

Babcock DS, Kaufman L, Cosnow I (1978). Ultrasound diagnosis of hydatid disease (echinococcosis) in two cases. *Am J Roentgenol* **131**: 895–7.

Bekhti A, Schaaps J-P, Capron M, *et al.* (1977). Treatment of hepatic hydatid disease with mebendazole: preliminary results in four cases. *Br Med J* **2**: 1047–51.

Brigden ML, Pattullo AL (1999). Prevention and management of overwhelming post-splenectomy infection: an update. *Crit Care Med* **27**: 836–42.

Brunetti E, Filice C (2008). Echinococcosis hydatid cyst. www.emedicine.com/med/topic629.htm.

Chatterjee KD (1973). *Parasitology in Relation to Clinical Medicine*. Calcutta: KD Chatterjee.

Evans DMD (2003). *Special Tests: The Procedure and Meaning of the Commoner Tests in Hospitals*. New York: Mosby.

Filice C, Pirola F, Brunetti E, *et al.* (1990). A new therapeutic approach for hydatid liver cysts: aspiration and alcohol injection under sonographic guidance. *Gastroenterology* **98**: 1366–8.

Garabedian GA, Matossian RM, Suidan FG (1959). A correlative study of immunological tests for the diagnosis of hydatid disease. *Am J Trop Med Hyg* **8**: 67–71.

Handa U, Bal A, Mohan H (2005). Cytomorphology of hydatid disease. *Internet J Trop Med* 2005. **2**(1).

Health Protection Agency (2007). Hydatid disease (Echinococcosis). www.hpa.org.uk/infections/topics_az/zoonoses/hydatid/gen_info.htm.

Heath DD, Christie MJ, Chevis RAF (1975). The lethal effect of mebendazole on secondary *Ecchinococcus granulosus*, cysticerci of *Tenia pisiformis* and tetrathyridia of *Mesocestoides corti*. *Parasitology* **70**: 273–85.

Karawi MAA, Yasawi MI, Mohammad ARE (1995). A study on combination of praziquantel and albendazole in the treatment of hydatid disease. *JK Practitioner* **2**: 25–6.

Khuroo MS (2002). Hydatid disease: current status and recent advances. *Ann Saudi Med* **22**: 1–2.

Kune GA (1985). Hydatid disease. In: Maingot R, Schwartz SI, Ellis H, Husser WC. *Maingot's Abdominal Operations*, 8th edn. Norwalk, CT: Appleton-Century-Crofts.

Lipman HM (2005). Preventing severe infection after splenectomy. *Br Med J* **331**: 417–18.

MayoClinic.com (2008). Drugs and supplements: praziquantel (oral route). www.mayoclinic.com health/drug-information/DR601147.

Morris DL, Dykes PW, Dickson B, *et al.* (1983). Albendazole in hydatid disease. *Br Med J* **286**: 103–4.

Orloff MJ (1978). The liver. In: Sabiston DC (ed.) *Davis-Christopher Textbook of Surgery: The Biological Basis of Modern Surgical Practice*, 11th edn. Philadelphia, PA: WB Saunders Co., pp. 1149–207.

Saidi F, Nazarian T (1971). Surgical treatment of hydatid cysts by freezing of cyst wall and instillation of 0.5% silver nitrate solution. *N Engl J Med* **284**: 1346.

Singh H, Qasim M, Chugh JC, *et al.* (1995). Albendazole therapy in liver hydatidosis. *Indian Pediatr* **32**: 1105–6.

Taori KB, Mahajan SM, Hirawe SR, *et al.* (2004). Hydatid disease of breast. *Ind J Radiol Imaging* **14**: 57–60.

Wilson JP, Rausch RL (1980). Alveolar hydatid disease: a review of clinical features of indigenous cases of *Echinococcus multilocularis* infection in Alaskan Eskimos. *Am J Trop Med Hyg* **29**: 1341.

Working Party of the British Committee for Standards in Haematology Clinical haematology Task Force (1996). Guidelines for the prevention and treatment of infection in patients with an absent or dysfunctional spleen. *Br Med J* **312**: 430–34.

29 Surgical considerations in schistosomiasis and filariasis

Refaat Kamel and Munther I Aldoori

A. SCHISTOSOMIASIS

● INTRODUCTION

Schistosomiasis is a major global public health problem, affecting more than 200 million people worldwide. About 600 million people are at risk globally.

Schistosomes are trematode blood flukes that require snail intermediate hosts living in water. Snails can be contaminated by the faeces or urine of infected people. The snails then release the infective stage (cercariae), which penetrate the skin of human hosts, passing to the circulation and finally settling in the portal vein, where they mature into adult worms. The adult male and female worms swim against the direction of the bloodstream to reach their final habitat either in the mesenteric plexus of veins (*Schistosoma mansoni*, *Schistosoma japonicum*) or in the vesical plexus of veins (*Schistosoma haematobium*).

Schistosomiasis is the most common cause of (pre-sinusoidal) portal hypertension worldwide (Kamel, 2004).

> ■ KEY POINT
> Schistosomiasis is the most common cause of (pre-sinusoidal) portal hypertension worldwide.

● CLINICAL PICTURE BASED ON PATHOLOGY

The pathology of schistosomiasis is produced as a reaction to dead worms or living ova, with granuloma formation (Figure 29.1) and subsequent fibrotic reaction (cf. periportal fibrosis). Dead ova are calcified, as in the case of calcified urinary bladder.

> ■ KEY POINT
> The pathology of schistosomiasis is due to a tissue reaction to the dead worms or living ova, with subsequent fibrosis.

Figure 29.1 ● Section of the liver showing bilharzial granuloma around *Schistosoma mansoni* egg: hepatocytes appear normal and the lobular architecture is usually intact.

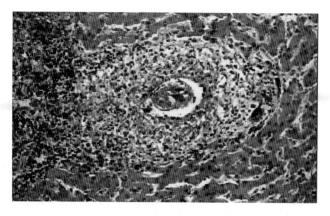

Schistosomiasis presents as two separate diseases: hepato-intestinal and urogenital (either separately or combined). Multisystem involvement is mostly hepato-intestinal, splenic and urogenital (male and female). Other systems can be affected, including the cardiopulmonary, endocrine and cerebrospinal systems and the skin.

> ■ KEY POINT
>
> Multisystem involvement is mostly hepato-intestinal, splenic and urogenital, although cardiopulmonary, endocrine, cerebrospinal and skin may also be affected.

Multiple diagnoses are common in the tropics, and this should always be kept in mind. Unlike in Western countries, where one tries to make a single diagnosis and all findings usually fit together, in the Tropics it is more common to find multiple pathologies. This can result in difficulty in diagnosis and management.

Hepato-intestinal and hepatosplenic schistosomiasis are mostly caused by *S. mansoni* and *S. japonicum*. *S. mansoni* eggs and granulomas have been found throughout the gastrointestinal tract, including the stomach, small and large intestines, pancreas, gallbladder, peritoneum and liver.

The basic pathology in the liver is granuloma formation around the portal tract, producing periportal fibrosis that looks in cut section like clay pipe ('pipe-stem appearance'). The hepatic parenchyma is not affected, and so it is a fibrotic, not cirrhotic, lesion. Portal hypertension is pre-sinusoidal.

Splenic enlargement is caused by both portal hypertension (congestive splenomegaly) and reticuloendothelial hyperplasia due to toxins of the parasite.

Hepato-intestinal and hepatosplenic schistosomiasis present with hepatomegaly, splenomegaly, and colonic and rectal polyposis (bilharzial granulomata) and should be differentiated from other types of polyposis and neoplastic lesions. It is not uncommon to present with dysenteric manifestations (Kamel, 2005).

Left colon and rectal strictures may cause acute colonic obstruction, but this is rare. Colon strictures up to 20 cm in length may be demonstrated on emergency barium enema examination and may be difficult to differentiate from other colonic lesions.

● HEPATOSPLENIC SCHISTOSOMIASIS

Classification

- *Group I:* bilharzial splenomegaly without varices or ascites
- *Group II:* bilharzial splenomegaly with varices but no ascites:

- With no history of haematemesis
- With history of haematemesis
- *Group III*: bilharzial splenomegaly with ascites (controllable or not by medical treatment) but no varices
- *Group IV*: bilharzial splenomegaly combined with varices and ascites.

Ascites

Many ascetic patients show no marked hypoalbuminaemia or gross portal hypertension sufficient to account for irreversible ascites. Post-sinusoidal veno-occlusive portal hypertension (Budd–Chiari syndrome) has been described in many endemic areas of schistosomiasis in children and young people.

Ascites raises the intra-abdominal pressure (increasing the risk of herniae, especially umbilical and para-umbilical herniae) and is dealt with by the usual classic treatment for similar lesions, but preferably using graft to reduce the risk of recurrence. Hernia in these cases is not only due to increased intra-abdominal pressure but also due to deficient collagen in the supporting abdominal wall.

Management

The general principles of management of schistosomal variceal haemorrhage are similar to those for portal hypertension and include the following:

- Sclerotherapy or banding
- Gastro-oesophageal devasularisation plus total or segmental splenectomy
- Portosystemic shunts and other allied procedures
- Transjugular intrahepatic portosystemic shunting (TIPSS)
- Splenectomy – total or segmental, either alone or combined with other techniques for variceal control (Kamel, 2004).

As the hepatocytes are usually spared in pure schistosomiasis, liver transplantation is rarely needed.

> ■ KEY POINT
> The hepatocytes are usually spared in pure schistosomiasis, liver transplantation is rarely needed.

● UROGENITAL SCHISTOSOMIASIS

Urogenital schistosomiasis may present with urinary calculosis (kidneys, ureters, bladder), hydronephrosis, pyonephrosis, and calcification of the urinary bladder. Bladder-neck obstruction, ulcers, chronic cystitis, contracted bladder and cancer of the urinary bladder are also frequently encountered in endemic areas.

Urogenital schistosomiasis usually starts with terminal, painful haematuria due to deposition of bilharzial ova in the trigone. Other bilharzial lesions include sandy patches, ulcers and leucoplakia and may be complicated with malignancy.

> ■ KEY POINT
> Terminal painful haematuria is a common presentation of urogenital schistosomiasis.

Ureteric lesions include ureteritis cystica and usually affect the lower third, which may be followed by stricture of the ureter, hydro-ureter with dilated elongated tortuous sacculated ureter, hydronephrosis (secondary to ureteric affection) and possibly pyonephrosis, which may end in renal failure.

Carcinoma of the urinary bladder is a not uncommon sequel of urinary bilharziasis.

Management

Cancer of the urinary bladder may be treated by radical cystectomy and some forms of urinary diversion.

Contracted urinary bladder, ureteric stricture, hydronephrosis and pyonephrosis are treated as similar conditions elsewhere.

In early-stage schistosomiasis of the prostate and seminal vesicles, treatment with anti-bilharzial drugs is beneficial. In the chronic stage, however, symptomatic treatment of the pain and combating of the associated bacterial infection usually succeeds.

CARDIOPULMONARY SCHISTOSOMIASIS

The lesion results from deposition of eggs in pulmonary arterioles and capillaries. It is commonly seen in *Schistosoma haematobium* and forms 7 per cent of pulmonary affections. In such cases many segmental pulmonary arteries and their arterioles suffer from endothelial proliferation resulting in endarteritis obliterans. This leads to pulmonary hypertension, pulmonary artery dilatation, hypertrophy of the right ventricle to be followed later by right-sided heart failure (Tag El-Din, 2004).

MALIGNANCY IN ASSOCIATION WITH SCHISTOSOMIASIS

Hepatocellular carcinoma associated with schistosomiasis is a consequence of associated post-hepatitis and is not related to the schistosomiasis itself. Carcinoma of the urinary bladder, however, is a common association with *S. haematobium*, which is strongly suspected to be pathogenic. Colorectal carcinoma is claimed to be associated with *S. japonicum*.

A hugely enlarged spleen should raise suspicion of the rare association with lymphoma.

DIAGNOSIS OF SCHISTOSOMIASIS

- Stool examination for active *S. mansoni* or *S. japonicum* infection.
- Urine examination for *S. haematobium* infection.
- Examination of rectal mucosa sample.
- A number of immunological tests have been used as epidemiologic tools in the diagnosis of schistosomiasis.
- Periportal fibrosis can be detected by ultrasonography and can be used for field screening of hepatic schistosomiasis in endemic areas.

DIFFERENTIAL DIAGNOSIS

Hepatosplenic schistosomiasis has to be differentiated from malaria, which may give rise to hyper-reactive malarial splenomegaly and from portal venous thrombosis, Kala-azar, lymphoma, and Laennec's and post-necrotic cirrhosis.

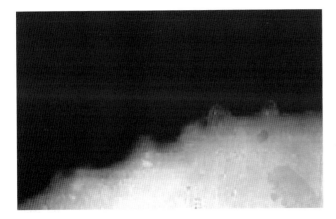

Figure 29.2 ● *Schistosoma mansoni* worm recovered from a patient with salmonella infection stained with antiserum to *Salmonella paratyphi* A and fluorescein-labelled conjugate.

INFECTIONS COMMONLY ASSOCIATED WITH SCHISTOSOMIASIS

- Chronic salmonellosis (Figure 29.2)
- Viral hepatitis B and C.

SUMMARY

- Schistosomiasis is a major global public health problem, affecting more than 200 million people. About 600 million people are at risk globally.
- Schistosomiasis is the most common cause of pre-sinusoidal portal hypertension.
- The pathology of schistosomiasis is a result of reaction to the dead worms or living ova, with granuloma formation and subsequent periportal fibrosis.
- Schistosomiasis presents as two separate diseases: hepato-intestinal and urogenital (either separate or combined).
- Hepato-intestinal and splenic schistosomiasis is usually caused by S. *mansoni* and S. *japonicum* eggs. It is a multisystem infection, involving the hepato-intestinal, splenic, urogenital, cardiopulmonary, endocrine, cerebrospinal and skin systems.
- As the hepatocytes are usually spared in pure schistosomiasis, liver transplantation is rarely needed.
- Hepato-intestinal and splenic schistosomiasis present with hepatomegaly, splenomegaly, colonic and rectal polyposis (bilharzial granulomata).
- Terminal painful haematuria is a common presentation of urogenital schistosomiasis.
- Carcinoma of the urinary bladder is a not uncommon sequel of urinary bilharziasis.
- Hepatocellular carcinoma associated with schistosomiasis is a consequence of associated posthepatitis and is not related to the schistosomiasis itself, unlike carcinoma of the urinary bladder.
- Infections commonly associated with schistosomiasis include chronic salmonellosis and viral hepatitis B and C.
- Hepatosplenic schistosomiasis has to be differentiated from malaria, portal venous thrombosis, Kala-azar, lymphoma, and Laennec's and post-necrotic cirrhosis.

QUESTIONS

1 Discuss the pathology of schistosomiasis.
2 What are the surgical complications of schistosomiasis in different systems?

3 Discuss the management of variceal haemorrhage in schistosomiasis.
4 Discuss the management of portal hypertension in schistosomiasis.
5 Discuss the clinical manifestations of schistosomiasis in various sites.
6 What are the most common infections associated with schistosomiasis?
7 Is schistosomiasis a common indication for liver transplantation?

● REFERENCES

Cook GC (2003). Schistosomiasis. In: Cook GC (ed.). *Manson's Tropical Diseases*, Vol. 3. London: WB Saunders.

Kamel R (2004). Schistosomiasis. In: Kamel R, Lumley J (eds). *Textbook of Tropical Surgery*. London: Westminster Publishing Group, pp. 1064–77.

Kamel R (2005). Benign diseases of the spleen. In: Fielding JWL, Hallissey MT (eds). *Upper Gastrointestinal Surgery*. New York: Springer, pp. 127–54.

Silva-Neto WB, Cavarzan A, Herman P (2004). Intra-operative evaluation of portal pressure and immediate results of surgical treatment of portal hypertension in schistosomotic patients submitted to esophagogastric devascularization with splenectomy. *Arq Gastroenterol* **41**: 150–54.

Strickland GT (2000). Schistosomiasis. In: Hunter GW, Strickland GT, Magill AJ (eds). *Hunter's Tropical Diseases*, 8th edn. Philadelphia, PA: WB Saunders.

Tag El-Din MA (2004). Pulmonary disease. In: Kamel R, Lumley J (eds). *Textbook of Tropical Surgery*. London: Westminster Publishing Group, pp. 394–415.

B. SURGERY OF BANCROFTIAN FILARIASIS AND LYMPHOEDEMA

- Introduction
- Lymphatic filariasis: incidence and epidemiology
- Clinical picture
- Acute retroperitoneal lymphangitis
- Chronic obstructive lesions
- Grading of Chronic Lymphoedema and Elephantiasis
- Chyluria and Lymphuria
- Chylothorax and chylous ascites

INTRODUCTION

Filariasis includes many parasitic infections, such as onchocerciasis, loiasis and bancroftian filariasis with different endemicity and clinical manifestations. The most commonly recognized type is bancroftian filariasis, which affects the lymphatic system.

Lymphatic filariasis, caused by the mosquito-borne, lymphatic-dwelling nematodes Wuchereria bancrofti and Brugia malayi, is still a common tropical parasitic disease. It is estimated that about 120 million people are affected by this disease and approximately one billion people at risk in more than 75 countries worldwide (Anitha and Shenoy, 2001).

Adult filariae may live in the lymphatics, the females produce microfilariae which live in the bloodstream or skin.

The adult worms live in lymphatics whereas their microfilariae live in blood. Adult worms may show in the dilated lymphatics by ultrasonography.

> ■ KEY POINT
> The adult filarial worms live in lymphatics whereas their microfilariae live in blood.

CLINICAL PICTURE OF FILARIASIS

The clinical manifestations may be divided into two stages:

- Acute inflammatory lesions (acute lymphangitis and lymphadenitis).
- Chronic obstructive lesions.

> ■ KEY POINT
> The clinical presentations may be divided into two stages: acute inflammatory lesions (acute lymphangitis and lymphadenitis) and chronic obstructive lesions.

Acute inflammatory adeno-lymphangitis (ADL)

The acute attacks are periodic and occur about once or twice a month. The acute lymphangitis and lymphadenitis may subside completely or leave residual thickening which will increase with the periodic exacerbation (Strickland, 2000).

Acute retroperitoneal lymphangitis

This is a rare but important complication that may be confused with acute abdominal emergency and lead to unnecessary and possibly dangerous surgery.

The onset is usually sudden with acute pain over a large area of the abdomen associated with shock and collapse. Profound toxaemia develops and the picture resembles acute peritonitis but the board-like rigidity is usually absent or not evident. In spite of energetic treatment, the mortality rate is high.

In less severe cases, there is a subacute course with slow onset; chills and rigors are less marked followed by remittent fever with pain referred to the back.

If laparotomy is performed, the findings are red oedamatous retroperitoneal tissues, especially in the midline of lower abdomen.

A residual abscess may develop as well as thrombophlebitis of the deep big veins. Treatment is conservative with antibiotics, plus the specific anti-filarial treatment (e.g. DEC citrate) in adequate dosage.

DEC acts on microfilariae but not on the adult worm. Treatment starts with 2 mg/kg body weight given three times a day for 3 weeks. The dose should be repeated at intervals of 10 days for at least 3 months.

Surgery may be indicated. Drainage or aspiration may be needed to evacuate fluid or pus collections (Kamel, 2004).

> ■ KEY POINT
> Acute retroperitoneal lymphangitis is a rare but important complication that may be confused with acute abdominal emergency and lead to unnecessary and possibly dangerous surgery.

Chronic obstructive lesions

These are caused by an adult worm lying in the cortical sinuses of lymph glands and the large lymphatics draining into them. At one end of the spectrum, perilymphangitis, lymphangitis and fibrosis may develop into intraglandular infiltration and possibly abscess formation.

The chronic stage of filariasis usually develops 10–15 years after the onset of the first acute attack. The incidence and severity of chronic clinical manifestations tend to increase with age.

Great enlargement of the lymphatic glands with fibrotic changes is common in chronic filariasis. The glands are enlarged to 5–7.5 cm in diameter and may form permanent swellings. On section they resemble an unripe pear, the central portion being fibrotic and the peripheral being glandular. They may contain numerous coiled-up adult worms.

Chronic Lymphoedema and Elephantiasis

There are four grades of chronic lymphoedema as follows:

1 Grade I: oedema which increases periodically with each attack of acute inflammation and subsides in the intervening period.
2 Grade II: oedema becomes permanent but still pits on pressure.
3 Grade III: the skin becomes hard with non-pitting oedema.
4 Grade IV: warts and varicosities and ulcers may develop on the top.

When the skin becomes chronically thickened it can be called elephantiasis and is associated with hypertrophy and fibrous hyperplasia of the subcutaneous tissues. In 95% of cases the lower extremities (either one or both), alone or in combination with the scrotum, or arms are affected. Circumscribed portions of the integuments of the upper limbs or the trunk may occur (Sharma, 2004).

■ KEY POINT
Elephantiasis mostly affects the lower extremities either alone or in combination with the scrotum. Foot, ankle, thigh, breast and vulva are rarely affected alone.

Small chemical particles found in the soil may enter the skin through the bare feet. These particles lodge in the lymphatic tissues and produce irritating effects. The traumatized tissue is then vulnerable to streptococcal infection (Kamel, 2004).

Elephantiasis neuromatosa is a rare congenital variant. It can affect any part of the body (pachydermatocele).

Obstructive lymphatic lesions occur most commonly in the lower limb, scrotum and penis. The result is elephantiasis that may reach gigantic dimensions. It is claimed that idiopathic hydrocele in endemic areas is related to filariasis. It can also affect the breast and the upper limb (Manokaran, 2005).

Lymphatic obstruction of inguinal and scrotal lymphatics can be detected by ultrasonography.

The occult syndromes are: Tropical Pulmonary Eosinophilia (TPE), filarial arthritis, filarial breast abscess, and filarial-associated immune-complex glomerulonephritis.

In filarial funiculitis, the large lymphatics associated with spermatic cord may be dilated and associated with thrombophlebitis, leading to the development of a firm indurated swollen cord, associated with hydrocele. Involvement of the penile skin is very common and prepuce escapes, as does the body of the penis. This is unlike schistosomiasis, where the body of the penis is the main site of spread of the granulomatous bilharzial tissue from the floor of the urethra, which is possibly complicated by urinary fistula. The involvement of the spermatic cord ends in matting of the tissues and the vas becomes inseparable from the rest of the cord (an important clinical finding for diagnosing filarial involvement of the cord).

The prostate and seminal vesicles are free from involvement (cf. schistosomiasis, where they are commonly involved and inguinoscrotal swellings) (Kamel, 2004).

Treatment of elephantiasis, although not really successful, is based on principles of plastic surgery.

Chyluria and Lymphuria

Lymphuria is discharge or escape of lymph into the urine. When the level of obstruction is proximal to cysterna chyli, the clinicopathological manifestation can be associated with chylous hydrocele, chyluria, chylothorax and chyloperitoneum, chylous ascites and chyloarthritis.

Chyluria may also be caused by ascariasis, malaria, tumour and tuberculosis, and the differential diagnosis includes gross pyuria, phosphaturia and caseous material from renal tuberculosis.

Prolonged chyluria may result in the loss of fat in the urine amounting to 15% of lymphatic drainage of the gut. Chyluria will have the same metabolic effects as malabsorption and causes considerable loss of weight with vitamin, electrolyte and other deficiencies. The protein loss in lymphuria and chyluria may lead to edema secondary to hypoalbuminemia.

Chylothorax and chylous ascites

Filariasis is not an uncommon cause, unlike other countries where aetiology varies and includes malignancy and trauma (Anitha and Shenoy, 2001).

● NON FILARIAL CAUSES OF LYMPHOEDEMA

It is classified into primary and secondary lymphoedema (Box 1) (Bradbury, 2002).

Box 29.1 Causes of lymphoedema other than Filariasis	
Primary causes	*Secondary causes*
Congenital lymphoedema (Milroy's disease) (5%). It develops from birth or during the first year. More common in males and usually bilateral.	Primary and secondary malignancy (Hodgkin's and non-Hodgkin's lymphoma, melanoma, pelvic and genital malignancy).
	Surgery (excision of draining lymph nodes).
Lymphoedema praecox (65%). It develops from age one to 35 years. Three times more common in females. The peak incidence is shortly after menarche.	Radiotherapy
	Bacterial infection (cellulitis)
	Fungal infection (tinea pedis) (predispose to cellulitis)
Lymphoedema tarda (30%) usually develops after the age of 35. It is associated with obesity.	Trauma, especially degloving injury
	Venous disease, thrombophlebitis and deep vein thrombosis (DVT)

Figure 29.3 ● Primary lymphoedema

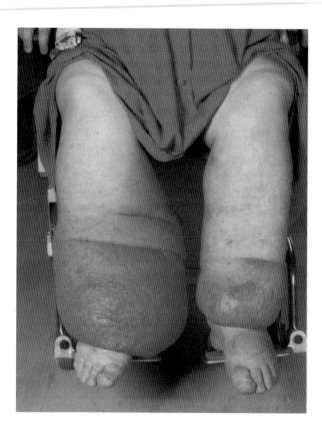

- Primary lymphoedema (Figure 29.3) is caused by inherited underlying lymphatic defects such as, hypoplasia, aplasia and hyperplasia; the latter is due to valvular insufficiency and lymphatic dilation.
- In some patients this inherited predisposition can only lead to clinically apparent disease following exposure to the environmental factors which trigger it (such as venous disease, surgery, cellulitis and trauma).
- Malignancy should be excluded in those who develop lymphoedema for the first time in their late life (especially pelvic and genital malignancy). Such lymphoedema usually starts in the thigh and progresses distally.

● SUMMARY

- Lymphatic Filariasis is commonly caused by nematodes called *wuchereria bancrofti*.
- In endemic areas beware of acute retroperitoneal lymphangitis, which could mimic acute abdomin. Lymphoedema developing for the first time in later life should prompt a thorough search for underlying malignancy.

● QUESTIONS

1 What part of human body is the habitat for microfilariae?
2 Describe the clinical picture of filariasis.
3 Describe the pathological picture of chronic obstructive lesion in filariasis.
4 How would you classify the causes of lower limb lymphoedema?

● REFERENCES

Anitha K, Shenoy. Treatment of lymphatic filariasis: Current trends. *Indian J Dermatol Venereol Leprol* 2001; **67**: 60-65.

Bradbury A. Lymphoedema. In Cuschieri A, Steele RJC, Moosa AR. *Essential surgical practice*. 2002 Arnold: London.

Kamel R. Surgery of Filariasis. In Kamel R, Lumley J (eds). *Textbook of Tropical Surgery*. 2004 Westminster Publishing Group: London.

Manokaran G. Management of genital manifestations of lymphatic filariasis. *Indian J Urol* 2005; **21**:39-43

Sharma AK. Filarial Elephantiasis. In Kamel R, Lumley J (eds). *Textbook of Tropical Surgery*. 2004 Westminster Publishing Group: London.

Strickland GT. Filariasis. In Strickland GT. *Hunter's Tropical Diseases* 8th Ed. 2000. W.B. Saunders Company: Philadelphia.

30 Surgical considerations in tuberculosis

Vikram J Anand

● INTRODUCTION

Tuberculosis (TB) is a contagious disease. It spreads by droplets from a person carrying cavitary disease in the lung and coughing out TB bacilli. The disease can also spread from infected animals to humans. Bovine TB is common in developing countries and is caused by *Mycobacterium bovis*, which infects humans primarily by ingestion of raw (unpasteurised) milk or dairy products and through aerosols containing TB bacteria coming from diseased livestock.

It is estimated that 1.6 million deaths resulted from TB in 2005. The highest number of deaths and the highest mortality per capita are in Africa. Africa and South East Asia lead the world in incidence, prevalence and mortality due to TB. According to the World Health Organization (WHO) (2007), someone in the world is newly infected with TB bacilli every second. Tuberculosis is becoming a worldwide problem because of the spread of human immunodeficiency virus (HIV): together, HIV and TB form a lethal combination, each speeding the other's progress.

> ■ KEY POINT
> TB is becoming a worldwide problem because of the spread of HIV. TB and HIV form a lethal combination, each speeding the other's progress.

It is believed that approximately 2 in every 100 cases of abdominal TB present with small bowel obstruction due to stricture in the terminal ileum or ileocaecal region.

● CAUSATIVE ORGANISMS

Tuberculosis can involve any organ in the human body and is caused by *Mycobacterium tuberculosis*. Other mycobacteria (called non-tuberculous mycobacteria, NTM), such as *Mycobacterium kansasii*, can produce a similar clinical and pathological appearance of the disease. *Mycobacterium avium-intracellulare* (MAI) is seen in patients with immunocompromised conditions such as acquired immunodeficiency syndrome (AIDS). Table 30.1 shows the medical classification of mycobacteria.

Table 30.1 Medical classification of mycobacteria

Mycobacterium tuberculosis	Causes TB. The organisms included are *M. tuberculosis, M. bovis, M. africanum, M. microti* and *M. canetti*
Mycobacterium leprae	Causes leprosy (Hensen's disease)
Non-tuberculous mycobacteria (NTM)*, or atypical TB – there are about 20 different strains of non-tuberculous mycobacteria	Include all the other mycobacteria that can cause pulmonary disease resembling TB, lymphadenitis, skin disease or disseminated disease. Pulmonary infections are caused by *Mycobacterium* avian complex (MAC), which includes *M. avium* and *M. intracellulare. Mycobacterium scrofulaceum* frequently causes cervical lymphadenitis in children. Risk for NTM infection is significantly increased in patients with HIV

*Unlike TB and leprosy, which are primarily spread by human-to-human contact, NTM are believed to be contracted from the environment, hence its alternative label 'environmental bacteria'. NTM are believed to exist naturally in soil and water. NTM do not take up a Gram stain (Gram-neutral).
HIV, human immunodeficiency virus; TB, tuberculosis.

Mycobacterium tuberculosis is an acid-fast bacillus (AFB). An acid-fast stain (Ziehl–Neelsen) shows the organisms as slender red rods. The inflammatory response initiated by M. *tuberculosis* is mediated by a type IV hypersensitivity reaction (see below).

Hypersensitivity reactions

There are four types of hypersensitivity reaction. These were first highlighted by Gell and Coombs (1963). Reaction types I–III are antibody-mediated, whereas type IV reactions are T-cell-mediated. The reactions are summarised in the following list and in Table 30.2:

- *Hypersensitivity type I:* also known as immediate or anaphylactic hypersensitivity. Mediated by immunoglobulin E (IgE). As well as causing anaphylaxis, the reaction may involve the skin (urticaria, eczema), eyes (conjunctivitis), nasopharynx (rhinorrhoea, rhinitis), lungs (asthma) and intestinal tract (gastroenteritis). The reaction usually takes 2–30 min from the time of exposure to the antigen. The primary cellular component is the mast cell or basophil.
- *Hypersensitivity type II:* also known as cytotoxic hypersensitivity. Mediated by immunoglobulin M (IgM) or immunoglobulin (IgG). The antigens are normally endogenous, although sometimes exogenous chemicals lead to type II hypersensitivity. Drug-induced haemolytic anaemia, granulocytopenia and thrombocytopenia are examples. The reaction time is minutes to hours.
- *Hypersensitivity type III:* also known as immune complex hypersensitivity. Mediated by IgG. The reaction may be general (serum sickness) or may involve individual organs, including the skin (systemic lupus erythematosus (SLE), Arthus reaction), kidneys (lupus nephritis), lungs (aspergillosis), blood vessels (polyarteritis) and joints (rheumatoid arthritis).
- *Hypersensitivity type IV:* also known as cell-mediated or delayed type hypersensitivity. The classic example is the tuberculin (Mantoux test) reaction, which takes 48–72 h after injection of antigen (purified protein derivative (PPD) or old tuberculin) to produce localised induration and erythema. Type IV hypersensitivity is involved in the pathogenesis of many autoimmune and infectious diseases, including TB, leprosy, blastomycosis, histoplasmosis, toxoplasmosis and leishmaniasis, and in the pathogenesis of granulomas due to infections and foreign antigens. Contact dermatitis due to, for example, heavy metals, poison ivy or chemicals is another example. Type IV hypersensitivity can be further subdivided into three categories on the basis of the time of onset and the clinical and histological presentation.

Table 30.2 Summary of hypersensitivity reactions

Type	Descriptive name	Time of onset	Mechanism of action	Examples
I	IgE-mediated hypersensitivity	2–30 min	Antigen induces cross-linking of IgE bound to mast cells, with release of vasoactive mediators	Systemic anaphylaxis, hay fever, asthma, eczema
II	Antibody-mediated cytotoxic hypersensitivity	5–8 h	Antibody directed against cell-surface antigens mediates cell destruction	Blood transfusion reactions, haemolytic disease of the newborn, autoimmune haemolytic anaemia
III	Immune-complex mediated hypersensitivity	2–8 h	Antigen–antibody complex deposited at various sites induces mast cell degranulation, with consequent damage to tissue	SLE, polyarteritis, Arthus reaction, disseminated rash, rheumatoid arthritis, glomerulonephritis
IV	T-cell-mediated hypersensitivity	24–72 h	Helper T-cells release cytokines that recruit and activate macrophages	Tubercular lesions, contact dermatitis

IgE, immunoglobulin E; SLE, systemic lupus erythematosus.

PATTERNS OF INFECTION

There are two major disease patterns in TB:

- *Primary TB – the Ghon complex:* this is usually seen in children as an initial infection. The initial focus of infection is a small subpleural granuloma accompanied by granulomatous hilar lymph node infection. Together, these make up the Ghon complex. In nearly all cases, these granulomas resolve due to good body defences.
- *Secondary TB – reactivation TB or fresh infection:* this is seen mostly in adults due to reactivation of previous infection or due to re-infection, which occurs due to poor health status. Typically, the upper lung lobes are most affected, and cavitation can occur. For anatomical reasons, the right apex has a higher chance of being involved than the left apex.

Miliary TB occurs within the lung when the body resistance is very poor. There are a large number of small millet-seed-sized (1–3 mm) granulomas in the lungs or other organs such as the liver or spleen. A chest X-ray shows multiple small areas of consolidation throughout the lung parenchyma on both sides (Figure 30.1).

Primary or reactivation TB can develop into an extensive area of consolidation called a *tuberculoma*. The tuberculoma usually presents as a nodule 10–15 mm in size. Tuberculomas can be found anywhere in the lung, but they are most commonly located in the apical region:

- There is relative underperfusion of the apex of lung. This allows the tubercle bacilli to accumulate in high concentration in the upper lobes. This facilitates tissue necrosis and cavity formation.
- There is a relatively high oxygen concentration in the upper lobes, which favours proliferation of the tubercle bacilli.

Figure 30.1 ● Chest X-ray showing miliary tuberculosis.

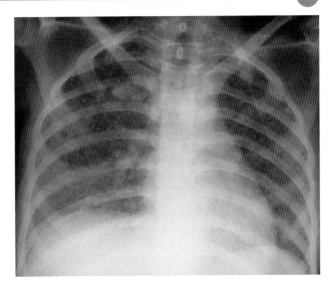

Figure 30.2 ● Chest X-ray showing cavitary tuberculosis on both sides in the upper zone. The right sided cavity shows a prominent patch of tuberculous pneumonia surrounding the cavity.

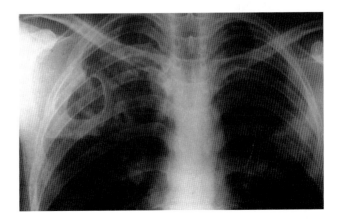

Cavitary TB, tuberculous empyema (pyopneumothorax) and *collapse of the lung* are late seque-lae and are potentially fatal if not attended to adequately. Patients with cavity in the lung due to TB (Figure 30.2) throw out TB bacilli as droplets during bouts of coughing, which then infect others.

> ■ KEY POINT
> Cavitary TB, tuberculous empyema (pyopneumothorax) and collapse of the lung are late sequelae and are potentially fatal if not attended to adequately.

Calcified nodule in the lung represents a chronically healed end stage of the disease in the lung. *Calcified nodes* represent the end stage of the disease in lymph nodes.

● PATHOLOGICAL FEATURES

Microscopically, the inflammation produced with TB infection is a granuloma with epithelioid cells, macrophages and Langhans giant cells. There are lymphocytes, plasma cells, fibroblasts with collagen, and characteristic caseous necrosis in the centre.

● ORGANS INVOLVED

Any organ in the body can be involved with TB.

Lymph node involvement

In Asia and Africa, involvement of the cervical and abdominal lymph nodes is a common occurrence. The presence of a solitary node in the posterior triangle of the neck is typical of TB. Alternatively, there may be a mass of firm, multiple, matted nodes in the submandibular group of nodes (compared with the firm, discrete, mobile individual nodes of lymphoma). Untreated, this leads to formation of chronic fistulous tracts arising from the lymph nodes and leading to the overlying skin. M. *scrofulaceum* is responsible for this picture (see Table 30.1). Patients present with palpable, non-tender or minimally tender nodes with an evening rise of temperature. Table 30.3 shows the stages of spread of TB in a lymph node.

Involved abdominal nodes can cause chronic central abdominal pain and mild tenderness in the paramedian position in the abdomen. This is due to the involvement of para-aortic or mesenteric groups of nodes. The patient has a mild fever that increases to 37 °C in the evenings. The patient is run-down, emaciated, hypoproteinaemic and anaemic.

Gastrointestinal tuberculosis

Gastrointestinal TB is uncommon in Western countries, but involvement of the small intestine remains common in Africa and Asia. The patient presents with vomiting preceded by severe intestinal colic. Intestinal peristalsis is visible in well-established cases (Figure 30.3). Vomiting may be projectile if the jejunum is involved with the disease process.

Table 30.3 Stages of spread of tuberculous infection in a lymph node

Stage	Features
1	Nodes are discrete initially, due to absence of periadenitis
2	Periadenitis develops, leading to matting of the nodes
3	Cold abscess forms in the nodes due to caseation; this causes the nodes to become fluctuant
	If the node is situated deep to the deep fascia of the neck, a collar-stud abscess develops; the abscess is narrow in the middle at the level of the deep fascia and has a wide body deep to and superficial to the deep fascia of the neck
	A caseous lymph node may burst on to the skin, leading to the formation of chronic sinus (or sinuses if multiple nodes are involved); this usually occurs in the deep-seated nodes
	A superficially located node may burst on to the skin, forming a tuberculous ulcer with typically undermined edges
	Often, all of these features at various stages are found in the same patient

Figure 30.3 ● Visible peristalsis in a patient with multiple ileal strictures due to tuberculosis.

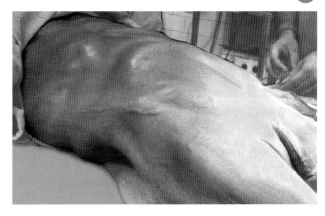

Figure 30.4 ● Tuberculous stricture of the small intestine with grossly dilated proximal segment of ileum. This 26 year old female presented with recurrent bouts of vomiting during the preceeding three months.

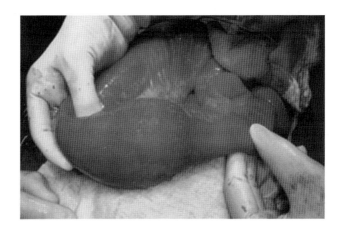

A common mode of transmission takes place when M. *tuberculosis* bacilli coughed up in sputum are swallowed into the gastrointestinal tract. The classic lesions are circumferential ulcerations with stricture of the small intestine. The patient presents with visible peristalsis (Figure 30.3) and grossly increased bowel sounds. There is a predilection for involvement of the terminal ileum and the ileocaecal regions because of the abundant lymphoid tissue and slower rate of passage of luminal contents. Figure 30.4 shows a typical stricture of the terminal ileum.

Urinary tract tuberculosis

In urinary tract TB, typically the patient presents with sterile pyuria with the persistent presence of white cells in urine. Urine culture for bacterial infection is negative. There is progressive destruction of the renal parenchyma. Involvement of the ureter can lead to ureteral stricture. The end stage of urinary bladder involvement is a small-capacity bladder, which causes severe frequency of maturation.

Skeletal tuberculosis

Tuberculous osteomyelitis involves mainly the thoracic and lumbar vertebrae and leads to Pott's disease of the spine. There is necrosis and bony destruction, with compressed fractures of the vertebrae producing kyphosis. Spread into the psoas muscles produces a psoas abscess (cold abscess). Psoas abscesses track down to the inguinal areas and produce a soft swelling, which is one of the considerations in differential diagnosis from a femoral hernia.

Genital tract tuberculosis

The fallopian tubes and the endometrium are commonly involved. Female patients present with irregular menstrual bleeding and infertility. In males, genital tract TB most commonly involves the epididymis and the patient presents with a mildly tender epididymal nodule, which fine-needle cytology shows to be TB. The prostate gland is occasionally involved.

Central nervous system tuberculosis

A common presentation of central nervous system (CNS) involvement is a solitary granuloma, or tuberculoma, which causes seizures or altered behaviour in a patient. Computed tomography (CT) scanning of the brain clinches the diagnosis. Tuberculous meningitis is frequently lethal. Involvement of the base of the brain leads to the presence of various cranial nerve signs. The abducent nerve (sixth cranial nerve) is one of the most commonly involved nerves because of its long intracranial route.

Cerebrospinal fluid (CSF) in tuberculous meningitis typically shows a white cell count of 500–2500, cells with a mononuclear predominance, high protein and low sugar. Since the disease evolves over a period of a few days, a repeat examination of CSF is advisable when the condition is suspected. Table 30.4 shows the evolving changes in CSF in tubercular meningitis.

Table 30.4 Evolving changes in cerebrospinal fluid in a patient with tuberculous meningitis

Presentation	White cell count	Polymorphs (%)	Mononuclear cells (%)	Protein	Sugar
Day 1	15	–	–	+	Nil
Day 2	200	70	30	++	Nil
Days 4–5	500–2500	20–25	75–80	+++	Nil

Adrenal gland tuberculosis

Spread of TB to the adrenal glands is usually bilateral, leading to the enlargement of both glands. Progressive destruction of the glands leads to Addison's disease. If the existence of the disease is not recognised, the patient may present with an addisonian crisis when the body is under stress.

Cardiac and pericardial tuberculosis

This is an uncommon condition, even in the parts of the world where TB abounds. The rich blood supply to the pericardium and the cardiac muscle is the likely cause. The pericardium is the usual site for tuberculous infection of the heart, resulting in granulomatous pericarditis. There may be haemorrhage in the pericardium. If not diagnosed and treated, fibrosis with calcification can lead to end-stage constrictive pericarditis.

CLINICAL PRESENTATION

Clinical presentation depends on the organs involved. Some of the symptomatology has been discussed above, with respect to specific organs. Listed below are some of the common clinical presentations:

- *Chronic cough with no response to antibiotics and other supportive medication for more than 3 weeks:* a common presentation in pulmonary TB. The cough is unproductive in the early stages but subsequently becomes productive. Cavitation in the lung makes the patient infective to others.
- *Pyrexia of unknown origin (PUO):* TB anywhere in the body may present as PUO. When no apparent cause is found for PUO, TB should be suspected in sites such as the abdominal nodes, urinary tract, genital tract, testis and epididymis.
- *Emaciated state with weight loss, anaemia and hypoproteinaemia:* patients with undiagnosed TB may present in an emaciated state with accompanying signs such as weight loss, anaemia, hypoproteinaemia and wasted muscles.
- *Palpable nodes:* in this common presentation, the nodes are palpable in the posterior triangle of the neck but can involve any group. The nodes are usually multiple and matted. Other sequelae such as sinus formation or ulceration with undermined edges may be present in advanced cases (see Table 30.3).
- *Abdominal ascites:* this is a common presentation of abdominal TB. According to one series, 60 per cent of patients with abdominal TB have ascites.
- *Small bowel obstruction:* this occurs late in the disease process. According to one series, 2 per cent of patients with abdominal TB present with small bowel obstruction due to strictures in the terminal ileum or the ileocaecal region.
- *Perianal fistulae:* TB is one of the most common causes of multiple perianal fistulae in Africa and Asia. In Western countries, one would consider Crohn's disease or a malignant process (mucinous adenocarcinoma) as the first causes for multiple perianal fistulae.

DIAGNOSIS

The following tests are used to help diagnose TB:

- *Haemoglobin (Hb) and white cell count (WCC):* Hb is often low, although patients have normal Hb in early stages of the disease. There is lymphocytosis with a raised WCC. These tests are not diagnostic for TB.
- *Erythrocyte sedimentation rate (ESR):* raised, but not specific to TB.
- *Mantoux test (tuberculin skin test):* the skin is pricked with antigens from M. *tuberculosis.* The test cannot clearly distinguish between people who have received a vaccine against TB and those who have a true infection.
- *Chest X-ray:* it is accepted practice to obtain a chest X-ray in patients whose cough fails to respond to antibiotics and other supportive treatment over a 3-week period. It is also essential to perform a chest X-ray in patients suspected of having TB anywhere else in the body.
- *Tissue biopsy:* see Table 30.5.
- *Diagnostic tapping of ascitic or pleural fluid:* tapped fluid is examined for biochemistry, cell cytology and adenosine deaminase (ADA) levels if facilities are available for such examination. The ascitic fluid in TB is an exudate.
- *Polymerase chain reaction (PCR):* a useful test based on amplification of mycobacterial deoxyribonucleic acid (DNA).
- *ADA levels in pleural and peritoneal fluids and CSF:* significantly raised in TB compared with non-tuberculous causes. Estimation of ADA can help in differentiating tuberculous effusions and

Table 30.5 Methods of obtaining tissue for histological examination

Method of biopsy	Features
FNAC	Quick, cheapest method; provides cytological details but does not provide histological details such as grade of tissue if the tissue turns out to be malignant
Core-needle biopsy using Trucut® needle	Uses a special spring-loaded needle to obtain a small, cylindrical core of tissue for histological examination
Wedge biopsy from skin ulcer margins	Tuberculous ulcers are typically undermined; biopsy from the margin of the ulcer confirms the pathology
Incisional biopsy	A small slice of the lump is removed; may be used to remove a part of the lymph node in a group of matted nodes
Excisional biopsy of lymph node	One of the best and quickest methods of diagnosis; if abdominal TB is suspected and the patient has palpable nodes in the neck, biopsy of one of the nodes gives away the diagnosis
Punch biopsy	A punch biopsy forceps is used to obtain tissue for examination from a lymph node or skin ulcer
Endoscopy to obtain biopsy material	A variety of endoscopy procedures can be used to obtain tissue for examination, including gastrointestinal endoscopy, bronchoscopy, thoracoscopy, mediastinoscopy and cystoscopy
Diagnostic laparoscopy	Provides tissue for histological diagnosis
Ultrasound- or CT-guided biopsy	For deep-seated lesions, ultrasound or CT is used to guide the needle to its destination accurately in order to obtain tissue for histological examination

CT, computed tomography; FNAC, fine-needle aspiration cytology.

meningitis from non-tuberculous effusions and aseptic meningitis respectively (Sontakke *et al.*, 1989).

- *Interferon gamma (IFN-γ) response test:* IFN-γ has been considered to be a critical protective immunomodulatory component against M. *tuberculosis* infection. The US Food and Drug Administration (FDA) approved the test QuantiFERON-TB-Gold® in 2005. The test measures IFN-γ release from whole blood. It shows the same sensitivity as the routine Mantoux skin test and is more specific to the presence of latent TB in the body. Unlike the Mantoux skin test, the IFN-γ test requires only one visit from the patient.

MEDICAL TREATMENT

Table 30.6 shows the current drug regimens for TB. Table 30.7 gives the dosages of first-line anti-TB drugs and their major adverse effects (Chan and Iseman, 2002), while Table 30.8 gives the dosages for intermittent regimens used for directly observed therapy (DOT).

The following points should be noted:

- *Duration of treatment:* for pulmonary TB, the usual length of treatment is 6 months. For abdominal TB and TB in other sites, the usual length of treatment is 9–12 months.

Table 30.6 Current drug regimens for tuberculosis

Regimen	Initial phase	Continuation phase
Daily: for patients self-administering their drugs	2 months of isoniazid, rifampicin and pyrazinamide, with or without ethambutol	4 months of isoniazid and rifampicin
Intermittent: for directly observed therapy (DOT)	2 weeks of daily isoniazid, rifampicin, pyrazinamide and streptomycin or ethambutol	24 weeks of twice-weekly isoniazid and rifampicin

Table 30.7 Dosages of first-line anti-tuberculosis drugs and their major adverse effects

Drug	Daily dosage	Adverse effects
Isoniazid	5 mg/kg oral (maximum 300 mg)	Hepatitis, peripheral neuritis, drug-induced lupus, seizures, hypersensitivity with rash and fever; drug interactions with phenytoin and disulfiram
Rifampicin	10 mg/kg oral (maximum 600 mg)	Orange- or yellow-coloured urine, flu-like syndrome, hepatitis, thrombocytopenia, nausea, anorexia, diarrhoea, renal failure; multiple drug interactions
Pyrazinamide	25–30 mg/kg oral	Hyperuricaemia, hepatitis, rash, nausea, anorexia
Ethambutol	25 mg/kg for initial 2 months, then 15 mg/kg oral	Optic neuritis, gastrointestinal discomfort
Streptomycin	15 mg/kg intramuscularly (maximum 1 g) for 5 days a week	Ototoxicity, vestibular dysfunction, nephrotoxicity, rash, hypersensitivity reactions

Table 30.8 Dosages for intermittent regimens used for directly observed therapy

Drug	Regimen
Isoniazid	900 mg twice a week, or 600 mg three times a week
Rifampicin	10 mg/kg: 600 mg twice a week, or 600 mg three times a week
Pyrazinamide	30–35 mg/kg
Ethambutol	50 mg/kg twice a week, or 30 mg/kg three times a week
Streptomycin	15 mg/kg (maximum 1.5 g) two or three times a week

- *Supplement of pyridoxine (vitamin B6)*: suggested for patients taking isoniazid in order to prevent peripheral neuritis and isoniazid psychosis (the patient may become violent). These side effects are uncommon. The recommended dose of pyridoxine is 6 mg/day (Joint Tuberculosis Committee of the British Thoracic Society, 1998).
- *Pretreatment liver function tests*: should be normal. Periodic monitoring of liver function tests is advocated in view of the potential hepatotoxicity of isoniazid, rifampicin and pyrazinamide.
- *Renal function*: should be checked before treatment with streptomycin or ethambutol. These drugs are best avoided in renal failure.

- *Ethambutol and visual acuity:* because of the possible toxic effects of ethambutol on the eye, visual acuity should be tested before the drug is prescribed. The drug should be used only in patients who have reasonable visual acuity. Patients should be advised to report any visual disturbances during treatment.
- *HIV and TB:* patients with HIV may fail to properly absorb anti-TB drugs, which may increase the risk of treatment failure, relapses, acquired drug resistance and toxicity (Peloquin *et al.*, 1989). Interactions between HIV and anti-TB drugs may compromise antiretroviral and anti-TB treatment.
- *Multidrug-resistant TB:* occurs when TB strains are resistant to at least isoniazid and rifampicin. It is agreed that DOT reduces the development of multidrug resistance. Once multidrug resistance is suspected, it is important to determine the sensitivity of the bacteria to the commonly used drugs. At least four drugs to which the organisms are sensitive should be used. Inclusion of one injectable drug is preferred; the injectable drug may be an aminoglycoside or streptomycin. The treatment may need to be continued for more than a year.

> ■ KEY POINT
> Ethambutol should be used only in patients who have reasonable visual acuity. Patients should be advised to report any visual disturbances during treatment.

● SURGERY IN TUBERCULOSIS

There are two main indications for surgery in abdominal tuberculosis: diagnostic and therapeutic.

Diagnostic surgery

Diagnostic laparotomy or laparoscopy is often required for histopathological and microbiological diagnosis when peritoneal or lymph node TB is suspect. Diagnostic biopsy is the priority when abdominal TB is suspected (Singh-Ranger *et al.*, 1999). Several more recent studies confirm that laparoscopy with tissue biopsy provides rapid and correct diagnosis of abdominal TB (Safarpor *et al.*, 2007).

Therapeutic surgery

Therapeutic surgery is indicated for complications such as intestinal obstruction (acute, acute-on-chronic, chronic), perforation and peritonitis (Kapoor, 1991). Commonly performed therapeutic procedures include the following:

- *Stricturoplasty:* usually done for one to three strictures, provided that they are not very close to each other. The bowel is incised longitudinally at the site of the stricture and then sutured transversally so that the area of the stricture opens up completely.
- *Resection anastomosis:* performed when there are multiple strictures close to each other. The patient in Figure 30.3 (see page 407) had several strictures over a small length of the ileum.
- *Segmental resection:* performed when there is very limited involvement of the terminal ileum close to the caecum. In this situation, segmental resection of the terminal ileum along with about 5 cm of the ascending colon is done and anastomosis made between the healthy terminal ileum and the ascending colon.
- *Right hemicolectomy:* performed when there is gross involvement of the terminal ileum and caecum. About 15–20 cm of the ileum is removed, incorporating all the diseased area, along with the caecum, appendix, ascending colon, hepatic flexure and right half of the transverse colon. An anastomosis is made between the healthy terminal ileum and the transverse colon (ileotransverse anastomosis).

- *Bypass surgery – ileotransverse anastomosis:* performed in unfit patients with advanced disease. The procedure is less traumatic than a right hemicolectomy to the patient. Intestinal obstruction is most often at the ileocaecal region.
- *Excision of lymph nodal mass:* if there is a lymph node mass in the abdomen (found on exploratory laparotomy or when dealing with bowel involvement), it is best excised, provided that it is technically safe to do so. Often the mesenteric nodes are involved and may be the seat of cold abscess formation.

SUMMARY

The chapter begins with a perspective on the incidence of tuberculosis in the world with approximately 1.6 million deaths due to tuberculosis in the year 2005. Medical classification highlights different types on mycobacteria. Different types of hypersensitivity reactions are elaborated with reference to tuberculosis. Primary and secondary tuberculosis are explained. Reasons for frequent involvement of the apical region of the lung are explained and it is stated that cavitary tuberculosis causes spread to other humans by droplets. Different stages of spread of tuberculosis in a lymph node are explained. There is a description of the involvement of various systems of the body with tuberculosis and the key lesions produced in each system. Diagnostic techniques for tuberculosis and their relative merits are discussed, including a list of methods of obtaining tissue for histological examination. Medical treatment and indications for surgical intervention are discussed.

QUESTIONS

1 How many types of mycobacteria do you know of?
2 Do you know roughly how many deaths occur due to tuberculosis across the world in a year?
3 How many types of hypersensitivity reactions do you know. Mantoux skin test is what type of hypersensitivity reaction?
4 What is Ghon complex?
5 Why is the apex of lung involved more frequently in pulmonary tuberculosis?
6 What are the stages of spread of tuberculosis in a lymph node?
7 What are the clinical presentations of tuberculosis?
8 Can you name the tests for diagnosing tuberculosis?
9 Name the commonly used drugs for medical treatment of tuberculosis and their common side effects.
10 Name the various techniques of obtaining tissue for histological examination.
11 What are the indications for surgical intervention in tuberculosis?

REFERENCES

Chan ED, Iseman MD (2002). Clinical review: current medical treatment of tuberculosis. *Br Med J* **325**: 1282–6.

Gell PGH, Coombs RRA (eds) (1963). *Clinical Aspects of Immunology.* Oxford: Blackwell.

Joint Tuberculosis Committee of the British Thoracic Society (1998). Chemotherapy and management of tuberculosis in the United Kingdom: recommendations 1998. *Thorax* **53**: 536–48.

Kapoor VK (1991). Abdominal tuberculosis: misconceptions, myths and facts. *Indian J Tuberc* **38**: 119.

Peloquin CA, Nitta AT, Burman WJ, *et al.* (1989). Low antituberculosis drug concentrations in patients with AIDS. *Ann Pharmacother* **30**: 919–25.

Safarpor F, Aghajanzade M, Kohsari MR, *et al.* (2007). Role of laparoscopy in the diagnosis of abdominal tuberculosis. *Saudi J Gastroenterol* **13**: 133–5.

Singh-Ranger D, Rockall T, Narward A-H, *et al.* (1999). Abdominal tuberculosis: the problem of diagnostic delay. *Scand J Infect Dis* **31**: 517.

Sontakke AN, Sinha R, Somani BL, Gopinathan VP (1989). Adenosine deaminase (ADA) levels in body fluids: a did in tuberculosis. *Armed Forces Med J India* **45**: 117–20.

World Health Organization (WHO) (2007). Tuberculosis. Fact sheet no. 104. Geneva: World Health Organization.

31 · Surgical considerations in typhoid

Vikram J Anand

● INTRODUCTION

Typhoid fever is a bacterial disease caused by *Salmonella typhi*. It is transmitted through ingestion of food or drink contaminated by the faeces or urine of an infected person. According to the World Health Organization (WHO, 2003), between 15 million and 20 million people suffer from typhoid fever annually worldwide. There are approximately 600 000 deaths from typhoid every year. The incidence of the disease is very low in developed countries due to the availability of good-quality drinking water and sanitation.

> ■ KEY POINT
> There are about 600 000 deaths from typhoid every year worldwide. The incidence of the disease is very low in developed countries due to the availability of good-quality drinking water and sanitation.

Each year, around 150–200 cases of typhoid are reported in England and Wales (NHS Direct, 2007). A total of 2412 cases were reported between 1980 and 1989; of these infections, at least 67 per cent were acquired abroad (Health Protection Agency, 2006). Although the number of reported cases decreased during the late 1990s, it has recently risen again, with a 69 per cent increase between 2002 (147 cases) and 2006 (248 cases).

● CAUSATIVE ORGANISMS

Typhoid fever is caused by *Salmonella typhi*, which belongs to the family of Enterobacteriaceae. The principal habitat of salmonella is the human intestinal tract. Salmonella is a Gram-negative rod-shaped bacterium with flagellae. The salmonella organism has three antigens, which are used for diagnosis or identification of the disease:

- Somatic (O) or cell-wall antigen
- Surface (envelope) antigen
- Flagellar (H) antigen.

PATHOGENESIS

Salmonella typhi enter the human intestine through contaminated food and water. They penetrate the intestinal mucosa at the site of Peyer's patches and are stopped in the mesenteric lymph nodes. There, the bacteria multiply. From the mesenteric lymph nodes, viable bacteria and endotoxin are released into the bloodstream, resulting in septicaemia. Release of endotoxin is responsible for cardiovascular collapse. Historically, the terms 'collapsus' and 'tuphos' were used to describe the stuporous state in typhoid. The name typhoid is derived from the term 'tuphos'.

About 5 per cent of patients, although clinically cured, remain typhoid carriers for months or even years. They have the potential to spread the disease.

> ■ KEY POINT
> About 5 per cent of patients, although clinically cured, remain typhoid carriers for months or even years. They have the potential to spread the disease.

In developing countries, the incidence of faecal contamination of water and food remains high, and so does the incidence of typhoid. The incidence of typhoid decreases when the level of development of a country increases, leading to, for example, controlled water and sewage systems and pasteurisation of milk.

> ■ KEY POINT
> The incidence of typhoid decreases when the level of development of a country increases.

CLINICAL PRESENTATION

The incubation period of typhoid is 1–2 weeks and depends on, among other things, how large a dose of bacteria has been taken in. Patients commonly present with the following features:

- Sudden onset of fever
- Severe headache
- Loss of appetite
- Nausea
- Sore throat
- Rash, usually on the chest
- Constipation or diarrhoea at times.

In the severe form of the disease, patients present with mental dullness, with an inability to think clearly and features of meningitis.

There are two phases of typical infection:

- *First phase:* this phase usually lasts a week. The patient's temperature rises gradually to 39°C. The patient's general condition becomes poor. There is headache, with bouts of sweating. The patient's appetite remains poor. Constipation and skin symptoms may be present. Towards the end of the first phase, the patient shows increasing listlessness and clouding of consciousness.
- *Second phase:* the fever continues to be high, and the patient has tachycardia. In the third week, constipation is replaced by diarrhoea. The faeces may contain blood. The patient's general condition begins to improve by about the fourth or fifth week.

Meningitis and intestinal perforation are both potentially fatal presentations of typhoid. In developing countries, patients often present with perforation of the small intestine and features of peritonitis. Since medical practitioners are not always monitored rigorously in developing countries, especially in rural areas, patients are often prescribed steroids in order to give symptomatic relief from undiagnosed fever. This results in a high rate of intestinal perforation and resultant mortality.

DIAGNOSIS

- *White cell count (WCC):* leucopenia (WCC < 4000/mm^3) is present in the majority of cases, even when perforation peritonitis is present. It may be due to bone marrow depression by enteric toxaemia (Beniwal *et al.*, 2003).
- *Widal test:* this has been used for more than 100 years for the diagnosis of typhoid fever (Grunbaum, 1896; Widal, 1896). The test measures agglutinating antibodies against the lipopolysaccharide O and protein flagellar H antigens of *S. typhi*. The serological diagnosis relies on the demonstration of a rising titre of antibodies 10–14 days apart. The earliest serological response in acute typhoid fever is a rise in the titre of the O antibody, with an elevation of the H-antibody titre developing more slowly but persisting for longer. The test should be ordered in patients who have a reasonable probability of having typhoid fever; however, a negative Widal test in a patient with a clinical history suggestive of typhoid does not exclude the disease (Parry *et al.*, 1999).
- *Blood culture:* the diagnostic test of choice. Antibiotic treatment before the blood culture may render the culture negative.
- *Stool and rectal swab cultures:* stool culture for diagnosis of typhoid is a useful test; however, the results are usually positive only after the first week of illness. Rectal swab culture can be done where it is not possible to obtain stool culture. A positive stool culture can occur in carriers as well as active cases (WHO, 2003).
- *Abdominal X-ray:* gas under the diaphragm in an X-ray of the abdomen in the standing position is an important finding that is diagnostic of intestinal perforation in a suspected case of typhoid.

PATHOLOGICAL FEATURES

There is proliferation of large mononuclear cells derived from reticuloendothelial tissue. As the bacteria invade, the Peyer's patches become hypertrophic. In some cases, intestinal lymphoid hyperplasia progresses to capillary thrombosis, causing necrosis of the overlying mucosa and characteristic ulcers along the long axis of the bowel. Although these intestinal ulcers are usually confined to the mucosa and submucosa, the muscular and serosal layers may be penetrated, causing intestinal perforation. The erosion of blood vessels in the lesions may occur, giving rise to intestinal haemorrhage.

The liver is enlarged during typhoid fever, with focal areas of necrosis and cloudy swelling of hepatic cells. The spleen and mesenteric lymph nodes are enlarged. There is hyperplasia of reticuloendothelial cells. Bronchitis is common and pneumonia may be present. The maculopapular skin rash is infiltrated with mononuclear cells. As well as the intestine, other tissues involved include the kidney, spleen, gallbladder, lymph nodes, lungs, liver, skin, bronchi and brain.

MEDICAL TREATMENT

The following drugs are used for the medical treatment of typhoid:

Table 31.1 Drug treatments for typhoid

Drug of choice in all age groups	Alternative
Uncomplicated disease:	
Ciprofloxacin for 7 days	Ceftriaxone for 10–14 days
15 mg/kg/day given in 2 divided doses	50–75 mg/kg/day in 1 or 2 divided doses
Adult dose usually 500–750 mg orally twice a day or 400 mg intravenous infusion every 12 h	
In pregnancy:	
Ceftriaxone for 7–14 days	Amoxicillin for 14 days
Adult dose 2 4 g daily (up to 2 g twice daily in severe disease)	75–100 mg/kg/day usually in 3 divided doses

Ciprofloxacin

Ciprofloxacin has several advantages:

- Convenient twice-daily dose
- Rapid relief of fever and other symptoms
- Shorter duration of treatment (Table 31.1)
- Usually given orally, unless major complications exist, when it is given parenterally.

Ciprofloxacin is not registered for use in children. Patients with severe disease or complications require parenteral dosing for 7–10 days.

Other drugs

Other drugs used in the treatment of typhoid include ceftriaxone, cefotaxime, ampicillin, amoxicillin and co-trimoxazole. These drugs can be used in children and pregnant women.

Ceftriaxone is used as short-term treatment and needs to be given intravenously. It is comparable to ciprofloxacin in clearance of the organisms from the gut and as a short-term treatment.

Co-trimoxazole, ampicillin and amoxicillin require treatment for at least 14 days. There may be difficulties with compliance. These drugs are not as effective in clearing the gut of typhoid organisms and therefore may contribute to a carrier state.

Chloramphenicol is a time-tested drug. It was once the drug of choice until drugs such as ciprofloxacin became available. In Western countries chloramphenicol fell out of favour primarily because of its side effects, which include aplastic anaemia and bone marrow suppression.

● COMPLICATIONS

The main complications of typhoid, all of which are potentially fatal, are:

- perforation of the small intestine, presenting as peritonitis;
- gastrointestinal bleeding;
- meningitis, presenting as neck stiffness and inability to think clearly.

> **Box 31.1 Use of catgut in surgery**
>
> Catgut is not used in Western countries because of the risk of transmission of Creutzfeldt–Jakob disease (CJD), a rare, but invariably fatal, disorder afflicting the brain. This disorder is the human form of bovine spongiform encephalopathy (BSE) in cattle, also known as 'mad cow disease'.
>
> Catgut continues to be used in Africa and South East Asia due to financial considerations. In India, over the period 1968–1997, the National Institute of Mental Health and Neurosciences (NIMHANS) in Bangalore recorded 69 cases of CJD from different parts of India in the CJD registry (Mehndiratta *et al.*, 2001). This translates to 2.3 cases per year in a population of about 1000 million.

● ROLE OF SURGERY IN MANAGEMENT

Surgical intervention is required for complications. The most frequent surgical complication is peritonitis due to perforation. Typically a patient who has had a fever for a few days (who may or may not have been diagnosed as having typhoid) presents with severe abdominal pain and features of abdominal guarding, board-like rigidity and masked liver dullness on percussion. X-ray of the abdomen shows gas under the diaphragm.

Exploratory laparotomy reveals perforation of the terminal ileum, with spillage of intestinal contents into the peritoneal cavity. A thorough lavage of the peritoneal cavity is required. The perforation is closed in two layers with 2-0 vicryl with a patch of omentum if necessary. Some surgeons use an inner layer of chromic catgut (Box 31.1) and an outer layer of black silk (Beniwal *et al.*, 2003). The abdomen is closed with one or two drains positioned suitably in the abdominal cavity. Simple repair of a perforation is the treatment of choice in enteric perforation and is quick, cost-effective and life-saving.

Resection–anastomosis is an extensive procedure and is best avoided. There are some situations, however, where it is necessary to resect the bowel and restore the continuity by anastomosis. An ileostomy is required in some cases. This procedure is time-consuming and requires reoperation in order to close the ileostomy. Postoperative faecal fistula formation due to an anastomotic leak is a potential complication of surgery in high-risk cases.

> ■ KEY POINT
> Resection–anastomosis is an extensive procedure and is best avoided.

Gastrointestinal bleeding is treated conservatively initially and usually settles without surgical intervention. If bleeding continues, surgical intervention becomes necessary. Resection of the involved bowel is the treatment of choice for an uncontrolled bleed due to typhoid ulcers.

● PREVENTION OF TYPHOID

Vaccines are available for the prevention of typhoid and can be given in a single dose or multiple doses.

● SUMMARY

The chapter gives a perspective on the incidence of typhoid across the world including figures for England and Wales. Nearly 600 000 deaths occur due to typhoid each year. Pathogenesis and clinical presentation are covered, including the significance of the carrier state. Significance of various diagnostic modalities has been highlighted. Pathological features and medical treatment is described. The medical treatment covers the newer drugs and makes a reference to older drugs like chloramphenicol. Management of surgical complications, which may be potentially fatal, is described. Special mention is made on the use of catgut in surgical management with reference to Creutzfeldt–Jakob disease, especially in the Indian context.

● QUESTIONS

1 State the name of the organism causing typhoid and name its antigens.
2 What is the significance of a person being a carrier of typhoid?
3 What are the possible clinical presentations of a patient with typhoid?
4 How can we make a definitive diagnosis of typhoid?
5 What is the commonly used drug to treat typhoid? What do you know about the use of chloramphenicol to treat typhoid?
6 Name some of the common complications of typhoid. Can you elaborate on the surgical management of typhoid perforation?

● REFERENCES

Beniwal U, Jindal D, Sharma J, *et al.* (2003). Comparative study of operative procedures in typhoid perforation. *Indian J Surg* **65**: 172–7.

Grunbaum AS (1896). Preliminary note on the use of the agglutinative action of human serum for the diagnosis of enteric fever. *Lancet* **ii**: 806–7.

Health Protection Agency (2006). *Salmonella typhi* and *Salmonella paratyphi* laboratory reports (cases only) reported to the Health Protection Agency Centre for Infections England and Wales, 1980–2006. London: Health Protection Agency. www.hpa.org.uk/webw/HPAweb&HPAwebStandard/HPAweb_C/1195733753804?p=1191942172078.

Mehndiratta MM, Bajaj BK, Gupta M, *et al.* (2001). Creutzfeldt–Jakob disease: report of 10 cases from North India. *Neurol India* **49**: 338–1.

NHS Direct (2007). Typhoid fever: introduction. www.nhsdirect.nhs.uk/articles/article.aspx?articleId=380.

Parry CM, Hoa NTT, Diep TS, *et al.* (1999). Value of a single-tube Widal test in diagnosis of typhoid fever in Vietnam. *J Clin Microbiol* **37**: 2882–6.

Widal F (1896). Serodiagnostic de la fièvre typhoide à-propos d'une modification par M. M. C. Nicolle et A. Halipre. *Bull Mem Soc Med Hop Paris* **13**: 561–6.

World Health Organization (WHO) (2003). *Background Document: The Diagnosis, Treatment and Prevention of Typhoid Fever.* Geneva: World Health Organization. www.who.int/vaccines-documents/DocsPDF03/www740.pdf.

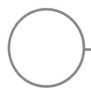

Index

Note: page numbers in *italics* refer to tables, those in **bold** to figures or boxes. Abbreviations used within the index are: CDAD = *Clostridium difficile*-associated disease; ERCP = endoscopic retrograde cholangiopancreatography; EUS = endoscopic ultrasound; PTC = percutaneous transhepatic cholangiography; SIRS = systemic inflammatory response syndrome; UGIB = upper gastrointestinal bleeding.